KV-127-917

MEDICINE

From Biblical Canaan to Modern Israel

EDITED BY

Stuart Stanton and Kenneth Collins

Presented by
Vallentine Mitchell
Publishers

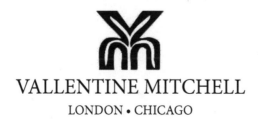

VALLENTINE MITCHELL

LONDON • CHICAGO

First published in 2021 by Vallentine Mitchell

Catalyst House,
720 Centennial Court,
Centennial Park, Elstree WD6 3SY, UK

814 N. Franklin Street,
Chicago, Illinois,
60610 USA

www.vmbooks.com

Copyright © Vallentine Mitchell 2021
Individual chapters © contributors 2021

British Library Cataloguing in Publication Data:
An entry can be found on request

ISBN 978 1 912676 73 6 (Cloth)
ISBN 978 1 912676 74 3 (Ebook)

Library of Congress Cataloging in Publication Data:
An entry can be found on request

All rights reserved. No part of this publication may be reproduced in any form or by any means, electronic, mechanical, photocopying, reading or otherwise, without the prior permission of Vallentine Mitchell & Co. Ltd.

Contents

Foreword

Leslie Turnberg

Israel has taken the lead in so many ways. It is making remarkable progress, from artificial intelligence to cyber-security and from research to innovation. It is hardly surprising then that in medicine and health care too it excels. Research in its institutions and universities is leading to novel diagnostic tools and treatments for disease.

Its health care system ensures that its whole population has access to high quality care, and it is based on the strong ethical principle of the sanctity of life regardless of religion or ethnicity. A visit to any hospital provides a heartening picture of the care being given to children and adults from Gaza, the West Bank and across the Middle East. The care system is at ready alert to cope with any emergency arising from war or terrorism. And its volunteer medical force is ready, at the drop of a hat, to fly out around the world to assist at scenes of devastation, as was the case in Haiti and Nepal in recent years.

Of course, Israeli medicine did not reach this enviable position overnight and this book, in a series of erudite and authoritative essays, lays out, in a clear and accessible way, the history of medicine in the Holy Land from the time of the Babylonians until today.

Jews have always been drawn to medicine. The combination of intellectual challenge together with a desire to assist those in need is a very Jewish characteristic and it is that which has led many into medicine. And that history has many towering figures, from Rabbi Abbaye in the third and fourth century CE who wrote of many therapies in the Talmud, to Moses Maimonides in twelfth-century Spain and Cairo, and on to recent Israeli medical Nobel Laureates: Daniel Kahneman, a psychologist/economist, Aharon Ciechanover and Avraham Hershko (both medical men, one a surgeon, but typically gained their prize in Chemistry). This is hardly unexpected, since the Jews were spread across the world in the diaspora for 2,000 years, that they imbibed much of their medical knowledge and practice from wherever they were.

The influence of the cultures of the Byzantines, the Persians, the Greeks and the Romans is clearly laid out here. There is so much of intriguing interest in this history of pre-Israeli medicine and I learnt so much of this period that I had not grasped before. And then, we come to the British influence during the Mandate period in the last century. But it is clear that the Zionists, valuing health and education above most else, relied on themselves using funds derived from the Jewish diaspora. They sought, and received, little from the Mandate Administration as they set up their clinics and hospitals.

There is much else of interest here. A chapter on 'Popular Medicine' as described in the Bible and Talmud is a revelation. It is fascinating to learn that the Talmud recommended that no wise person should live in a town where there was no doctor. For those unfamiliar with medical practice in the Ottoman period in the Middle East it has been generally assumed to be primitive and fatalistic. But Professor Shefer-Mossensohn disabuses us of that view in her description of a more sophisticated system of medicine gleaned from her analysis of Arabic and Ottoman sources.

The medical picture is brought right up to date in a series of chapters on modern medical practice in Israel. We are enlightened by essays on the modern health care system, on emergency and military medicine, on rehabilitation medicine and on the underlying ethical principles of medicine. It is a feast of information on ancient and recent history of medicine with clear expositions on the state of modern medicine in Israel today, describing in detail many of the innovations which have transformed aspects of medicine across the globe.

The editors are to be congratulated on gathering such a remarkably well informed and lucid group of authorities together in one volume.

Leslie Turnberg, Baron Turnberg of Cheadle, is a former Consultant Gastroenterologist, Professor of Medicine and Dean of the Medical Faculty at the University of Manchester. He is a former President of the Royal College of Physicians and was made a Life Peer in 2000.

Acknowledgements

We express our gratitude to the authors who have co-operated in the production of this book, which tells a story which we felt from the outset needs to be told. As editors we have enjoyed our contacts with the authors and our partnership has been one of effective co-operation. We have to thank Avi Ohry for bringing us together and helping us to take the important steps in defining the scope of the book.

We are delighted to thank David Dangoor for the sponsorship of Dangoor Education in the publication of this book. Dangoor Education is part of the philanthropy of the Exilarch's Foundation which provides support to major institutions in Britain and Israel, associated with health, education and interfaith activities, as well as to charities associated with Sephardi Jewish heritage and the story of the Jewish community of Iraq.

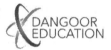

We are also grateful to David and Marion Cohen for their generous support. Eli Jaffe, Uriel Goldberg and Roman Sonkin gave us a guided tour of Magen David Adom headquarters in Jerusalem and provided an understanding of the complexity and efficiency of their organisation.

We would like to acknowledge the help of Eli Beer, Founder and President of United Hatzalah of Israel, Daniel Katzenstein, Director of International Donor Relations and Raphael Poch, International Media Spokesperson, for their help in compiling the material about United Hatzalah of Israel. We acknowledge permission of the Pharmaceutical Press to quote from an article on Jewish Traditional Medicine by Kenneth Collins, in Steven B. Kayne, *Traditional Medicine: A Global Perspective* (London: 2010).

It has been a great pleasure to work with the publishers Vallentine Mitchell as they have steered this book to publication. Our thanks to Toby Harris, Lisa Hyde and cover designer Jenni Tinson. We acknowledge permission of the Pharmaceutical Press to quote from an article on Jewish Traditional Medicine by Kenneth Collins, in Steven B. Kayne, *Traditional Medicine: A Global Perspective* (London: 2010).

Stuart Stanton dedicates this work to his parents Michael and Sarah Stanton, and to Julia, Claire, Talia, Jo, Tamara and Noah. Kenneth Collins dedicates this work to his parents, Dr. David and Dr. Hetty Collins.

Stuart Stanton and Kenneth Collins

List of Illustrations

List of Contributors

Aref Abu-Rafia is Professor Emeritus at Ben Gurion University of the Negev. He has successfully completed his administrative responsibilities as Chair of the Department of Middle Eastern Studies. His research has included anthropology and Public Health. His main publications are on traditional medicine, family customs, holy saints, education, cosmopolitanism, Sufism, Islamic medical law and ethics and alternative and complementary medicine. His research focuses on the Middle East, North Africa and Islamic communities. Based on this research and fellowship he has received several awards and honours, such as the Berelson Prize for Jewish-Arab Understanding and Co-Existence in Israel and has been a Greenberg Middle East Scholar and Fulbright Scholar for the Muslim World.

Nava Blum, BPT, MOccH., Ph.D (Haifa), has had fellowships in the Mayo Clinic and post-doctoral in the National Institute of Health, Bethesda, USA. Her area of expertise is in clinical rehabilitation, public health services and history of medicine. She was the Director of Rehabilitation and Physiotherapy, developing new services in a Rehabilitation Hospital and in Rehabilitation Centres in the Ministry of Health and the Clalit HMO. She is a Senior Lecturer at the Department of Health Systems Management at the Max Stern Academic College and directs courses related to public health, rehabilitation, occupational health, risk management and advanced new technologies. She has published a book, many chapters and articles in peer review journals and has been a keynote lecturer at national and international meetings.

Kenneth Collins, PhD FRCGP, was a general medical practitioner in Glasgow, Scotland for over 30 years. He served as Chairman of the Scottish Council of Jewish Communities and has been the Chairman of the Scottish Jewish Archives Centre since it was founded in 1987. He is Senior Research Fellow at the Centre for the History of Medicine, University of Glasgow and Visiting Professor, History of Medicine, at the Hebrew University of

Jerusalem. He was the Editor of *Vesalius: Journal of the International Society for the History of Medicine* (2009-2017) and has published widely on Jews and medicine in Scotland and co-edited works on Moses Maimonides and Isaac Israeli.

Nadav Davidovitch, MD, MPH, PhD, is an epidemiologist and public health physician He is a Full Professor and Director, School of Public Health at the Faculty of Health Sciences, Ben Gurion University of the Negev in Israel. His research interests are health policy, public health, vaccination policy, health/eco health, comparative health care systems, public health ethics and global health. Prof. Davidovitch serves on several international and national committees related to public health and environmental epidemiology. He has authored or co-authored over 140 papers and book chapters, co-edited six volumes and books and published his work in leading medical and health policy journals including the *New England Journal of Medicine, Lancet, Clinical Infectious Diseases, Emerging Infectious Diseases, Journal of Pediatrics, Vaccine, Social Science and Medicine* and *Law and Contemporary Problems.*

Eran Dolev is a graduate of the Hebrew University School of Medicine and Professor of Medicine at the Tel Aviv University School of Medicine. He was Surgeon General of the Israel Defence Forces (1979-1983), Head of the Department of Internal Medicine, Tel Aviv Medical Centre (1990-2005) and taught at the Tel-Hai College, Upper Galilee (2005-2017). Professor Dolev was Visiting Professor of Military Medicine, Uniformed Services University of the Health Sciences, Bethesda, USA and was Head of the Supreme Ethical Committee of the Israel Medical Association (IMA) from 1996 to 2002. He has many publications in the fields of Military Medicine, History of Medicine and Bone Diseases. His book *Allenby and Military Medicine* was published in 2007 (London: I.B. Tauris).

Markham J. Geller is Jewish Chronicle Professor at University College London (UCL), Department of Hebrew and Jewish Studies. From 2011-2018, he was on secondment from UCL as Professor für Wissensgeschichte at the Freie Universität, Berlin and Principal Investigator of a five-year European Research Council project, *BabMed*. He is currently a Fellow at the Max Planck Institut für Wissenschaftsgeschicht, Berlin and Institute for Advance Study, Paris (2020-21). He has held fellowships from the Alexander von Humboldt-Stiftung and was twice Fellow at the Netherlands Institute for Advanced Study, Wassenaar (NIAS). He is collaborator on a

British Museum Wellcome-funded project *NinMed* to produce an online edition of the Nineveh cuneiform medical library (2020-2022).

Shimon Glick received his MD degree at the Downstate Medical Center, New York. He specialized in internal medicine and endocrinology. At the Ben Gurion University Faculty of Health Sciences he served as Professor of Medicine and founding chairman of the Division of Medicine, and subsequently as Dean of the Faculty, as head of the Prywes Centre for Medical Education and as acting head of the Jakobovits Centre for Jewish Medical Ethics. For a decade he was the national Ombudsman for Israel's Ministry of Health.

Uriel Goldberg was born in London and educated at Hasmonean High School. In 2010, he travelled to Israel to take part in the Magen David Adom Overseas Programme after which he made Aliyah. Uriel joined the IDF in 2012 in the Combat Search and Rescue Brigade where he served for three years. Then he joined MDA Israel as an instructor in Emergency Medical courses and ran First Aid courses for the public. In 2018 after dedicating many hours to his studies, Uriel qualified as a Paramedic. He continues to work in International Relations, alongside being a Paramedic, driving ambulances and saving lives.

Eli Jaffe, Ph.D, is the Community Deputy Director and the Manager of Public Relations, Volunteers, Training and Fundraising division at Magen David Adom, Israel. Eli has a Ph.D in Public Administration from the University of Haifa, and a Ph.D in Medical Sciences from Ben Gurion University of the Negev. In addition to his role in MDA Dr. Jaffe teaches in various academic programmes in the field of pre-hospital emergency medicine and preparedness to disasters.

Samuel Kottek is Emeritus Professor of the History of Medicine at the Hebrew University of Jerusalem. He is the Editor of *Korot: Journal of the Israel Society for the History of Medicine* and has published widely on topics related to Jews and the history of medicine, including writings on medicine in the Bible, *Medicine and Hygiene in the Works of Flavius Josephus*, (Leiden: Brill, 1994) and *La Bible la santé and l'hygiène* (Paris: Editions Glyphe, 2012, French).

Menachem Oberbaum, MD (Vienna), is the founder and current Director of the Centre of Integrated Complementary Medicine, Shaare Zedek

Medical Centre, Jerusalem, and the Director of Complementary and Alternative Medicine at the Faculty of Medicine of the Hebrew University of Jerusalem. He was Vice President and a founding member of the International Research Group on High Dilution Research (1991-1993) and its President (1993-1995). He holds the Hans Reckeweg Award for achievements in homo-toxicological research (2005) and is a Fellow of the British Faculty of Homeopathy. He founded Israel's first medical school course on Complementary Medicine at the Ben Gurion University, Beersheva. Oberbaum is a Deputy Editor of *Homeopathy*, the only homeopathic peer-reviewed journal, and has authored and co-authored over 70 publications and written five book chapters.

Avi Ohry, MD, was born in Israel in 1948. He is Emeritus Professor of Rehabilitation Medicine, Faculty of Medicine, Tel Aviv University and former Director of the Section of Rehabilitation Medicine, Reuth Medical Centre, Tel Aviv. In 2005, he was selected to be featured in the *Caring Physicians of the World* publication, by the World Medical Association. His main topics of research are neuro-rehabilitation, medical humanities, bio-ethics, history of medicine, the Jewish-Polish medical infrastructure between the two World-Wars, the Holocaust and medicine and the long-term effects of disability and captivity.

Miri Shefer-Mossensohn is an Associate Professor at the Department of Middle Eastern & African History at Tel Aviv University, and heads the Zvi Yavetz School of Historical Studies in the same institution. She is a historian of the Ottoman Empire, focusing on medicine, health and well-being in the Arabic and Turkish regions of the Middle East. Her books include *Ottoman Medicine: Healing and Medical Institutions 1500-1700* (New York: State University of New York Press, 2009; Turkish edition in 2014) and *Science among the Ottomans: The Cultural Creation and Exchange of Knowledge* (University of Texas Press, 2015, Turkish and Arabic editions in 2018).

Judy Siegel-Itzkovich, a veteran US-born medical and science journalist, moved to Israel after receiving her Bachelor's degree (Brooklyn College) and Master's degree (Columbia University). She was Health and Science editor of *The Jerusalem Post* for nearly 35 years and, after leaving in 2018, became health and science editor of the *Breaking Israel News* website and a translator from Hebrew to English. She has received numerous awards for her efforts to improve public health in Israel and for fighting against cigarette smoking. She has an honorary doctorate from Ben Gurion University of the Negev in Beersheva.

Roman Sonkin is a senior paramedic and instructor at Magen David Adom. Working in the Community Division as well as an active paramedic team-leader on the Mobile Intensive Care Units, Roman began as a volunteer at the Mitzpe-Ramon MDA station when he was fifteen. During his volunteering he took leadership, instructors and volunteer management courses among other training. He holds a bachelor's degree in Emergency Medicine (BEMS) from Ben Gurion University of the Negev. In addition to his work at MDA, Roman is a medical student in Silesia Medical University, Poland and is due to graduate in 2021.

Stuart Stanton FRCS (England and Edinburgh), FRCOG, FRANZCOG (Hon), is retired Professor of Urogynaecology, London University. He was educated at the City of London School and qualified in medicine in 1961 at the London Hospital Medical School, University of London. In 1984 he established the Department of Pelvic Floor Reconstruction and Urogynaecology at St. Georges Hospital, London and in 1997 was awarded a personal Chair there in Urogynaecology. He has authored or co-authored thirteen textbooks and over 230 peer-reviewed papers on gynaecology. He has served on six Charitable Foundations and twelve Editorial Boards.

Introduction

Medicine – From Biblical Canaan to Modern Israel

For Jews medicine has often been described as an obsession with the Yiddish farewell message זײַ געזונט *Zai Gezunt!* (Be Well!) seen as much an imperative as a formal leave-taking. The association of Jews with medicine began in earliest times and has continued through the millennia with physicians and patients, healers and carers, midwives and magic workers sometimes working together and at other times seen in fierce competition. Famous Jewish physicians worked in a variety of settings in many different cultures, often exemplified by the life of Maimonides (1138-1204) which began in Toledo and flowered as a rabbi, physician and community leader in Cairo.

This book covers that part of the Jewish story of medicine, health and healing as focused in the Holy Land from earliest times up to the present. It looks at the early influences which have influenced the Jewish practice of medicine requiring an understanding of the context in which this practice emerged and can be seen today in the ethical and religious underpinning of certain medical precepts. We begin with Babylonia, although it lies beyond the historic Holy Land, because of the profound influence of its medicine on the Babylonian Talmud, the largest corpus of early Jewish rabbinic thought developed over half a millennium in Israel and Babylon. In its analysis of medicine in the Holy Land and Israel from earliest times it covers many key topics in the understanding of health and illness. With its beginnings in Babylonia to present-day developments in Israel, covering both the Jewish and Arab populations, this book will coalesce with publications in the field of history, social science, anthropology and Islamic medicine.

It is more than 20 years since Manfred Waserman and Samuel Kottek edited *Health and Disease in the Holy Land: Ancient to Present* (Edward Mellen Press, 1996), an historical and scholarly review covering some of the ground of this book. However, it is now dated, and its focus was primarily concerned with public health and hygiene and so does not cover many of the areas we touch on: medical ethics, medical innovations, rehabilitation medicine and emergency care. Other recent works which touch on aspects of the story include Yosef Perry and Efraim Lev, *Modern Medicine in the Holy Land (1825-1920): Pioneering Studies in Late Ottoman Palestine* (Tauris Academic Studies, UK, 2007) and the writings of Shifra Shvarts on the Israeli Health Care System: *The Workers' Health Fund in Eretz Israel, Kupat Holim 1911-1937* (University of Rochester Press, 2002); *Health and Zionism: Israeli Healthcare System 1948-1960* (University of Rochester Press, 2008), Kenneth Collins, Guest Editor, *Korot: Israel Journal of the History of Medicine and Science*: 'Special Issue on Infectious Disease and Epidemics in the Land of Israel: 19th-20th centuries' (Magnus Press of the Hebrew University of Jerusalem, vol.21, 2011-2012). Finally, the immense contribution of Fred Rosner should be noted, in his *Medicine in the Bible and the Talmud* (New Jersey: Ktav Publishing, 1995) and his English translation of the classic Julius Preuss, *Biblical and Talmudic Medicine* (New York: Sanhedrin Press, 1978).

In Chapter 1, Professor Mark Geller, Professor of Hebrew and Jewish Studies, University College London, points out that as the last *dated* cuneiform tablets were composed in the late first century CE, it would be reasonable to assume that cuneiform writing lasted at least as long as Egyptian hieroglyphs, until the fourth century CE, providing ample opportunity for Aramaic and Syriac healers to meet and converse with experts who could still read the ancient scripts of Babylonia. Thus, he quotes a Vademecum in the Babylonian Talmud, in Tractate Gittin (68b-70a): a head-to-foot medical handbook in Aramaic with no attributed author, loaded with prescriptions containing Akkadian loanwords and calques, although with virtually no Greek technical terms.[1]

Geller considers that the particular strength of Babylonian medicine was its rigorous systematic arrangement of its data. While he notes that the logic of 'physiognomic omens' remains problematic, the results of symptom gathering in reference to progress of a disease or its prognosis could have been influenced by extensive experience of observing the course of fevers, infections or even patterns of pain by generations of physicians and healers.[2] Geller points out that the bulk of our knowledge of Babylonian medicine comes from the large number of prescriptions or medical recipes, which are distributed among numerous cuneiform tablets. An ancient medical catalogue, a tablet originating in the city of Assur in the eighth to seventh century BCE, predates Hippocratic influence.[3]

In Chapter 2, Professor Samuel Kottek, Emeritus Professor of History of Medicine, Hebrew University of Jerusalem, looks at surgery in the Bible and Talmud giving instances of some of the scenarios where the wounds, injuries and other accidents occurred. Thus, for example, he describes the death of Abimelech, the son of Yerubaal, as written in the Book of Judges. Abimelech was besieging a tower when a millstone was thrown by a woman from the top of the tower, which crushed his skull. The fracture of the skull was not immediately fatal; the King did not lose consciousness but he realized that he would not recover so he called for his armour-bearer to kill him so that his pride as a soldier would not be diminished by being killed by a woman.

Kenneth Collins, Visiting Professor, History of Medicine, Hebrew University of Jerusalem, outlines the story of Jewish popular medicine in the religious tradition using sources from the Bible and Talmud. He notes that the Land of Israel was strategically placed on the trade routes of antiquity and was especially open to the medical practices and traditions of its many neighbours, especially Egypt and Babylon/Mesopotamia. The Talmud, with its encyclopaedic view of the Jewish world spanning many centuries of Jewish life both in the Land of Israel and the Babylonian Diaspora, lent itself to coverage of a wide variety of traditional medical themes including folk remedies and health beliefs. From Talmudic times it was recommended that no wise person should live in a town which did not have a doctor and it was required for a patient to seek help for healing even on the Sabbath when religious restrictions might be set aside if there is any possible danger to health.

Professor Collins points out that some of the popular medicine tradition recorded in the Talmud will naturally seem strange, even outlandish, to the modern mind, but we should remember that in mediaeval Europe as late as the sixteenth century the apothecary was legally required to keep woodlice, ants, vipers, scorpions, crabs, sparrow brains and fox lungs in stock.[4] Leading rabbis of the Talmudic period, such as Abbaye and Raba, did have concerns about the use of magic and charms but, mindful of contemporary sentiment, accepted that whatever is done for therapeutic purposes is not to be regarded as superstitious.[5]

In Chapter 3 Professor Aref Abu-Rabia, Department of Middle Eastern Studies, Ben Gurion University of the Negev, Beersheba, provides the background for understanding Islamic medicine, as practised in the area for centuries until the beginnings of Ottoman rule. He shows the influences of the many local cultures and civilisations, including Byzantine, Persian, Greek and Roman. Included among the impressive array of physicians he describes, working across the whole of the Muslim world, are the outstanding Jewish physicians, *Sulayman al-Isra'ili* (Isaac Israeli) who practised in Kairouan, in modern Tunisia and *Musa ibn Maymon* (Moses Maimonides), physician in Fostat (Old Cairo).

Abu-Rabia considers that the main achievements of medieval Arabic-Islamic medicine were in five areas: systematization, hospitals, pharmacology, surgery and ophthalmology. The development of Arabic medical literature involved the constant reshaping of the Greek heritage by commenting on and systematizing ancient source material as exemplified by Ibn-Sina's (Avicenna) masterpiece the *Canon of Medicine (al-Qānūnfī al-tibb)* completed in 1025. In a brief review of Prophetic Medicine, Abu-Rafia asks for fresh thinking about a synthesis between Arabic-Islamic and Western medicine for their mutual benefit.

No account of medicine in the Holy Land would be complete without examining Islamic and Jewish Traditional Medicine. This has often been dismissed as representing primitive 'folk' customs but many of these beliefs have been persistent and affect medical care to the present day. In his Section on Islamic Traditional Medicine in Chapter 4, Professor Abu-Rabia outlines its role, indicating that its aim is to deter the causes of illness by hanging amulets or talismans on a person, making vows, visiting the tombs of saints, or using stratagems to mislead the sources of the disease, such as the influence of the evil eye, which can be a psychological idiom for the fear of misfortune.

Traditional healers among Palestinians/Arabs in Israel have used local plants for a variety of ailments, such as a brew of eucalyptus bark to treat influenza. For a serious cold or backache, cupping, the placing of hot cups on the patient's back, is employed. Lacerations are then made in the swollen areas to allow the malady to be eliminated. Professor Abu-Rabia notes that as modern medicine has become more effective, the need for popular or folk medicine for essentially physical problems is declining. Yet, when modern medicine fails to offer a solution to a problem, there is a tendency to turn to healers in the hopes that they can succeed where modern medicine has failed. Traditional medicine, sometimes also referred to as popular or folk-medicine, occupies the ground between the use of natural medicinal substances and the traditional religious quest for the victory of the forces of good in an uncertain world. Though the pharmacology of Biblical and Talmudic medicine, as well as that of medieval Jewish practitioners, may seem strange to the modern health consumer Jewish folk practices have remained remarkably persistent surviving to the present day.

In the Section on Jewish Traditional Medicine, Professor Kenneth Collins notes that this has often been seen as the superstitious and primitive legacy of the encounter between Jews and their neighbours, especially in the medieval Christian and Arab worlds, over millennia of dispersion. However, in recent years, especially following the movement of the previously marginalised Jews from eastern communities into the political mainstream in Israel, there have been serious attempts to understand this folk medicine culture in its proper context.[6]

Professor Collins notes that the rabbinic *Responsa* literature of the Middle Ages contains much of medical interest. Here we see the attitudes of people distressed by illness, to healing practices and what they had recourse to in the hope of returning to full health. Indeed, the efficacy of many plant medicines has long been understood for simple symptom control and to this day there are many plant based remedies in official national pharmacopoeias which have stood the test of time and have met the criteria of randomised control trials.[7] However, Lev and Amar relate that the commercial field for the sale of traditional medicines in Israel is declining and businesses have closed and the inventory of medicines has diminished.[8] Their work in documenting the decline of this sector is a window into the medieval world, using philology, comparisons across Levantine cultures and comparisons with Biblical and Talmudic medicine.

In Chapter 5 Emeritus Professor Eran Dolev, Department of Internal Medicine, Tel Aviv University, shows how Military Medicine is a unique discipline of the medical profession. While doctors in general, are committed only to their patients, military doctors are also committed to the organisation and to its missions. Wars and their concomitant injuries can be identified from the Biblical Era though there is no indication, whatsoever, that Biblical armies had the support of doctors. While wartime trauma was identified in Greek culture it was not until Roman times that armies enjoyed the support of medical personnel.

Professor Dolev follows the development of military medicine through Byzantine and Crusader and times until the well-documented French campaign under Napoleon Bonaparte at Acre (Akko) in 1798, which he describes in detail. The Palestine Campaigns of the British Army from 1916 to 1918 were fought by a British Expeditionary Force against the Ottoman army in the Sinai desert, in the Holy Land, especially at Gaza and Beersheva and ending in Damascus. The cardinal lessons that the British had learned from the Boer War in South Africa, such as the need to protect the troops from infectious diseases, measures to control blood loss, surgery under anaesthesia and the introduction of field ambulances, were applied to the

Palestine Campaigns. Finally, he discusses the medical lessons learned in the various wars in Israel since Independence in 1948.

In Chapter 6, which covers Health and Medical Services in Ottoman Eretz Israel, Professor Miri Shefer-Mossensohn, Middle Eastern and African History, Tel Aviv University, uses extensive local Arabic and Ottoman sources which show the inhabitants of this Ottoman province as active players in the realm of health and medicine, signifying a level of complexity that many Jewish and European sources have missed, perhaps through a lack of familiarity with Arabic and Turkish. These have emphasised the backwardness of the area indicating that no real understanding of diseases existed, and that fatalism was the norm.

However, Professor Shefer-Mossensohn shows that in addition to the dirt and disease, the Arabic and Ottoman sources reveal that time was taken to understand disease and that action was taken to ward off illness. She shows that the building blocks of the Ottoman medical system were folk, or traditional, medicine, religious or 'Prophetic' medicine and classic medicine based on Galen's four humours. Shefer-Mossensohn notes that there were also female healers, not only midwives (*dayas*) and wet nurses (*qabilas*), who enjoyed formal training with the expertise to deal with male and female patients and colleagues alike. The use of original source material allows for proper consideration of the diseases, infections and plagues, and the stories of real lives in the maelstrom of illness during the Ottoman centuries.

Kenneth Collins provides an account of Medicine during the British Mandate in Chapter 7. When the British arrived, there were some health clinics and hospital facilities, sometimes provided by European religious societies, only available in the larger towns, especially in Jerusalem. However, in general, health care was often undeveloped with low life expectancy, high infant mortality and a significant susceptibility to diseases such as malaria, trachoma and leprosy. Collins examines health policy, developments in the delivery of care and changes in medical outcomes during the roughly 30 years of the British Mandate for Palestine.

While health services improved during the three decades of British rule, Government funding for health was not seen as a priority. Developments in the Jewish community were often funded by the Jews themselves or were supported by Jewish communities abroad, especially in the United States. Rural Arabs tended to rely on traditional folk healers, while in larger towns they had to accept the lower level of health care provision which was provided by the Mandate Government. This inevitably led to health inequalities between the Jewish and Arab populations especially as, within the Jewish sector, there was from the start an emphasis on health improvement as an early priority of the Zionist movement to create a healthier and fitter Jew. The Mandate years saw the extensive development of health services in the Jewish community which were ready to form the nucleus of health care when the State of Israel was born.

In his Health Schemes and Health in Israel, in Chapter 8, Professor Nadav Davidovitch, Department of Public Health Medicine, Ben Gurion University, Beersheva, describes the development of services since the establishment of the State. Alongside the spread and growth of the population the health infrastructure steadily expanded, building on services that served the pre-State Jewish population. The Israeli healthcare system combines certain characteristics of centralised control, and a market economy. The political ideological composition of health organisations constituted unique features of the healthcare system, and they continue to shape its nature today.

Professor Davidovitch notes the factors which produced the National Health Insurance Law in 1995. This means that medical care in Israel is to be provided on the basis of medical need, independently of the financial means of the insured. The law also defined a uniform basket of medical services that the health providers (HMOs) must give their subscribers with government oversight over their operations. At the same time, the responsibility for managing the Ministry of Health's budget was delegated to the Ministry of Finance. Davidovitch goes on to outline the major diseases, cardiovascular, cancer and diabetes, and the risk factors, including smoking and obesity, across the Jewish and Arab communities. He points to possible changes in the medical services to adapt to evolving needs, as life expectancy increases and medical innovations add to growing costs, and all this in a current system chronically under-funded and needing additional personnel. Thus, the need to reduce health inequities, sustaining a strong healthcare system available for all, as envisioned in the Israeli National Health Insurance Law, is one of the major challenges of Israeli society.

In Chapter 9, on Rehabilitation Medicine in Israel, Professor Avi Ohry, Former Director of Rehabilitation Medicine at Reuth Medical and Rehabilitation Centre, Tel Aviv and Dr. Nava Blum, Senior Lecturer, Director of the Rehabilitation Program, Max Stern Academic College, Emek Jezreel, define rehabilitation medicine as a medical branch concerned with the diagnosis, treatment and long-term follow up that aims to enhance and restore, where possible, functional ability and quality of life to people with disabilities in all ages. They note that neither the medical establishment during the British Mandate, nor the medical care provided during the four centuries of Ottomans rule, could cope with existing medical or psychiatric disabilities and they outline the basis of the strides made in rehabilitation medicine in Israel in recent decades, often emerging from the limited facilities that existed within the Jewish community in the pre-State period.

Professor Ohry and Dr. Blum focus on developments in Physical Medicine and Rehabilitation in the first ten years of the State of Israel, as it faced the problem of thousands of handicapped people following the War of Independence, and thousands of injured or handicapped immigrants. It also had to deal with a polio epidemic, mainly affecting children. They show how comprehensive rehabilitation services were introduced into Israel which continue to serve the population to this day.

In Chapter 10, on Emergency Care in Israel and Abroad, Roman Sonkin, Uriel Goldberg and Eli Jaffe of Magen David Adom (MDA) describe the history and development of the organisation from its establishment in 1930 with volunteer recruitment and first aid training to its advanced status today. Magen David Adom, the Israeli Emergency Pre-Hospital Medical Services is a national, statutory non-governmental organisation supervised by the Ministry of Health. In 1950, MDA was entrusted by the Israeli Parliament (the Knesset) to be the national ambulance service, blood bank and the Israeli Red Cross organisation.

Today it has a fleet of over 1,100 fully equipped ambulances, over 750 first response Medi-Cycles, as well as two helicopters, a Jet-ski and a rescue boat which are used on the Sea of Galilee. They are stationed across the country to allow for an average response time of less than five minutes for first responders and less than 8.7 minutes for ambulances and Mobile Intensive Care Units. Sonkin, Goldberg and Jaffe describe the innovative technology which enhances MDA care and show how it operates in time of peace and war while able to take part in international emergency operations.

Complementing the care of emergencies in Israel is United Hatzalah, a volunteer-based organisation which has changed the way emergency care is both viewed and delivered. Over 5,000 volunteers each answer two or three emergency calls every day of the week using ambucycles, two-wheeled ambulance-motorcycle hybrids which have the fastest response times because they can weave in and out of heavy traffic and achieve an average response time of fewer than three minutes, covering every single city in Israel.

In Chapter 11 on Medical Ethics in Israel, Professor Shimon Glick, Faculty of Health Sciences, Ben Gurion University, Beersheba, describes the modern era of medical ethics as 'an era in formation, perhaps even as a unique, as yet unfinished, experiment'. While the chapter deals in the main with the Jewish ethos, he notes that in all areas of public debate on bio-ethical issues an effort is made to receive and include input from the non-Jewish population. As the Muslim position on many bio-ethical issues is quite close to that of the Jewish view, the major differences of opinion in many bio-ethical issues in Israel are rather between religious and secular viewpoints.

Professor Glick notes that the major innovation and the dominant, almost revolutionary, feature among current Western bio-ethical principles has been the emphasis on autonomy. This prioritisation of autonomy represents a clear break with the dominant spirit of 'paternalism' dating back on the part of the physician to the days of Hippocrates. Sanctity of human life is not included in the current secular Western list of values but is a central value in the Jewish tradition. Glick elaborates on the word 'mitzvah', which literally means a religious commandment but has a general meaning closer to 'incumbent obligation' which occupies a place equivalent in evocative force to the American legal system's 'rights'. This seemingly minor difference in the presentation of the issues has significant implications in the field of medical ethics. This naturally leads into his coverage of such issues as patient's rights and historical controversies involving abortion, euthanasia, autopsies, transplantation and fertility treatments. In fact, the area of assisted reproduction is highly developed in Israel with more centres per unit population than any country in the Western world.

In Chapter 12 on Complementary and Alternative Medicine, CAM, Dr. Menachem Oberbaum, Director of the Centre for Integrative and Complementary Medicine, Shaare Zedek Medical Centre, Jerusalem, identifies and describes three broad periods which can be distinguished in the history of CAM in Palestine/Israel. The first ended with the establishment of mainstream, bio-medical medicine in Palestine in the mid-twentieth century. The second, which lasted for about a generation, was practised by a group of 'celebrity' CAM therapists and their followers. The third period, which began in the 1980s and continues into the present, is one in which CAM is struggling for recognition, legalization and integration into the mainstream of conventional medicine.

Dr. Oberbaum believes that in the longer view, however, the gradual entry of CAM into bio-medicine cannot be ignored. He points to profound and lasting changes in the status of CAM in Israel without endangering the primacy of conventional medicine. CAM has progressed from being seen as a relic of the Middle Ages to the stage where almost all Israeli hospitals have CAM units. However, he cautions that this expansion may be following growing consumer demand, economic factors and market competition.

The book concludes with a chapter on medicine in Israel today. It has looked on the many influences which have shaped that medicine as the area has been settled and fought over for the past three millennia. Standing at a strategic crossroad between Babylon and Egypt political and military conquerors have crossed its borders many times and traces of their presence form part of the medical story. There is a national Israeli openness to new and sometimes alternative ways of achieving the best health-care outcomes and this has been exemplified by Israel's description as the 'Start-Up' nation with very many more new start-ups than many larger industrialised nations. A lack of natural resources and positive funding initiatives allied to a skilled and well-educated workforce has driven many fields of innovation forward. This ability to think and react in a creative way has extended into every advanced technological area including medicine and health care.[9] This chapter focuses on some key areas of medical research, and the practical procedures and therapies it has produced.

We have followed the path of Waserman and Kottek in their *Health and Disease in the Holy Land*, combining studies which extensively use original research with those that review and re-interpret previous scholarship. The region of the Holy Land, the Land of Israel, has a rich history and its medical story has been a source of fascination throughout the ages. Our story of medicine in the Land of Israel gives an overview of the influences which have affected it, from Babylonia and the Islamic World, to the Roman, Greek, Byzantine, Crusader and Ottoman links seen in various chapters of the story.

We trust that this work, which concentrates on a geographical area which has contributed so much to humanity through the legacy of the three Abrahamic faiths, fully tackles many of the topics which illustrate the broad canvas that the subject demands.

Notes

1.   Few rabbis in the Talmud are credited with medical knowledge. One who stands out from the rest is the third-fourth century scholar Abbaye, who contributed 27 medical prescriptions to Talmudic discourse, almost all of which were erroneously attributed to his mother, who died in childbirth. Abbaye's source for such technical knowledge was likely to have been a Babylonian expert, since many of Abbaye's prescriptions contained technical Akkadian loanwords and calques.

2. E.g. death of a wife, becoming rich or poor, etc.

3. Babylonian rabbis or Amoraim knew no Greek nor read Greek texts such as Aristotle or Hippocrates. Many of the Greek terms found in the Babylonian Talmud were introduced via the Mishnah and other writings brought over from Roman Palestine, and these Greek terms were often grossly misunderstood and misused. A remarkable pattern appears in the Talmud, that Greek loanwords usually appear within Hebrew contexts and Akkadian words appear in Jewish Babylonian Aramaic, and this applies to medical passages in the Talmud.

4. Rosner, F. (ed. and trans.), *Julius Preuss' Biblical and Talmudic Medicine* (New York, Sanhedrin Press, 1978), p.433.

5. Epstein, I., *The Talmud*, Shabbat 67a and Hullin 77b.

6. Matras, H., *Jewish Folk Medicine in the 19th and 20th Centuries* (Tel Aviv, Bet HaTfutsot, 1995), pp.113-135.

7. There is an extensive contemporary literature relating botanical species and modern pharmacological research. See, for example, Lansky, E.P., Paavilainen, H.M., Pawlus, A.D., and Newman, R.A., Ficus spp. (fig): 'Ethnobotany and potential as anticancer and anti-inflammatory agents', *Journal of Ethnopharmacology*, 2008, 119, pp.195-213.

8. Lev, E. and Amar, Z., 'Ethnopharmacological Survey of Traditional Drugs Sold in Israel at the end of the 20th Century', *Journal of Ethnopharmacoly*, 200; 72. pp.191-205.

9. https://www.israel21c.org/topic/health/ accessed 18/5/2020.

1

Introduction to Theory in Babylonian Medicine

Markham J. Geller

Ancient Babylonian medicine was essentially an extensive pharmaceutical or drug-based system of therapy based upon externally observable symptoms, with little in the way of surgery.[1] Medical interventions consisted largely of ingesting drugs orally, clysters applied through the rectum, external application of bandages and massage, combined with the use of amulets suspended from the body, fumigation and other kinds of psychologically-oriented procedures. There is no evidence for phlebotomy, nor a theory of humours on the Greek model. Treatment for disease, however, was not limited to drugs and manipulation, but could also involve

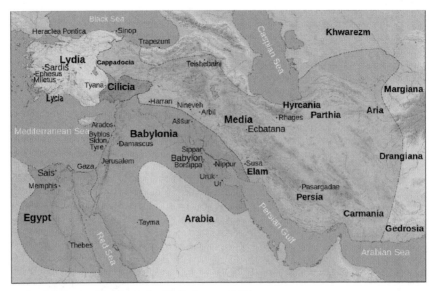

1. The Babylonian Empire in the Sixth Century BCE.

the use of incantations and magical rituals; on the level of practice, these professions were involved in the administration of healing measures, involving both physical contact and participation in activities intended to affect the patient's state of mind. Unlike Greek, Chinese, or Ayurvedic medicine, it is difficult to discern any specific Babylonian medical theory, partly because Babylonian scribal culture had no tradition of promulgating theory in written form, since such topics were the subject of oral commentaries within academies. This in no way implies that Babylonians avoided medical theory, but rather that it must be inferred from the large corpus of texts dealing with many different forms of therapy, diagnosis and prognosis, as well as academic works on anatomy and pharmacology. As we will see below, in some instances one has to look at later sources and languages from Mesopotamia to reconstruct medical theories from this region.

It is important, for comparative purposes, to think of medicine in the ancient world in terms of 'systems' of medicine, falling into major groups, e.g. Greco-Roman medicine, Mesopotamian medicine,[2] Egyptian medicine and later Arabic medicine. An ancient system of medicine often consisted of sub-corpora, such as Hippocratic treatises, or of Diocles (the fourth century BCE Greek physician whose works were mostly lost but have been reconstructed from quotations in later authors, especially Galen, see van der Eijk, 2000-2001), as well as Greek medical philosophies (e.g. Methodists, Empiricists, Dogmatists), culminating in the works of Galen, but the inherent similarities allow us to view these as components of a single comprehensive system of medicine. So far, however, no one has proposed similarly distinctive Babylonian medical 'philosophies' or theoretical approaches comparable to these competing Greek schools of thought, but this may be due to the nature of our sources. Even though the modern view of Babylonian medicine is largely monolithic, in fact Babylonian medicine incorporated quite different approaches to healing and treatments, depending upon the orientation of practitioners.[3] One area of potential conflict was in the relative role of gods and divine influences (including demons and ghosts) within diagnosis and therapy, since it seems plausible that in some quarters, expressions like the 'hand of a god' in a medical context may have implied personal divine involvement in a patient's health (see Heeßel 2000, 49-54), although ancient scholars may have used this expression as a technical term for disease (as suggested by van der Toorn 1985: 199, and see now Schmidtchen 2018, 211-219). The same applies to the activities of the ghost-induced roaring in a patient's ear, which could either be interpreted literally or as a metaphor for anxiety or psychogenic diseases, usually requiring magical interventions.[4] The main healing professions – the *āšipu*-exorcist and *asû*-physician – also reflect different approaches to healing, primarily contrasting appeals for divine help versus technology (recipes), and both of their traditional approaches were later challenged by the introduction of astral-medicine, dependent upon zodiac or planetary influences on the body and disease.

The particular strength of Babylonian medicine was its rigorous systematic arrangement of its data, implying limited technical knowledge available to the Babylonian physician, despite the lack of instruments or technology. This can best be seen in Babylonian knowledge of anatomy, which was rudimentary at best, especially as far as internal anatomy is concerned. Little was known about the function of organs such as the heart (thought to be an organ of cognition, Westenholz and Sigrist 2006), versus the brain (usually understood as bone marrow), and there is little evidence to demonstrate that Babylonians associated lungs with respiration. Nevertheless, Babylonian scholars generally understood the components and functions of the urinary tract, probably based upon studies of animal anatomy, since there is virtually no evidence for autopsies or studies of morbid anatomy. On the other hand, except for a brief period in third century BCE Alexandria,[5] Greek medicine also resisted autopsy. The exception to this rule was, of course, mummification in Egypt, but since this was treated as a mortuary rather than medical science, it is unclear how much anatomical knowledge processed through mummification filtered through to Egyptian physicians.

However, the absence of dissection did not deter Babylonian scholars from producing detailed academic studies of anatomy preserved in so-called lexical lists, which listed human bodily organs as well as diseases. The interesting feature of these lists, known as UGU.MU,[6] is the many divergences from anatomical nomenclature known from medical prescriptions and diagnostic texts, with the supposition being that such lists represented academic or 'theoretical' anatomy which differed from the practical anatomy of medical prescriptions. These lists demonstrate an early interest in anatomy, since many examples come from school texts, known mainly from the scribal centre of Nippur in Mesopotamia and from the Hittite capital, Hattuša (Cohen, 2012). An example of the relationship between these academic lists and medical texts can be seen in the following extract (MSL 9, p. 67):

kir$_4$.mu	= *ap-pi* 'my nose'
pa.an.ta kir$_4$.mu	= *na-pi-iš ap-pi-ia* 'breathing of my nose'[7]
pa.ág kir$_4$.mu	= *na-hi-ir ap-pi-ia* 'snoring of my nose'[8]

im kir$_4$.mu	= *ša-ar ap-pi-ia* 'inhaling (lit. wind) of my nose'
sag kir$_4$.mu	= **re-eš ap-pi-ia** 'top of my nose'
šakir$_4$.mu	= **li-ib-bi ap-pi-ia** 'middle of my nose'
bùru kir$_4$.mu	= *pi-li-iš ap-pi-[ia]* 'nostril (lit. perforation) of my nose'
síg kir$_4$.mu	= *ha-an-zar-ar-ti ap-pi-ia* 'slime (lit. green wool) of my nose'[9]
[bad] kir$_4$.mu	= *du-ur ap-pi-ia* 'wall of my nose'

The terminology marked in bold indicates Akkadian phrases which either appear or are likely to appear in medical recipes, while the other terms are more exotic and hence would only appear in recipes exceptionally. This pattern repeats itself throughout the text of UGU.MU, in which many terms are not commonly found in medical recipes.

Surprisingly, the anatomical lists appear to have dropped out of scholarly interest in the first millennium BCE. This is not true for a comparable list of diseases, which existed in both unilingual Sumerian and bilingual Sumerian-Akkadian formats, which were actively copied and studied in Assurbanipal's Royal Library in Nineveh (MSL 9, p. 90-102).[10] The same pattern emerges, that the lists preserve rare or unusual names for diseases not known from medical recipes, and moreover that the disease list was intended to match descriptive Akkadian disease terms with their Sumerian counterparts, as a work of philology rather than medical science (see MSL 9, p. 95 and DCCLT):

giš.giš.g[íd]	= [*pa*]-*ṣa-du* 'to smash'
gìri h[um]	= [*ha*]-*ma-šu* 'to snap off' (the foot)
gìri tag	= *še-pa ha-miš-tu* 'deformed foot' (see PBS 12, 13)
gìri.gába.an.du	= (*še-pi*) *i-te-eq-lip-pu-u* (<*neqelpû*) 'my drifting foot'[11] (MSL 9 78: 110, 95: 103)
níg.na.me.eš e$_{11}$.da	= *mim-ma i-li-a-šum* 'anything (pl.) going up it' (MSL 9 p. 79)
gìri al.g[ilim]	= (*še-pa*) [*i*]*t-te-né-gi-ir* 'the foot gets twisted'
gìr [peš$_6$.peš$_6$]	= *še-pa ub-bu-ṭa-tu* 'swollen' (foot)
[gìr ....]	= (*še-pa*) *nu-pu-ha-tu* 'inflamed' (foot)
[gìr.du.du.ur].hi.	= (*še-pa*) *na-mu-ši-ša-tu* 'dead (foot)'

Like the extract from UGU.MU given above, this list offers another example of descriptions of pathologies which hardly occur as medical symptoms, and it is likely that this list is not based on medical literature. The disease list in its entirety appears to represent an independent non-therapeutic study of medical conditions and disabilities.[12]

Medicinal Plants

A similar argument can be made for the academic study of medicinal plants, herbs, and minerals, in a series of tablets containing much more complex lists under the heading of Uruanna. These lists serve as precursors to the later and more extensive works of Theophrastus and Dioscorides, but Uruanna nevertheless contains valuable information on roughly 400 medical ingredients regularly used in Mesopotamian therapeutic prescriptions. In addition to giving names with brief descriptions, the Uruanna treatise also provides information on *Dreckapotheke* or disagreeable recipe ingredients (such as animal faeces), which mostly turn out to be secret names for ordinary plants (cf. Geller, 2015: 39-40, 43):

25	'fruit'-plant	*Deckname*: human testicle (gloss: mankind)
26	field-plant (gloss: clod)	*Deckname*: mountain *galgaltu*[13]
27	camelthorn (*ašāgu*)	*Deckname*: ditto of donkey crotch[14]
28	*illūru*	*Deckname*: bedbugs
29	'shepherd's crook'	*Deckname*: [human] thigh-bone

The purpose of this section of the plant list is to explain secret names (*Deckname*), usually of a prurient character, which happen to represent quite ordinary ingredients, perhaps to prevent non-specialists or laymen from trying to reproduce medical recipes. Hence a reference to 'human testicle' in a prescription actually refers to a harmless 'fruit'-plant, an ordinary fruit ingredient. A 'field'-plant turns out to be a clod of earth from a field, which may be useful to counteract moistness in a medical symptom, but this may also be represented by a nickname for insects, 'mountain hunger', reflecting the voracious activity of such pests. A similar gloss, 'donkey's crotch', is probably another nickname for an insect or parasite associated with this particular beast, as a secret name for a common thorn plant. A similar term for bedbugs (*išid bukāni*) refers to the reddish *illuru*-plant, while the unsavoury ingredient of human bone in a recipe actually refers to a common plant known as 'shepherd's crook'.

Finally, the plant and mineral lists are accompanied by explanatory treatises known as Šammu šikinšu and Abnu šikinšu (lit. 'a plant – its properties, a mineral – its properties'), describing the inherent characteristics and uses of medicinal plants and minerals.[15] The existence of such texts – not necessarily composed by doctors – within libraries and archives indicates independent study of topics related to medicine but not strictly for the use of doctors, in a somewhat similar manner in which later Greek philosophers (including Aristotle) made use of medical knowledge in their studies of nature and the cosmos (see for example Stadhouders, 2011: 25, Stadhouders, 2012: 11 [IIIa 5]):

> *šammu šikinšu kīma urnê inibšu kīma ašāgi ṣalim šammu šū murru*
> *šumšu ana šuburri damiq arqūssu ana šuburrīšu tašakkanma iballuṭ,*
> The plant – its nature is like *urnû*-mint, its fruit is black like a thorn: that plant has (as) its name – *murru*. Good for the anus, you should administer (it) while it is fresh into his rectum, and he should get well.

This concise statement informs us that a medicinal plant called *murru* ('bitter') has the properties of mint and its fruit is black (or dark) like thorns. Since the drug is beneficial for rectal disease, the practitioner should insert the plant while freshly picked into the patient's anus.

The *Šammu šikinšu* commentary on *materia medica* is not alone as an example of explanatory lists of drugs. A similar explanatory lexical text, a therapeutic vademecum, reads as follows, as a typical example of this kind of instruction (BAM 1, see Attia and Buisson, 2012: 27 ii 7-8):

> *kukru*-plant / a drug for *ašû*-disease / ditto (pound and rub in fat)
> The plant(s): *kukru, burāšu*-juniper, *kamantu, nikiptu, hûratu, qudru*-seed,
> put all these plants into fat, cook in a fire and while it is hot rub into his head.
> *kamantu*-plant / a drug for flatulence / pound and rub in fat

The purpose of this vademecum is to combine several kinds of data into a single list, identifying which drugs are useful against which disease, and it provides typical preparations or use of the drug in a recipe. In other words, the vademecum provides all minimal requirements for making a standard recipe. A recipe likewise takes two distinct forms. It can either be a *simplicium* consisting of a single drug being prescribed against a single symptom, or a 'compound' recipe containing numerous ingredients, similar to a theriac in Roman medicine. The *simplicia* might reflect theoretical pharmacology as well as pharmaceutics.[16] Here are examples of *simplicia* found in renal disease (see BAM 7, pp. 4-5):

plant ingredients:

ajar-kaspi	'silver-rosette'-plant
baluhhu	(aromatic tree) (mixed with pressed oil)
imhur-līm	'it confronted a thousand(diseases)'-plant
hašû	thyme(?)
irrû	cucumber
karān šēlibi	'fox-vine'
kasû and *mê kasî*	juice of tamarind or the plant itself
kurkānû	(a 'duck-like' plant)
lišān kalbi	'dog's-tongue'-plant
maštakal	(used in beer in rectal disease texts)
murru	'bitter'-plant (mixed in tavern beer)
uhhahu	thorn
zēr bīni	tamarisk seed
šaman erēni	cedar oil (mixed with vinegar)
šammu peṣû	'white plant'

Since relatively few of these *simplicia* can be identified with modern botanical names, it remains difficult to assess the value of these ingredients, especially since we have little information regarding dosage and amounts prescribed for individual conditions. Nevertheless, once the entire Babylonia pharmacopeia is reconstructed, the next important step will be to compare the *simplicia* to similar substances used in other systems of medicine (e.g. Greek and Arabic medicine), to determine whether continuities existed within ancient systems of therapy.

Diagnostic Handbook

Another example of systematic thinking can be seen in the so-called *Diagnostic Handbook*, which is a lengthy list of several thousand individual symptoms organised from head to foot.[17] The format and structure of this synonym list is based upon the standard casuistic 'if P then Q' logic of divination,[18] such as

> If (a patient's) head is hot, the veins of his temples, his hands and his feet throb together, his feet are cold up to his shins, the top of his nose is black, moles on his fingers are spotted yellow, the middle of his eyes are spotted yellow and white, both eyelids are affected … and breathing in his nose is affected, (then as) breath escapes from his mouth, it promotes death into his life ….

(TDP III, 61-62; cf. Scurlock, 2014, 15, 21, l. 61-62; see Rutz 2011: 301)

The symptomatic indicators are similar to what is known from Hippocratic medicine, with parts of human anatomy being labelled as hot or cold, or coloured (black, white, yellow), or pulsating, all used as diagnostic indicators of impending death. Other passages relate whether the patient's body is moist or dry, such as the following extract from the same work (TDP XXII 33, see Heeßel, 2000, 254; Scurlock, 2014, 187):

> If a man's epigastrium is thoroughly dried up, his epigastrium pains him but is not burning hot, he urinates blood, that man is 'loosened' and suffers from *li'bu*-fever disease.

Moreover, the opening two 'tablets' (or chapters) of the *Handbook* are modelled on classic mantic procedures, listing good or bad omens which the therapist might see en route to visiting the patient, such as seeing a pregnant woman or pig;[19] in effect, the character of the symptoms in the *Diagnostic Handbook* can arguably be described as representing diagnostic theory, since they do not reflect actual symptoms appearing in medical prescriptions.[20] One of the other key differences between the *Diagnostic Handbook* and medical prescriptions is that the former collection of symptoms often provides prognoses on whether the patient would be likely to live, die, or suffer chronic illness, reflecting the mantic nature of the symptoms as omens; in contrast to this, medical prescriptions rarely offer prognoses, but most often affirm that the patient will recover. The interesting question is how the symptom data was gathered and how it was then used. Mesopotamian science was attuned to mantic observation (protasis) combined with a possible result or interpretation of the sign or omen (apodosis), although the actual basis for interpretations is often unclear. The criteria for determining results from omens and signs within major types of omens (from entrails of animals, movements of celestial bodies, prodigies and terrestrial omens, or dreams) differ for each genre, and a modern understanding of omens is hampered by the lack of any ancient guidelines for interpreting the system.

The same applies to diagnostic omens or symptoms, which resemble divination in certain respects, although with some possible modifications. Whereas the logical relationship between the protasis and apodosis of general omens is often obscure,[21] omens dealing with symptoms had certain obvious advantages. First of all, the genres of diagnostic and physiognomic omens were considered by Mesopotamian scholarship to be closely related (see Steinert, 2018: 4), which meant that all physical characteristics and behaviour of the human body were systematised, scrutinised and recorded. Second, symptoms which led to the prediction of a specific result (e.g. death or chronic illness) could be checked empirically, which is not necessarily the case with other types of omens.

Although the logic of physiognomic omens remains problematic,[22] the results of symptom gathering in reference to progress of a disease or its prognosis could have been influenced by extensive experience of observing the course of fevers, infections or even patterns of pain by generations of physicians and healers. Furthermore, a theoretical element was also generated by the symptom lists, which distinguished between parts of the body being hot, cold, wet, or dry, or reflecting four diagnostic colours of red, white, black, or yellow, and these criteria were occasionally also applied to internal organs as well, which would not have been observed.

The highly systematic nature of symptom lists, e.g. from head to foot, made ample use of symptoms as a general study of semiotics of disease, but this work was clearly not designed as a diagnostic tool in the modern sense. For one thing, the symptoms are not drawn from specific case histories but from many patients suffering from a particular disease. At the same time, we have to wonder why ancient scholars never thought of recording individual symptoms from a specific disease, in order to better identify these. Under the present arrangement, each individual disease symptom would have been assigned its place in the list according to which body part it affected, rather than as a collection of symptoms referring to a single patient. Although from our point of view, this entire system looks cumbersome and impractical, it might be worth turning the clock back and trying to understand why the *Diagnostic Handbook* was created in this way.

First of all, it seems clear that the *Diagnostic Handbook* (like its Hippocratic counterparts) dealt with acute diseases, not common colds. For this reason, every symptom was considered to be potentially decisive as the basis of a prognosis, i.e. whether the patient would live or die. Second, all divination and forecasting in Mesopotamia was based upon single-omen prognoses, rather than combinations of different omens used to determine what would happen in future. Finally, the end user of the *Diagnostic Handbook* would probably know the text by heart and in any case know where to find the symptoms, if listed according to human anatomy. In any case, anatomy-based symptoms would have been easier to detect and comment upon in a world without instruments (thermometers or microscopes, etc.), while disease-based symptomology may not have rendered more accurate or reliable diagnoses, because of differences between patients in regard to age, general health, and any other diseases they might have had. In fact, the *Diagnostic Handbook* has the advantage of being somewhat neutral and observational, in assigning a specific symptom to a part of the body rather than to an assumed illness. So what looks like a medically useless endeavour from the standpoint of modern medicine may have had practical applications as well as offering theoretical perspectives on ancient diseases.

The bulk of our knowledge, however, of Babylonian medicine comes from numerous prescriptions or medical recipes, which are distributed among a number of specific treatises or 'series' of cuneiform tablets devoted to a particular theme. Most of our information regarding the overall structure of texts containing medical prescriptions comes from an ancient medical catalogue, a tablet originating in the city of Assur in the eighth-seventh century which is now known from fragments in New Haven (Yale) and Chicago (The Oriental Institute). This ancient catalogue of some ninety medical treatises compiled by Assyrian and Babylonian scholars became widely known, with treatises listed by their titles from head to foot, as well as listing general pathologies which had no specific anatomical connections. The obverse of this Assur Medical Catalogue defined twelve areas or regions of the body which became the subjects of medical works and these have conveniently been labelled as follows:

'Cranium' deals with diseases of the head, consisting of five tablets
'Eyes' deals with eye problems and diseases.[23]
'Ears' (a single-tablet treatise) deals with ear diseases.[24]
'Neck' probably consisted of six tablets dealing with neck problems predominantly attributed to ghosts.
'Nosebleed' is very fragmentary and only the colophon of one manuscript has survived.[25]
'Teeth' consisted of at least two tablets dealing with diseases of the mouth.[26]
'Bronchia' consisted of six tablets dealing with respiratory and lung disease.[27]
'Stomach' consisted of five tablets dealing with digestive problems.[28]
'Epigastrium / Abdomen' may have consisted of as many as eight tablets and deals with diseases of the chest and belly.
'Kidney' may have comprised three tablets and deals with renal and urinary problems, including kidney stones and male sexual dysfunction.[29]

'Anus' consists of five tablets dealing with rectal problems and haemorrhoids.[30]

'Hamstrung' probably consisted of at least four tablets and deals with leg and foot problems.[31]

'Other Diseases'

While these texts deal with diseases affecting specific areas of human anatomy, another listing on the reverse side of the Assur Medical Catalogue provides the opening lines (incipits) of texts dealing with diseases not associated with any particular body organ. These are associated with 'skin' lesions, 'hazards' (e.g. being attacked by lion, epilepsy, stroke, paralysis), 'evil powers' (manifested by twitching or aphasia), 'divine anger' (indicated by severe anxiety, etc.), 'oracles' (with poor medical predictions), 'mental illness', 'impotence' and 'sexual dysfunction', 'pregnancy' and 'childbirth', and finally with 'veterinary medicine' (see Steinert, ed., 2018: 203-291). The general taxonomy of disease has a different orientation than that found in later Greco-Roman medicine, partly because of an older tradition in Mesopotamia of attributing diseases such as epilepsy, stroke, and neurological disorders to divine wrath.[32] However, gods are not specifically referenced in the Assur Medical Catalogue as primary causes of disease, with the exception of the god Anu, the remote god of heaven who has no clearly defined role within magic and medicine; the reference to the wrath of Anu is a metaphor for general divine anger.

It is noteworthy that the medical corpus as a whole, as redacted by the royal scribes of King Assurbanipal in the seventh century BCE for his Nineveh library, appears to adhere to the organisational principles characteristic of the Assur Medical Catalogue. However, medical prescriptions also had a characteristic organisational template, as exemplified by the following Late Babylonian text from Uruk:

SBTU I No. 46 (p. 57)

If a man has (symptoms of) stroke in the face, he blinks, day and night (his eyes) stare and he cannot sleep, he should not cease from massaging his face in honey and ghee, he should keep eating *maštakal* on an empty stomach, and he will improve.

Incantation ....

Recited spell (from the composition) 'if a man's nose had been seized by a Bailiff-demon'

Its ritual (medical procedure): he should put dust from the crossroad into well water, wash his nose and recite the incantation.

The four Sumerograms which regularly appear in this sequence in Akkadian therapeutic texts, DIŠ NA ('if a man'), ÉN ('incantation'), KA.INIM.MA ('recited spell'), and DÙ.DÙ.BI or KÌD.KÌD.BI ('its ritual' – medical procedure), all serve to label specific therapeutic functions which comprise a medical recipe.

Medical Incantations and Ritual Procedures (ÉN and KA.INIM.MA)

One of the characteristics of Babylonian medicine is the regular presence of 'incantations', which left the impression among historians of medicine that Babylonian medicine was essential magical rather than medical (usually in comparison with Hippocratic writings). The remarkable feature about 'incantations' in the medical corpus is that they differ considerably from other genres of incantation literature, which normally appeal for protection for suffering patients and clients from demons, while adjurations demand that demons remain at a distance from the victim.[33] This pattern is not shared by medical incantations, which tend to offer allegorical explanations for disease or suggest natural causes, in contrast to demons and angry gods of non-medical incantations. Examples of a medical incantation occur frequently in eye-disease texts, such as the following extract:

> Incantation: the open eye is a staring eye, the opened eye stares, the reddish eye is a crimson eye, the opened eye is crimson. The open eye is drowsy, the open eye is *weak*, the open eye is harmed. O cloudy eyes, blurred eyes (vision). [The (eye) blood vessel] is porous. The eyes are suffused with blood like a slaughtered sheep, they (= the eyes) are spotted like the (muddy) water of a lagoon with *alapû*-algae, they (= the eyes) are spotted like a vinegar-jar with a film. (IGI I 89'-92', see Geller and Panayotov, 2020: 81)

The point of this passage (marked with the label ÉN, 'incantation') within eye-disease prescriptions is to provide additional or collateral pathological data which does not correspond exactly to symptoms or signs of disease. In this particular case, the eye is described as being fixated, bloodshot, lazy ('drowsy'), or with blurred vision, and these features are explained with comparisons to a slaughtered sheep, murky water, or a film-covered container. There is virtually nothing magical in this passage, but the medical incantations provide insights into non-technical descriptions of pathologies which are not identical with treatable symptoms.

Medical Recipes

The prescription usually begins with a typical format, e.g. 'if a man suffers from...',[34] which can then be followed by a second or third clause providing further descriptive data regarding the nature of the symptoms or disease. The descriptions of symptoms in therapeutic texts do *not* resemble the head-to-foot descriptions of symptoms of the *Diagnostic Handbook*. One might assume, in the interests of economy, that medical recipes would have simply copied the symptom descriptions from diagnostic omens, and the fact that the symptom-descriptions of recipes differ tell us two things. 1) The medical prescriptions and the *Diagnostic Handbook* originated from two different professional guilds or practitioners, who may not have communicated with each other regularly. 2) While recipes represented the practice of medicine on patients (applied medicine), the *Diagnostic Handbook* was more of a work of theory, exploring all possible aspects of prognosis and diagnosis in relation to disease without specific reference to individual patients.

Example of a Prescription

The prescription for a sick spleen was an important topic, since the recipe was the subject of a medical commentary from the mid-first century BCE. The following extract is preserved on two cuneiform tablets from seventh century BCE Assur (BAM 77 and 78, see Scurlock, 2014: 532), with further information in a medical commentary from Nippur (Civil, 1974: 336).

> BAM 77 (variants BAM 78):
> If a person's spleen[35] hurts him, he cannot sleep day or night, his body contains fever, his drinking beer and consuming bread is diminished; that man, when seeking out a 'Marduk sanctuary', can improve. Pound together..., *tarmuš*, black obsidian, tamarisk seed, and alum,

mix (them) in mountain honey, he should lick them on an empty stomach. Your dry out and pound ox liver and [*decoct*] it into tavern-beer and he should chew it while hot. Put... into a litre of beer and colocynth-fat...He should move his bowels and afterwards you pour oil and beer (into his anus) and he will improve.

This recipe enumerates the main symptoms associated with a sick spleen, being sleeplessness, fever and loss of appetite, but unusually adds a marginal note, that when the patient looks for a 'Marduk sanctuary' (*ašrat Marduk*), he may improve. This notation was clearly difficult to understand even for ancient physicians, since a late commentary from Nippur cites this passage and adds a notation:

> ᵈSAG.ME.GAR : ŠÀ.GIG : *ṭu-li-mu,*
> 'Jupiter' = black (internal) organ = the spleen'

According to this interpretation, Jupiter is the planet associated with Marduk and which influences the 'black' (or sick) internal organ, which is the spleen (see Reiner 1995: 58-59). The likely point of this notation is that the correct diagnosis of the patient's spleen illness may be found in astral medicine (the planet Jupiter's power over the spleen) and awareness of this may help the patient improve, even before drugs or treatment are recommended.

A second somewhat unusual instruction in this recipe (BAM 77, see above) is that the patient should 'lick' (*unaṣṣab*) the ingredients, consisting of crushed minerals (obsidium, alum) and organic substances (e.g. tamarisk seed) mixed into mountain honey. As we shall see below, since one aim of spleen recipes was to dry out the spleen, the administering of medication through a drink may have been thought counter-productive, and hence 'licking' was recommended.

> If a person's spleen hurts him and it is constantly present,[36] dry out, crush, and sieve a field-clod,[37] stir it into canal water and have him keep drinking it on an empty stomach, and he should improve.
>
> If a person's spleen hurts him and it is constantly present, boil the spleen of a dog (or) weasel, the nickname of which is 'restoring' (*tašlamtu*), let him eat (it) for three days on an empty stomach and drink the liquid,[38] and he should get better.
>
> If a person's spleen hurts him and it is constantly present, [you dry out] the spleen of a black dog (and) *induhallātu* lizard of the

desert — the nickname of which is 'restoring' (*tašlamtu*), you pound *šumuttu* and mix (it) in its blood, you boil these spleens and for three days *he eats it on an empty stomach.*

If ditto, dry out and pound (the spleen) of an *induhallātu*-lizard, *decoct* it in beer, he should keep chewing it while hot.[39]

[If a person's spleen] is present, [you dry out] the spleen of a black dog (or) *induhallātu*-lizard of the desert — the nickname of which is 'restoring' (*tašlamtu*), pound... and mix (it) in its blood, remove (the spleens) and boil (the mixture) and he should get better.

This group of recipes all involve treating the patient with the spleen of a desert lizard or weasel, although the spleen of a dog is a useful substitute in case these might not be available. The lizard or weasel, with an exotic nickname, provides the substitute spleen from a desert environment for the patient to devour, as a way of sympathetically drying his own spleen.

This prescription illustrates the multi-layered nature of Babylonian medical therapy, which includes substances drawn from minerals, plants, and animal viscera. Nevertheless, the logic behind the treatment is not obvious, nor did Babylonian physicians leave us with explanatory guidelines, since the underlying theoretical suppositions behind the medicine are never explained in a prescription (nor would one expect them to be). Hence, we are forced to look outside the corpus of cuneiform medicine for explanations, and we are lucky to have spleen disease discussed in the Babylonian Talmud and Syriac *Book of Medicines*, both based on earlier Akkadian prescriptions.

The Aramaic prescription in the Babylonian Talmud is remarkably reminiscent of the Akkadian prototype (BT Gittin 69b):

For a (sick) spleen: let one take *black cumin*[40] (infused in) water and dry it in the shade[41] and let him (the patient) drink (the water) two or three times each day in wine.

If not,[42] let one take the spleen of a virgin kid[43] and smear it on an oven and let him stand near it and let him say, 'just as this one spleen is dried up, may that spleen of So-and-so dry up.'

And if not, let one smear it between the brick layers of a new house.

If not, let one search for a corpse of one who expired on the Sabbath, and let him one take his hand and put it on his (the corpse's) spleen and say, 'Just like this had dried up, may the spleen of So-and-so dry up'.

The clear idea from Talmud references is that the sick spleen is moist and needs to be dried out in order for the problem to be remedied.[44] The Talmud strategy to this effect is to take a drug and dry it out, and subsequently to be ground up (not mentioned) and imbibed in wine. The alternative recipe is to take a goat spleen and dry it in an oven, as a sympathetic ritual act. In either case, the overall strategy is similar to that of the Akkadian recipe, which calls for the drying out and pounding of the spleen of a typical desert creature, a lizard or gecko, the body of which was to be used to prepare the medication. The underlying idea (emphasised in the alternative recipes) is that whatever these creatures are, they will have a drying effect upon the patient's spleen.

The other comparison between the Talmud and the Akkadian prescription is the very next Aramaic recipe quoted in the Talmud in connection with spleen-disease:

> And if not, let one take a *creature* and roast it in a forge and let him (the patient) eat it in water of a forge and let him drink from the water of a forge. A certain goat was drinking from the water of a forge and when slaughtered, its spleen was not found.

The patient should eat the animal-ingredient (not specified clearly) once it is cooked in wastewater from a forge, and then the patient should drink the wastewater (once the creature is removed). However, the results to be achieved were tested on a goat, which was found to have no spleen after drinking forge-water, a positive sign.

This anecdote about the goat's spleen illustrates an aspect of the Akkadian text which has not been fully understood. The usual translation of the Akkadian phrase is, *šumma amēlu ṭulīmšu ittanazzaz,* 'if a person's spleen continually stands,' without a clear picture of what 'standing' designates.[45] A similar expression also occurs in omens resulting from examining entrails of animals.[46] The meaning of the verb *izuzzu,* however, means 'to be present' as well as 'to stand,' and this now becomes more understandable in the light of the goat anecdote in the Talmud. The presence of the spleen (with its logogram [uzu]ŠÀ.GIG, lit. the black organ, translated in a lexical list as *irru ṣalmu,* the 'black intestine'), was considered in itself to be a bad sign. The aim of the treatments was not to heal the spleen, but to make it disappear, which would in effect cure the problem, and the treatment involved drying the spleen, presumably to make it shrivel up.[47] Ancient physicians may have concluded – for the wrong reasons – that a sick spleen would be best if no longer present in the body, which doctors today would mostly agree with as correct.[48]

The final section of the Syriac *Book of Medicines* (567:15-568: 9) confirms the information from the Talmud. Apart from plant-based remedies, the Syriac recipe calls for the eating of rabbit spleen or fumigating the patient with the spleen of a fox. Most similar to the Talmud is the instruction to 'let a spleen which is dried up be suspended on his left side for three days, and on the fourth day release and hang (it) over the hearth and when it dries, also the spleen dries.' A further comment in the *Syriac Book of Medicines* refers to the lungs of a raven, that eating it will dry out the spleen (SBM 592: 22). The idea reoccurs that the unhealthy spleen is moist and drying it is the best way to remedy the situation. Moreover, one Syriac instruction involves imbibing swallow blood in wine, and ' if he drank all of it, nothing at all from his (the patient's) spleen remains,' which reinforces the idea that the purpose of the prescription is to make the spleen disappear or no longer be present in the body. This may reflect the Akkadian symptom that the sick spleen is constantly 'present', as noted above.

The parallels between Aramaic and Syriac recipes with earlier Akkadian medicine raise important methodological questions regarding the survival of cuneiform and whether Akkadian was still legible in Late Antiquity, contemporary with the Talmud or *Syriac Book of Medicines*. Since the last *dated* cuneiform tablets were composed (not just copied) in the late first century CE, it would be reasonable to assume that cuneiform writing lasted at least as long as Egyptian hieroglyphs, until the fourth century CE, providing ample opportunity for Aramaic and Syriac-speaking healers to meet and converse with experts who could still read the ancient scripts of Babylonia.

A Note on Aramaic/Syriac Medicine

There is evidence for cross-language knowledge transfer in Late Antiquity in Mesopotamia. A Vademecum in the Babylonian Talmud, in Tractate *Gittin* (68b-70a), is a head-to-foot medical handbook in Aramaic with no attributed author,[49] loaded with prescriptions containing Akkadian loanwords and calques. There are virtually no Greek technical terms and no evidence of Hippocratic influence.[50] The *Gittin* Vademecum reflects a late version of local Babylonian medicine, a brand of cuneiform medicine originating in

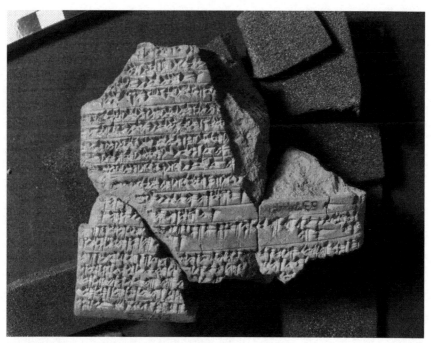

2. Babylonian cuneiform medical text. (F. Badalanova Geller)

Mesopotamia from within Babylonian culture and eventually transmitted to rabbis in the Talmud.[51] This interesting and unique medical handbook preserved within the Babylonian Talmud has a very distinctive format. The *Gittin* text lists illnesses from head to foot, with each illness or symptom being introduced by Aramaic *lamed* meaning 'to' or 'for': for example, *ldm' drš'*, 'for blood from the head'. Each illness can simply be designated by the anatomical organ which it affects, so that 'for the spleen' really means, 'for an illness of the spleen', which is also characteristic for labelling diseases in Akkadian medicine. Each entry for an illness is then followed by one or more medical prescriptions or procedures, some of which appear to be magic (as in Akkadian medicine), but the Vademecum as an entity is clearly medical, not magical. Moreover, the drugs in *Gittin* recipes are not simply drawn randomly from cuneiform literature, but they can also be found in Akkadian medical prescriptions. Second, there is no theoretical discussion in the Gittin Vademecum of bodily humours or the use of bloodletting, or even diet and regime, all of which are signature themes of Greek medicine.[52]

The question remains *how* exactly cuneiform medicine inscribed on clay tablets was somehow translated into Aramaic medicine and eventually found its way into the Babylonian Talmud. One possibility is that this process took place over a long period of time, since Aramaic had been an official language of the Assyrian Empire and later became more widely used as the official *lingua franca* of the enormous Achaemenid Empire, which extended from India to Ethiopia. What is missing, however, is any evidence for a major Aramaic or Syriac library under royal patronage, similar to the Royal Library of Nineveh or the great Library of Alexandria, which might help explain the slow process of transition from Akkadian into Aramaic medicine. Instead, we must look to Syriac medical compendia to bridge the gap between Akkadian and Aramaic medicine, such as the *Syriac Book of Medicines* (cited above in connection with a diseased spleen).[53]

The *Syriac Book of Medicines* spans the ancient world, since the first part is essentially a Syriac translation of Galen, with the second part being devoted to astrology, while the third section is a large collection of individual prescriptions for various ailments, with strong affinities to the Talmud's *Gittin* Vademecum while also containing many Akkadian loanwords and calques, but relatively few Greek or Persian loanwords.[54] The connections between Akkadian and Syriac medicine can easily be detected in the following example of eye disease recipes from both sources, with the first example coming from a damaged compendium of Akkadian eye disease prescriptions (Geller and Panayotov 2020: 25):

> .... you prick their eyes with a needle ....(you take) the plants which the raven took to its young

Here is a fragmentary but still comprehensible recipe instruction: blind the eyes of a small bird and wait for its mother to come back to the nest; whatever healing root the mother bird brings to her injured chick will be the plant to choose for eye therapy. The eminent British scholar Reginald Campbell Thompson in 1926 unassumingly pointed out in a brief footnote (Thompson, 1926: 32 n. 8) a significant parallel in an eye-disease recipe from the *Syriac Book of Medicines* (SBM 558: 5ff.):

> Take the chick of a swallow (= Akk. *sinuntu*) and pull out its eyes and bind a sign on it and leave it for three days. When its mother comes and sees it that it is blind, she goes and brings a certain root and places it on its eyes and they open.

There can be no doubt about the shared features of two recipes, both from eye disease compendia, and both recommending a cure stemming from a mother bird healing its young, intentionally blinded by the physician-researcher.

Conclusion

The origins of Babylonian medicine have been poorly understood, because of confusion over the roles of magic within medicine and therapy. Treatments for illness were mainly divided between two professions, the 'exorcist' (*āšipu*) and 'physician' (*asû*), each with their own healing strategies involving incantations and medical prescriptions. The practice of Babylonian medicine, known best from numerous prescriptions redacted into major medical treatises, relied upon a theoretical framework based on studies of anatomy, *materia medica,* and symptoms, preserved in *Listenwissenschaften* formats along with some surviving commentaries; these represent the skeletal remains of Mesopotamian science, which was primarily conducted through oral instructions. In some instances, however, the theoretical bases for Babylonian diagnosis and treatment can be reconstructed from later Aramaic medical recipes, which developed from earlier Akkadian prototypes, and the process of combining this medical data from earlier and later periods from Mesopotamia can lead to a fuller appreciation and understanding of the system of medicine from this part of the world.

Bibliography

Attia and Buisson, 2012 = Attia, A. and Buisson, G., 'BAM 1 et consorts en transcription', *Le Journal des Médecines Cunéiformes,* 19, pp. 20-50.

Civil, 1974 = Civil, M., 'Medical Commentaries from Nippur', *Journal of Near Eastern Studies,* 33, pp.329-338.

Civil, 2010 = Civil, M., *The Lexical Texts in the Schoyen Collection* (CUSAS 12, Bethesda: CDL Press).

Cohen, 2012 = Cohen, Y., 'The Ugu-mu Fragment from Hattuša/BogazköyKBo 13.2', *The Journal of Near Eastern Studies,* 71, pp.1-12.

van der Eijk, 2000/2001 = van der Eijk, P., *Diocese of Carystus, a collection of fragments with translation and commentary* (Leiden/Boston: Brill).

Eypper, 2016 = Eypper, S.C., 'Diseases of the Feet in Babylonian-Assyrian Medicine A Study of Text K.67+', *Le Journal des Médecines Cunéiformes,* 27, pp.1-58.

Geller, 2015 = Geller, M., ''Encyclopaedias and Commentaries', in Johnson, J.C. (Ed.), *In the Wake of the Compendia* (Berlin: de Gruyter), pp.31-46.

Geller and Panayotov, 2020 = Geller, M. and Panayotov, S., *Mesopotamian Eye Disease Texts. Die Babylonisch-assyrische Medizin in Texten und Untersuchungen,* X (Berlin: de Gruyter).

George, 1991 = George, A.R., 'Babylonian Texts from the Folios of Sidney Smith. Part Two: Prognostic and Diagnostic Omens, Tablet I', *Revue d'assyriologie* 85: pp. 137–63.

Heeßel, 2000 = Heeßel, N., *Babylonisch-assyrische Diagnostik* (Münster: Ugarit Verlag).
Jeyes, 1989 = Jeyes, U., *Old Babylonian Extispicy, Omen Texts in the British Museum* (Leiden: NINO).
Reiner, 1995 = Reiner, E., *Astral Magic in Babylonia* (Philadelphia: American Philosophical Society).
Rochberg, 2004 = Rochberg, F., *The Heavenly Writing* (Cambridge: Cambridge University Press).
Rochberg, 2010 = Rochberg, F., *In the Path of the Moon* (Leiden/Boston: Brill).
Rutz, 2011 = Rutz, M.T., 'Threads for Esagil-kīn-apli. The Medical Diagnostic-Prognostic Series in Middle Babylonian Nippur,' *Zeitschrift für Assyriologie* 101, pp.294-308.
Schmidtchen, 2018 = Schmidtchen, E., *Mesopotamische Diagnostik: die diagnostisch-prognostische Standardserie Sakikkû alse in Kernbereich des Beschwörungs-experten sowie eine Neu edition des zweiten Kapitels* (unpubl. Ph.D dissertation, Freie Univ. Berlin).
Schramm, 2001 = Schramm, W., *Bann, Bann! Eine sumerisch-akkadische Beschwörungsserie* (Göttingen).
Schuster-Brandis, 2008 = Schuster-Brandis, A., *Steine als Schutz- und Heilmittel. Untersuchung zu ihrer Verwendung in der Beschwörungskunst Mesopotamiens im 1. Jt. v. Chr.* (Münster: Ugarit Verlag).
Scurlock, 2005 = Scurlock, J., *Magico-medical Means of Treating Ghost-induced Illnesses in Ancient Mesopotamia* (Leiden/Boston: Brill).
Scurlock, 2014 = Scurlock, J., *Sourcebook for Ancient Mesopotamian Medicine* (Atlanta: SBL Press).
von Staden, 1989 = von Staden, H., *The Art of Medicine in Early Alexandria* (Cambridge: Cambridge University Press).
Stadhouders, 2011 = Stadhouders, H., 'The Pharmacopoeial Handbook *Šammu šikinšu* – An Edition,' *Le Journal des Médecines Cunéiformes*, 18, pp.3-51.
Stadhouders, 2012 = Stadhouders, H., 'The Pharmacopoeial Handbook *Šammu šikinšu* – A Translation,' *Le Journal des Médecines Cunéiformes*, 19, pp.1-52.
Stadhouders and Johnson, 2018 = Stadhouders, H. and Johnson, J.C., 'A Time to Extract and a Time to Compile: The Therapeutic Compendium Tablet BM 78963', in Panayotov, S.V. and Vacín, L. (Eds), *Mesopotamian Magic and Medicine, Studies in Honor of Markham J. Geller*, (Leiden/Boston: Brill), pp.556-622.
Steinert, 2018 = Steinert, U., *Assyrian and Babylonian Scholarly Text Catalogues: Medicine, Magic and Divination* (Berlin: de Gruyter).
Thompson, 1926 = Thompson, R.C., 'Assyrian Medical Texts', *Proceedings of the Royal Society of Medicine*, pp.29-78.
Uehlinger, 2016 = Uehlinger, C., 'From "Heaven" to "Nature": Some Afterthoughts', in K. Schmid, K. and Uehlinger, C. (Eds), *Laws of Heaven – Laws of Nature, Legal Interpretations of Cosmic Phenomena in the Ancient World*, (Orbis Biblicus et Orientalis 276, Freibourg / Göttingen), pp. 162-171.
Van der Toorn, 1985 = van der Toorn, K., *Sin and Samnction in Israel and Mesopotamia* (Assen: von Gorcum).
Westenholz and Sigrist, 2006 = Westenholz, J.G. and Sigrist, M., 'The Brain, the Marrow, and the Seat of Cognition in Mesopotamian Tradition', *Le Journal des Médecines Cunéiformes* 7, pp.1-10.

Westenholz, 2010 = Westenholz, J.G., 'The Tale of Two Little Organs: the Spleen and the Pancreas', *Le Journal des Médecines Cunéiformes,* 15, pp.2-24.

de Zorzi, 2011 = de Zorzi, N., ' The omen series *Šumma izbu*: Internal Structure and Hermeneutic Strategies', *KASKAL,* 8, pp.43-75.

Notes

1. Work on this article was carried out under the auspices of a European Research Council Advanced Grant Project No. 323596 *BabMed*. An earlier version of this paper is planned to appear in French under the title, 'Origins of Babylonian Medicine', in a volume edited by V. Boudon-Millot.

    Abbeviations used:

    MSL = Material for the Sumerian Lexicon

    BAM = *Die Babylonisch-assyrische Medizin in Texten und Untersuchungen*; BAM 7 = Geller, M.J., *Renal and Rectal Disease Texts* (Berlin: de Gruyter, 2005).

    CAD = Chicago Assyrian Dictionary

    PBS = Publications of the Babylonian Section of the University Museum of the University of Pennsylvania.

    DCCLT = Digital Corpus of Cuneiform Lexical Texts

    (http://oracc.museum.upenn.edu/dcclt/intro/lexical_intro.html)

    TDP = Labat, R., *Traité akkadien de diagnostics et pronosticsmédicaux*(Paris/Leiden: Brill, 1951).

    YOS 10 = Goetze, A., *Old Babylonian Omen Texts* (Yale Oriental Series 10, New Haven: Yale University Press, 1947).

    SBM = Wallis Budge, E.A., *The Syriac Book of Medicines* (London: 1913).

    SBTU = Spätbabylonische Texte aus Uruk

2. We use the designation Mesopotamian medicine to refer to medicine in any language from this region (Sumerian, Akkadian, Hittite, Aramaic and Syriac), while we use Babylonian medicine to refer to texts specifically in Akkadian.

3. In the absence of any third-party assessments of medical competence, or even of polemical comments between rival physicians, there is little opportunity to assess competitive theories of Babylonian medical knowledge or competing schools of thought, although it is likely that these existed.

4. See Scurlock, 2005: 14 for examples, and for a specific recipe, cf. BAM 503 I 20'-23' (Scurlock, 2014: 369):

    If a man has been affected by Hand of a Ghost, (so that) his ears roar: pound *murru*, arsenic? (*ašgigû*), (and) malachite? (*ešmekku*), wrap (them) into a wad of wool, sprinkle (them) in cedar resin (lit. 'blood'), recite the incantation...It is unclear whether the condition is perceived to be the result of a personal attack or resulting from a neurological condition, for which the treatment resembles magic (in modern terms) but in the form of a medical recipe.

5. Attributed to Herophilus and Erasistratos, see von Staden, 1989.

6. Literally 'my cranium/brain', published in MSL 9, pp.49-73, and Civil, 2010, pp.148-161. The anatomical lists are known both in Sumerian unilingual and Sumerian-Akkadian bilingual formats, translating Sumerian anatomical terminology.

7. The variant reading in Civil 2010: 155 (4:5) translates this phrase as *na-hi-[ir ap-pi-ia]*, 'snoring of my nose'.

8. Or: nostril of the nose, as interpreted by CAD N/1 136, but Civil's interpretation is to be preferred (Civil, 2010:, p.155).

9. Civil, 2010, p.149 (10) translates the Sum. as 'hair of my nose', but Akk. translation *haṣartu* refers to green wool and by extension to mucous. However, the Babylonian Talmud (Gittin, 69a) provides a recipe for nosebleed and recommends, 'let one take tufts of wool into a strand (*ptylt'* = Akk. *pitiltu*)' to be inserted into the nostrils. It may be that this line in UGU.MU could have originally referred to a treatment for nosebleed which was incorporated into descriptions of the nose.

10. It is unclear why anatomical lists ceased to be copied while disease names remained of later interest, although one cannot rule out the possibility that first millennium exemplars have not yet been found.

11. The term *neqelpû* 'to drift or float (downstream)' is an example of a literary term which occasionally appears in symptoms, but only exceptionally. See CAD N/2, p. 173.

12. The assumption is that such list entries served as topics for discussion within scribal academies, serving as the starting point rather than end-product of scholarly activity.

13. Perhaps an insect.

14. Possibly another insect.

15. See Schuster-Brandis, 2008 for a comprehensive study of minerals used in magico-medical applications.

16. The uses of *simplicia* have never been studied within the context of Babylonian medicine, but the results of such research could be promising, in highlighting which drugs were considered to be active ingredients within a compound recipe against a specific disease.

17. The *Diagnostic Handbook* was attributed to the exorcist (*āšipu*), which partially explains why symptoms described in this theoretical collection of symptoms do not often match the symptoms described in medical prescriptions, attributed to the physician (*asû*).

18. For a discussion of this standard omen format, see Rochberg, 2010, pp.376-382, and see now Uehlinger, 2016, p.163 (if A then B, expressing regularity or coincidence or periodic intervals). Rochberg, 2004, pp.58-60 for a clear review of if-clauses and their meaning in omen literature, although not including diagnostic or medical omens within her discussion.

19. See George, 1991, pp. 142f., publishing cuneiform commentaries on this passage of the *Diagnostic Handbook*, indicating that even ancient scribes had difficulty in understanding why these terrestrial omens, resembling other omen genres, were used to introduce diagnostic symptoms.

20. Kidney disease prescriptions provide colourful similes to describe the nature of urine, comparing it to the urine of an ass, or beer or wine dregs, or clear paint, with colours being yellow or white, etc. (BAM, 7, p.71), all indications of 'discharge' or a related disease. The *Diagnostic Handbook*, on the other hand, offers much more straightforward descriptions of urine within standard if-clauses, such as, 'if (his) urine is red / black / blocked up / like water / like wine, etc., with each entry accompanied by an apodosis predicting whether the patient will live or die (BAM, 7, p.251). The differences between these entries in prescriptions and the *Diagnostic Handbook* indicate that these texts were drafted in different workshops.

21. See, for instance, Šumma izbu omens drawn from malformed foetuses or miscarriages (both human and animal): 'if a woman gives birth and (the foetus) has two ears on the

right and none on the left – the gods (who were) angry will return to the land and the land will live in peace' (3: 18, translation de Zorzi, 2011, p.53). The logical connection between protasis and apodosis is not possible to reconstruct with any certainty.

22. E.g. death of a wife, becoming rich or poor, etc.

23. See Attia, 2017, for a translation and commentary from a French ophthalmologist who is also an authority on Babylonian medicine, and a recent critical textual edition is based upon three large Nineveh manuscripts (Geller and Panayotov, 2020).

24. See Scurlock, 2014, pp. 387ff.

25. See Scurlock, 2014, pp. 388ff.

26. See Scurlock, 2014, pp. 398-405, including the incantation of the tooth worm.

27. See Scurlock, 2014, pp. 469ff.

28. Edited and translated into French in an unpublished doctoral dissertation (Cadelli, 2000), with a forthcoming updated edition and translation by J. C. Johnson.

29. See BAM 7.

30. See BAM 7.

31. See Eypper, 2016.

32. The designation of epilepsy in the Hippocratic Corpus as the 'sacred disease' might reflect some older similar attitude within older pre-Hippocratic medicine from Greece.

33. See Schramm, 2001, pp.76-77: 'You (the demon) should not approach my body, you should not surround my face, nor should you return behind my back. You should not go where I go, you should not enter where I enter, you should not approach my house, you should not clamber onto my roof. In the incantation, the word of (the god) Ea, may nothing evil come near before me, may nothing unfavourable [approach] my body I adjure you by the great gods, so that you (the demon) goes away.'

34. The casuistic notation, 'if a man', was modelled on similar if-clauses (*šumma amēlu*) in legal compendia (such as the Codex Hammurabi) or in omen compendia. The symptom (or even a disease) is identified in this characteristic way.

35. Westenholz, 2010, argues for this organ to be the pancreas rather than the spleen, but the argument is not entirely convincing, since she has not taken into account the necessity of drying out the spleen. The pancreas does not usually feature in Greek anatomy.

36. See Westenholz, 2010, pp. 6-7, translating this phrase 'constantly stands up/protrudes', which she explains as referring to an enlarged organ, 'palpable when the abdomen was examined.'

37. The use of 'field-clod' as a medical ingredient might have been considered to be a drying agent.

38. The result of the boiling.

39. This text repeats the term *ba-a-a-ri* several times before the verb to 'chew' (*kasāsu*), which has prompted a translation of 'rawhide' for this text (Scurlock), but the easiest solution to this difficulty is to assume an unusual orthography for the common term *bahrû*, 'hot'.

40. The usual translation is seven leeches, although without solid evidence.

41. A calque on Akkadian *ina ṣilli tubbal*, you dry it in shade.

42. The equivalent of 'ditto' in Akkadian recipes.

43. Akkadian *unīqu lā petītu*, literally 'a kid not opened'.

44.   This idea of the spleen being 'moist' may be reflecting that this organ is full of blood as part of its function to filter the blood, although the function would have been unknown to the ancients. Nevertheless, the dark colour of the spleen was noted.

45.   The spleen being either 'present' or 'standing' may reflect a spleen pathology indicated by swelling in the abdomen, which is noticeable externally.

46.   See for convenience CAD, Ṭ, 124, quoting the Old Babylonian liver omen passage, *šumma ṭulīmum ina imitti karšim ittaziz*, 'if the spleen is present on the right of the stomach' (YOS, 10, 41:15). Other descriptions of the spleen as seen in hepatoscopy are that it is elongated (*ītarik*) or enlarged (*irabbi*), see CAD, Ṭ, 124, indicating that it is the size of the spleen which indicates abnormality, even in animals. See also Jeyes, 1989, 79, pp.170-173.

47.   An entry in the lexical List of Diseases discussed above (MSL 9 p. 93: 65) reads, šà.bur.šu.ná.a = *e-ri-a mu-ri-im*, 'naked in respect to the *mūru*'. The term *mūru* cannot be specifically associated with the spleen, but one Sumerian equivalent of this organ is uzu.*mu-ru*mur, which may well designate the liver or similar organ (CAD, M/2, 110). The absence (*erû* 'naked') of this *mūru* organ is described as a disease, which is the opposite of what was assumed for the spleen, which was best when not present.

48.   There is no treatment today for the spleen other than splenectomy, nor is the actual function of the spleen fully understood in modern medicine.

49.   Few rabbis in the Talmud are credited with medical knowledge. One who stands out from the rest is the third-fourth century scholar Abbaye, who contributed 27 medical prescriptions to Talmudic discourse, almost all of which were erroneously attributed to his mother, who died in childbirth. Abbaye's source for such technical knowledge was likely to have been a Babylonian expert, since many of Abbaye's prescriptions contained technical Akkadian loanwords and calques.

50.   Babylonian Rabbis or Amoraim knew no Greek nor read Greek texts, such as Aristotle or Hippocrates. Many of the Greek terms found in the Babylonian Talmud were introduced via the Mishnah and other writings brought over from Roman Palestine, and these Greek terms were often grossly misunderstood and misused. A pattern appears in the Talmud, that Greek loanwords usually appear within Hebrew contexts and Akkadian words appear in Jewish Babylonian Aramaic, and this applies to medical passages in the Talmud.

51.   Medicine in Roman Palestine was essentially Greek medicine, based mainly on Hippocratic principles of body humours. Medicine in Sassanian Babylonia, on the other hand, was Akkadian medicine, dating back to much earlier periods but still practiced locally. Babylonian medicine is not theory-driven but based primarily on careful observation of symptoms and pharmaceutical drugs, and not much surgery.

52.   Hippocratic medicine was innovative in recommending diet and regimen as part of medicine, giving advice about how to stay healthy: advice on healthy eating, as well as when to have meals, when to use the toilet, when to take exercise, when to drink wine, when to have sex, etc., but this kind of advice is completely unknown to Akkadian medicine. The Babylonian Talmud does contain advice on diet and regimen, but relevant passages are almost exclusively in Hebrew, not in Aramaic. This points to a particular characteristic of the Babylonian Talmud. Much of the raw material of the Babylonian Talmud was brought from Roman Palestine to Babylonia, and this includes the Mishnah and other texts, including medicine, all in Hebrew. These Palestinian and Babylonian (Aramaic) traditions become so mixed, that

passages and even sentences can appear in a mixture of both Hebrew and Aramaic, which means that Hebrew prescriptions from Greco-Roman Palestine frequently confronted local Aramaic recipes from Sassanian Babylonia, although these originated from very different systems of medicine. The *Gittin* Vademecum, however, is entirely in Aramaic and displays no evidence of Hebrew or influence from Graeco-Roman medicine from Palestine.

53. E. A. Wallis Budge writes about the Syriac manuscript which he brought back to the British Museum (cf. SBM, p.xl): 'The manuscript, from which my copy of the Book of Medicines...was made, was one of a small collection which belonged to a native of Mosul, the famous town on the Tigris opposite the ruins of Nineveh (Kuyunjik), and which he guarded jealously. After much talk he agreed to allow a copy of it to be made by one of his friends who was a scribe.'

54. Budge considered the prescriptions in the third section of the SBM to be medical folklore of little scholarly value, as he remarks (SBM, p.xi): 'The third section contains four hundred prescriptions, many of them of a most extraordinary character; these must have been written by "physicians" who were both ignorant and superstitious.'

2

Surgery and Medicine in the Bible and Talmud

A. Surgery

Samuel Kottek

Before focusing on surgery, it is in order to say a few words on Medicine in the Bible and Talmud. Julius Preuss (1861-1913), in his epochal work on this topic, first published in German in 1911, had a significant sub-title: 'Contributions to the History of Medicine and of Culture' more generally. In his Introduction, he states that there is no 'Medicine in the Talmud' that could be compared to the medicine of Galen, or Susruta or of the Egyptians or the Greeks.

In the Bible, the Lord is the [ultimate] healer (cf. *Exodus*15: 26). However, the physician has the right to perform his treatment, according to *Exodus* 21: 19 'And healing, he will heal!' In a few cases, Prophets may be effective as healers, for instance Elijah for the child of the woman in Sarepta (I Kings 17: 17-24), and Elisha for the Syrian general Naaman (II *Kings* 5: 14).

The main topic generally considered of medical interest in the Bible is in *Leviticus*, Chapters 13 and 14. It describes the skin disease called *tsara 'at,* usually translated as leprosy. Actually, in view of the symptoms described, it was not leprosy, but some complex skin disease, or rather skin diseases. The diagnosis was made by a priest (Hebrew: Cohen) and no physician is mentioned. The evolution of the 'disease' is taken into consideration: it may heal thoroughly or else cover the whole body. The Cohen will ultimately decide whether the 'patient' is pure or impure. This is the real subject matter of *tsara 'at.* The Talmudists saw this affliction as a punishment for several sins, mainly evil speech (Heb: *lashon ha-ra '*). The fact that the leper was excluded from the community is an adequate retribution for evil speech. Several biblical notables were temporarily stricken with *tsara 'at,* including

Moses, his sister Miriam, the Syrian general Naaman, King Uzziah and Geḥazi, the servant of Elisha. The last named was afflicted permanently, himself and his offspring.

Some data can be found on hygiene in the Bible and in the Talmud. Topics include the dietary Laws, sexual hygiene, Sabbath rest, baths and washing as well as death and burial. In the Talmud, we find a number of diseases, they are however lacking even minimal description though there are some exceptions – malformations are mentioned, in humans as well as in animals. There is more information on obstetrics and gynaecology both normal and pathological. Eye diseases, mental and neurological illnesses are also mentioned. Materia medica is often problematic, due to the difficulty to find the exact meaning of the names of drugs and plants in Aramaic. We cannot forget to mention the magic aspects of healing in the Talmud, such as incantations, amulets and demonology, which are nearly inescapable in the context of Babylonian medicine.

We shall close these brief introductory words with a summarized quotation from the second century BCE Jewish ethicist Ben Sira. His book has not been included in the Hebrew Bible. However, several of his maxims have been quoted in the Talmud.

> Give credit to the physician, even before you need [his help].
> Whenever you are sick, waste no time, pray the Lord that He would heal you
> Then make room for the physician, for he too is requisite
> He too will pray the Lord that his diagnosis and treatment be of help
> Whoever is haughty in front of the physician is a sinner before the Creator.

Surgery in the Bible

The passage in *Exodus* where medical care is clearly mentioned and on which human intervention is legally allowed is a surgical case, based on traumatology. One could ask the following question: Do we really need to be given permission to heal as the Talmudic Sages stated that saving a life is equivalent to saving a whole world? However, we read in *Exodus* 15: 26:

> If you listen to the voice of the Lord and do what is right in His eyes […] I shall not place on you the 'disease' (sic) I applied to Egypt, for I am the Lord, your healer (Heb. *rof'ekha*).

If the Lord is the Healer, we need to be shown another Biblical statement, which gives permission for human healing. This is the content of *Exodus* 21: 19:

> And if men strive together, and one smite another with a stone or with his fist, [so that] he dies not but keeps his bed, he that struck him will be acquitted; only he shall pay for the loss of his time and shall cause him to be thoroughly healed.

While it is true that we cannot find in Scripture any mention of a surgical practitioner, or of a military surgeon, the Hebrew term *rofé* might be understood as 'physician' as well as 'surgeon'. However, the servants of Joseph, called *rof'im* (physicians) were those who performed, or rather attended, the embalming of his father Jacob.[1] The prophet Jeremiah is in despair while describing the situation of the Jewish people. He deplores 'the hurt of the daughter of my people'; (*Jeremiah* 8: 21). The term translated as 'hurt' is (Heb.) *shever*, which means 'fracture' but also nervous breakdown, or in other words either a bone or a nervous balance is broken. And the prophet exclaims: 'Is there no balm in Gilead, is there no healer there?' (*Jeremiah* 8: 22). Obviously healing, or in other words 'repairing' or 'restoring' may be applied to medical, to surgical and even to mental practice.

We intend to offer in this overview on surgery in the Bible a description of wounds and fractures and their treatment, a number of war injuries, inflicted in particular to kings and high officials, and a brief excursus on the practice of anaesthesia.

Wounds and Fractures

Various terms are used in the Bible for wounds and injuries, such as *makkah, petsa'* or *haburah*. The three terms appear together in a verse of the prophet Isaiah describing the terrible state of the Children of Israel:

> From the sole of the foot even to the head there is no soundness in it; but wounds (Heb. *petsa'*) and bruises (Heb. *haburah*) and putrefying sores (Heb. *makkahteriyah*) [*Isaiah*. 1: 6].[2]

The last-mentioned term – *makkahteriyah* – deserves an explanation. *Teriyah* may also be translated as 'fresh', in other words a wound that remains wet with matter oozing out of it. An older wound would be progressively covered with a crust or a scar. Some commentators try to differentiate between the three terms: *petsa'* could be seen as a clear-cut wound caused for instance by a sword; *ḥaburah* would be a bruise without laceration and without blood having issued from it; and *Makkah teriyah* has often been considered as an infected wound. I would however rather see it as an active, granulating wound, from which serum oozes out. Be this as it may, this is only meant to explain the verse of Isaiah, not the general use of these terms in the Bible.

We read in *Psalms* (38: 6): 'My wounds stink; they fester because of my foolishness'. Here the term *ḥaburah* is selected, as it designates no doubt an infected wound. In *Proverbs* (20: 30) we read: 'Bruises and wounds purge away evil; so do stripes that reach the inward parts.' Here again we find in this brief verse the three terms found together in Isaiah: *ḥaburah* for 'bruise', *petsa'* for 'wound' and *Makkah* for 'stripe'.[3] Another type of wound mentioned several times in the Bible is a burn (Heb. *kevi'ah*). It is mentioned in the context of the Laws of Retaliation. For instance, in *Exodus* 21: 24-25, we read:

> Eye for eye, tooth for tooth, hand for hand, foot for foot, burning for burning, wound for wound (Heb. *petsah'*), bruise for bruise (Heb. *ḥaburah*).

We thus may remark that burns, which are cited first, were perhaps considered as being more serious than wounds. The ways of treatment for wounds are hinted at in several places in a allegoric aspect. The prophet Hosea has another term for 'wound'. We read [*Hosea* 5:13]:

> When Ephraim saw his sickness and Judah saw his wound (Heb. *mezor* - sic) then Ephraim went to Ashur and sent to King Yariv.[4] But he is unable to heal you, nor cure you from your wound (*mazor*).

Mazor appears also in Jeremiah; we quote from *Jeremiah* 30: 12-13:

> Thus, says the Lord: Your bruise (Heb. *shever*) is critical (i.e. incurable), your wound (Heb. *makkah*) is grievous. There is none to take up your case (Heb. *mazor*), to bind up the wound [...] For I have wounded you with the wound (Heb. *makkah*) of an enemy...

We have here a problem with the English translation, and with the meaning of *mazor*. It says literally 'There is none to judge your case toward *mazor*.'

This term is therefore to be understood in two different ways. It can be a 'bruise' or a 'healing'. It means 'bruise' in *Hosea* and 'healing' in Jeremiah.[5] *Mazor* comes from *zur* – to compress, or express [i.e. to press out]. One could therefore argue that 'compression' may lead to a sore and may also be a way to close a wound and to stop bleeding. And 'expression' could be applied to healing an abscess.

We would now like to come back to the term *makkah*. The Ten Plagues inflicted upon Egypt are well known in Hebrew as *esser makkot*.[6] However, this phrasing appears nowhere in Scripture. It was first introduced by the rabbis in the period of the *Mishnah* (second century BCE to beginning of third century CE).[7] The only occurrence of *makkah* in the same context is in I *Samuel* 4: 8. The Philistine army is going to fight the Israelites. They are afraid and exclaim:

> Woe to us! Who will deliver us out of the hands of these mighty gods? These are the gods who smote Egypt with all the plagues (Heb. *makkot*) in the wilderness.

It is striking to discover that this application of *makkah* to 'plague' is placed in the mouths of the Philistines. Let us also remark that in French the ten plagues are called *les Dix Plaies* – the word 'plaie' being the exact translation of 'wound'.

Treatment of Wounds

Isaiah's metaphoric description of wounds quoted above included three different kinds: *petsa' – ḥaburah –makkah*. Let us now quote what follows thereafter in the same verse *(Isaiah* 1: 6):

> They have not been pressed (Heb. *zoru*), neither bound up (Heb. *ḥubashu*), nor mollified with oil.

We find here the 'compression' mentioned above, then the bandaging (bound up), and the alleged treatment with oil, which was advocated in ancient medicine. It might have somewhat impeded bacterial infection and prevented the bandages to stick to the sores. But why 'mollified' (Hebrew: *rukekhah*)? I would have chosen one of the following translations: to soften, or soothe, or alleviate or buffer. I guess that this would have been more appropriate. We may also remember that during the Middle Ages war injuries were usually 'treated' with boiling oil, until Ambroise Paré (1510-

1590) replaced it with boiled water. In Ayurvedic medicine, Calendula Oil was used as a first-aid agent in the treatment of wounds.[8] In the Middle East, the oily resinous Balm of Gilead, mentioned earlier in this chapter, may well have been used in the treatment of wounds; this is, however, nowhere mentioned in Scripture.

Fractures

A fracture (Heb. *shever*) can be the result of an accident, or of a war injury, even as a blemish (Heb. *mum*). The term *shever* is cited about 40 times in the Bible. In most cases it is used in a metaphoric context and has a sense of disaster or of misfortune. For instance, we read in *Jeremiah* (8: 21): 'For the hurt (Heb. *shever*) of the daughter of my people I am broken, I am thrown into gloom.' When the prophet writes 'I am broken' (Hebrew *hoshbarti*), the literal meaning is 'I am fractured' and 'hurt' is literally a fracture. And the verse that comes just after our quote is:

> Is there no balm in Gilead, no physician there, why then, is not the health of the daughter of my people recovered? *(Jeremiah* 8: 22).

We may therefore (perhaps) infer from this that a physician would have been able to treat the 'fracture' with the 'Balm of Gilead'. Jeremiah had a special liking for *shever*, the term appears no less than twelve times in his book.

In the Biblical passage where blemishes that render priests unable to perform their duties in the Temple are reviewed, we read:

> A blind man, or a lame [...] or a man that is broken footed (Heb. *shever ragel*) or broken handed (Heb. *shever yad*) or crookbacked [...] shall not come to bring the offerings of the Lord... (*Leviticus* 21: 18-21).

It seems that such cases of deformation of arms and legs, which are included in the wording 'hands and feet' might well describe fractures which were in a displaced and/or non-aligned position. The idea was that a priest should not present any visible blemish while officiating. In other words, if a fracture had consolidated without deformity, the priest would not be put out of work, although this is not stated explicitly. In the *Lex Talionis*, as described in *Leviticus* 24: 19-20, we read that:

If a man maims his neighbour, as he has done so shall it be done to him: breach for breach (Hebrew *shever*) eye for eye, tooth for tooth.

In this quote the list of injuries does not go farther. These might have been considered as the most frequent cases of maiming.

A case of cervical fracture is featured in I *Samuel* 4: 18. The High Priest Eli was deeply struck when he learned that the Israelite army had been defeated by the Philistines, his two sons had died in battle and the Holy Ark had been taken from them. We read:

And it came to pass, when he mentioned the Arch of the Lord, that he fell from off the seat backwards by the side of the gate, and his neck was broken, and he died; for he was an old and heavy man.

It is worth noting that the old age and the heaviness of Eli were factors that could explain his falling down, although being seated. And it is known that a cervical fracture can often be fatal for old persons. When Job pleads his righteousness, he exclaims:

If I have lifted up my arm against the fatherless [...] then let my arm fall from my shoulder-blade and let my arm be broken (Hebrew: *tishaver*) from the bone; (*Job* 31: 22).

This is obviously no case of actual fracture, but it is considered as a punishment for lack of charity.

Wounds and fractures are also described in the prophecies of Isaiah (*Isaiah* 30: 26). 'The light of the moon will be as the light of the sun [...] on the day when the Lord will bind [Heb. *ḥavosh*] the breach [*shever*] of his people and heal the stroke of his [their] wound [Heb. *Makkah*].'

According to a commentator, when a fracture is associated with a wound, the condition is much more serious. Open fractures were often fatal in ancient times. First, the fracture must be fixed and bound, and then the wound will be cared for. The metaphor may account for internal, perhaps also psychic harms [fractures] and external or superficial sores [wounds], suffered by the Children of Israel.

Treatment of Fractures

We find here again the bandaging, or binding (Heb. *ḥavash*). This word can be found in that meaning some ten times in Scripture, several times in the book of *Ezekiel*. We shall quote two examples:

> You have not strengthened the weak, nor have you healed the sick, nor have you bound [Hebrew: *ḥavash*] the crippled [Hebrew: *nishbar* = 'broken'], nor have you brought back the strayed, nor have you sought that which was lost.(*Ezekiel* 34: 4)

Here 'crippled' seemed more appropriate to the translator than 'broken'. Some ten verses later, the prophet writes that the Lord 'will bind up the crippled' (*Isa.* 34: 16). In this metaphor, the prophet addresses the shepherds of the people, the latter being the sheep. We see that medical as well as surgical conditions are depicted in this metaphor.

Another quote is even more striking.

> The word of the Lord came to me, saying: Son of man, I have broken the arm of Pharaoh King of Egypt; and lo, it has not been bound up to be healed, to put a dressing to bind it, to make it strong to hold the sword.(*Ezekiel* 30: 21)

This quote deserves a detailed analysis; its translation may be slightly emended. 'The broken arm has not been bound up', that is, it has not been immobilized and dressed. To 'put a dressing to bind it' means to lay some medicines on the spot and cover it. The fact that 'dressing' is mentioned twice can be understood as accounting for two bandages, one to cover the sore and the drugs, the other to bind the fracture.

In *Psalms* 147: 3, the Lord is building again Jerusalem. We read:

> He gathers together the outcasts of Israel. He heals the broken-hearted [Hebrew: *shevurei lev*] and binds up [Hebrew: *ḥavash* – here *meḥabesh*] their wounds.

Here the text does not mean real wounds, but rather 'afflictions'. To sum up this brief account of fractures and wounds, the Bible mentions very few practical cases and very few anatomical details. It is clear however that these images of bruises and injuries are metaphorically quite common in the Bible, just as they are frequent and routine in human life and therefore ubiquitous in many languages and cultures.

War Injuries

Wars and battles are frequently featured in the Bible, however few details are given on the injuries suffered by soldiers. Nevertheless, whenever a King or a high commander was injured, one finds occasionally some interesting account. The weapons which were used in Biblical times are delineated several times. We read in II *Chronicles* 26: 14:

> Uzziah prepared for them throughout all the host shields, and spears, and helmets, and coats of mail, and bows, and stones for slinging.[9]

The prophet Ezekiel writes, toward the end of the war against Gog:

> Those that dwell in the cities of Israel shall go forth, and shall set fire to the weapons and burn them, both shields and bucklers, bows and arrows, and the staves, and the spears, and they shall make fires with them for seven years.(*Ezekiel* 39: 9)

We thus find in the Bible stones, arrows, spears, javelins, lances, swords and cudgels, whereas protection against them was provided by helmets, shields and coats of mail, in fact the normal ways in ancient times. A few cases may be singled out, where some description of the injury suffered in battle is offered.

Abimelekh, the son of Yerubaal,[10] while attacking a tower where a number of his enemies had taken refuge, was struck by a millstone thrown from the top of the tower. We read:

> And a woman cast an upper millstone upon Abimelekh's head and crushed his skull. Then he called hastily to the lad, his armour-bearer and said to him: 'Draw your sword and slay me, so that men should not say of me A woman slew him.' And his lad pierced him, and he died. (*Judges* 9: 53-54)

The fracture of the skull was not fatal at once, and the king did not even lose consciousness. He realised however that he would not recover and his pride as a soldier dictated this stratagem. During the war between the followers of David and those of Saul, Asael was pursuing Abner and succeeded in coming quite close to him. We read:

> And Abner said to Asael 'Turn aside from following me, why should I smite you to the ground? How then shall I be able to lift up my face to your brother Joab?' But he refused to turn aside. So, Abner stroke him in the belly with the butt end of the spear, so that the spear came

out behind him. And he fell down there and died in the same place. (II *Samuel* 2: 23-24)

There is in this description a problem regarding its translation. According to the *Koren* Bible Asael was smitten 'in the belly'. In the King James Version (the basic version for the *Koren* Bible) it says 'Under the fifth rib'. The Hebrew word which has been translated differently is *homesh*, which appears four times in the Bible. All four mentions are in II *Samuel* and in a similar context of war injury. Abner was struck somewhat later in the *homesh* by Joab, the brother of Asael [II *Samuel* 3: 27].The commentaries here say that this means 'at the fifth rib'. According to Rashi[11] this is where the gallbladder and the liver are situated and according to others (cf. *Metsudat David*) this is where the heart is situated.[12] Obviously, this translation relates *homesh* to *hamesh* (five).Those who translate with 'in the abdomen or belly' (cf. Gesenius) point out that in Syriac *humsha* designates the belly, the area between the ribs and the pelvis.

Joab also murdered his cousin Amasa, who had been at the head of the army of Avshalom, but later came back to David:

> And Joab took Amasa by the beard with his right hand [as if] to kiss him. But Amasa took no heed to the sword that was in Joab's hand; so he smote him with it in the belly [Hebrew*ba-homesh]* and he shed out his bowels to the ground, [...] and he died. (II *Samuel* 20: 9-10)

In this case, *homesh* was indeed the belly, as shown by the fact that Amasa's bowels 'poured'. It says further (20: 12) that 'Amasa was drenched in blood in the midst of the highway'; but someone removed his body to the field and threw a cloth over it. We are given less detail about the death of King Ahab during a war against the Syrian army. We read:

> And a certain man drew a bow at random and smote the king of Israel between the joints of the armour; so, he said to the driver of his chariot: 'Turn your hand and carry me out of the host, for I am badly wounded' (Heb. *hahaleyti*).[...] He died at evening. (I *Kings* 22: 34-35).

It says then that 'the blood ran out of the wound into the hollow of the chariot' (v. 35). This was most probably an arrow wound in the chest, which resulted in intense bleeding. There is no mention of any medical care, although the King remained in upright position in his chariot for some time, but he may well have been maintained artificially upright, in order not to discourage his army. Regarding the Hebrew term *haḥaleyti* – translated here as 'badly wounded' – it means rather something like 'I am debilitated'.[13] He was, however, no doubt 'badly wounded'!

Accidents

We shall not return to the fatal accident suffered by the High-Priest Eli described in our passage on fractures. As a matter of fact, he might well have lost consciousness from the shock caused by the terrible news, or even from a stroke, and therefore he fell down backwards. When the Patriarch Jacob wrestled with the 'man', according to tradition the Guardian Angel of his brother Esau, his hip joint was injured, or rather displaced:

> And when he [the 'man'] saw that he did not prevail against him, he touched the hollow of his thigh; and the hollow of Jacob's thigh was put out of joint as he wrestled with him [...] and he limped upon his thigh. (*Genesis* 32: 26, 32)

This translation is fairly literal, although rather problematic. How could Jacob walk back to his family and cross the ford of Penuel if his hip was dislocated, as it says (*Genesis* 32: 32): 'The sun rose upon him...and he limped upon his thigh'. This has been linked with a saying of the prophet Malachi:

> To you who fear my name the sun of righteousness will arise with healing in its wings; and you will go out and leap like calves from the stall. (*Malachi*, 3: 20)

It has thus been suggested that Jacob indeed limped, but as soon as the sun arose, he was cured.[14]

Aḥaziah, the son of king Aḥab reigned only two years.[15] We read that:

> ...he fell down through the lattice in his upper chamber [...] and was injured (II *Kings* 1: 2). Then Aḥaziah sent messengers to Baal-Zevuv, the 'god of Eqron' [a city of the Philistines], in order to ask whether he would recover from the 'disease' (Hebrew: *ḥoli*). The messengers were stopped by the prophet Elijah, who told them that Aḥaziah shall not come down from that couch to which you have gone up, for [he] will die. [II *Kings* 1: 4].

There is in this case no description of the injury, no mention of the treatment; the only interest is in the prognosis. The term *ḥoli* seems strange in this context to a modern reader; here it means 'infirmity' or 'lameness' – a dangerous condition.

Another incident, not really an accident, occurred to King Jeroboam. After the schism between the kingdom of Judah and that of Israel, Jeroboam decided to prevent his citizens from going to Jerusalem, capital of the Judah.[16] He therefore installed, in Dan and in Beth-El, idolatrous shrines with priests who were not Levites. He was himself performing a sacrifice in Beth-El, when a 'Man of God' arrived from Judah and rebuked him in public. He then became infuriated:

> And it came to pass, when the King heard the saying of the Man of God [...] that he put out his hand from the altar and said: 'Lay hold on him'. And his hand, which he put out against him, dried up (Heb. *va-tivashyado*) [...] and he could not draw it back to him. (I *Kings* 13: 4)

The king then begged the man to pray to 'his Lord' for recovery, which he did, 'and the king's hand was again restored to him (*I Kings* 13: 6). We may ask ourselves what kind of affliction is featured by his hand, in fact rather his arm, being 'dried up'. According to Gesenius, it became lifeless, in other words unresponsive or paralysed.[17] As a matter of fact, the idea is that the hand, or the arm, is the instrument of action; therefore, the king had to stop his sacrilegious action. We find a similar story, in a different context, in Zekhariah. In the so-called Prophecy of the Shepherds, this sentence is its conclusion:

> Woe to my worthless shepherd who forsakes the flock! The sword will be upon his arm and upon his right eye; his arm will be dried up [Heb. *yavosh tivash*] and his right eye will be darkened. (*Zekhariah* 11: 17)[18]

Without going into commentaries, the arm is again featuring action, whereas the eye is the evaluation of the situation. In the next chapter, the Lord is quoted by the prophet as follows:

> I shall open my eyes upon the house of Judah and will smite every horse of the nations with Blindness. (*Zechariah* 12: 4). 18

We remember that when the inhabitants of Sodom attacked Lot and wanted to break into his house, the two angels blinded the whole crowd and they were unable to find the door.(*Genesis* 19: 10-11)

Anaesthesia

Operating under special conditions including deep sleep is hinted at in the Bible, while describing the creation of Eve:

> And the Lord caused a deep sleep [Heb. *Tardémah*] to fall upon the man, and he slept. And He took one of his sides and closed up the flesh in its place. And of the side, which the Lord had taken from the man, He made a woman and brought her to the man. (*Genesis* 2: 21-22)

This 'deep sleep' can be seen as a pre-figuration of total unconsciousness during surgery. The term *tardémah* appears several times in Scripture, however never again in a surgical context. The fact that the Lord 'closed up the flesh in its place' may also be considered as a pre-figuration of a procedure allowing healing by 'primary intention'. This means that wound edges are put and maintained close together, thus allowing quick healing.

The Hebrew word *tséla'* translated as 'side' has been usually translated as 'rib' – which remains its meaning in Hebrew to this day. In the Bible however, it means often the 'side' of a building, for instance *Exodus* 26: 26-27: 'the side of the Tabernacle'. There is indeed an esoteric tradition that man and woman (Adam and Eve) were created attached side by side, the operation that followed was thus a separation.[19]

Surgery in the Talmud and Second Temple Period

We intend here to give an overview of sources related to surgery mentioned in the Talmud. They are mainly taken from the Babylonian Talmud, which was edited in the sixth century, but had been collected progressively since the third century. These statements are generally only brief and incidental records of events. We shall, as often as possible, try to look for comparable items in the Graeco-Roman and in the Babylonian medical literature. The surgeon in the Talmud was usually called *umman*, in Aramai *cummna*. It is clear that we find here the root 'man', which in many Hindu-European languages designs the hand.[20] The Greek term for surgery is *kheirurgia*: the action of the hand (*kheiron*). In fact, the main business of the *umman* was to perform venesection (bleeding). Such a surgeon, Abba Ummna, was known to, and praised by the rabbis of the Talmud. We are told that he did not treat men and women in the same room so that the modesty of women was preserved. He did not take payment, but put a box outside where the patients could put the fees, without causing shame to those who were poor and to whom he often gave some money in order to allow them to drink and eat, as was the rule after bloodletting (cf. Ta'anit 21b). The *umman* was however not always a practitioner particularly praised in the Talmud. He could not be appointed[21] King or High Priest or even head of a Jewish community.[22] In one especially disparaging statement, he is called *gara'* (in Latin *minutor*)[23] and is accused of being conceited, jealous, suspected of incorrect demeanour toward women, even on (unwilling) slaughter – if he draws too much blood (*Kiddushin* 82a).

Let us remark that these exaggerated accusations are stated as a comment to a previously noted and not less extreme indictment: 'the best of physicians to Gehenna!' It seems that the rabbis who made this comment refrained from vilifying physicians, so they shifted, therefore, their criticism toward the socially lower group of the 'surgeons'. The deprecating statement on physicians has been widely discussed by later commentators of the Talmud and we pick out one of them, who says 'The physician who considers himself as the best of physicians will be sent to Gehenna'.[24] Conceit has indeed been quite often attributed to physicians, who deal with problems of life and death.

Second Temple Period

We shall now give a few examples of surgeons, or surgical procedures in the works of two prominent Jewish authors, who were deeply immersed in their non-Jewish environment and who wrote in Greek. Both lived in the first century CE. Philo Judaeus (20BCE-50CE), lived in Alexandria in Hellenistic Egypt and Flavius Josephus (37CE-100CE) was living in Rome when he wrote his works. We read in Josephus' *Jewish Antiquities* XIII, 7, 1 (219):

> Not long after Demetrius had been taken captive, Tryphon, acting as the guardian of Alexander's son Antiochus, surnamed Theos, put him to death after he had reigned four years. And while he gave out that that Antiochus had died under the hands of the surgeon, he sent

his friends and intimates to go among the soldiers promising to give them large sums of money if they would elect him King.[25]

This needs some explanation. Tryphon was better known under the name Diodotus Tryphon, who killed King Alexander Balas' infant son Antiochus VI Dionysus, and declared himself king. Some historians derive the name Balas from *Bel* (Hebrew) – the Lord (hence *Theos*). Livy (Titus Livius, 59 BCE-17 CE) relates this episode in his *Epitome* (Latin *Periochae)* of his *History of Rome*, as follows:

> Antiochus the son of Alexander, King of Syria, who was a mere ten years old, was killed by the treachery of his tutor Diodotus, surnamed Tryphon. He had bribed the physicians, who declared that the boy had suffered severely from the stone, and killed him on the operating table. (Chap. 55, 11)

We hear from this, first that surgeons then operated for urinary calculus – although here with an alleged fatal outcome. Second, that these surgeons were subservient to the ruler who had corrupted them. It is known that Celsus (ca.25BCE – 50CE.) described in detail the operation for the stone.[26] Celsus was, like Philo and Josephus, not a practising physician. He was what can be called a *polyhistor* or a polymath, who knew how to gather excellent information. Another similar episode is briefly noted in Josephus' work the *Jewish War* (Book. I, 13, 10):

> According to another account, Phasael recovered from his self-inflicted blow, and a physician sent by Antigonos, ostensibly to attend him, injected noxious drugs into the wound and so killed him.

Phasael was the elder brother of Herod. The Parthians had accredited Antigonos, who was fiercely opposed to Hyrcanus and Phasael, as ruler in Judea, while these two were actually not less opposed to each other. All this happened some time before Herod was declared by the Roman Senate to be the King of the Jews.[27] Regarding Philo, there is, in his work *On the Contemplative Life* (44) a passage where he describes what may happen when people have been drinking wine without measure:[28]

> Those persons who a little while before came sane and sound to the banquet [...] depart in hostility and mutilated in their bodies. And

some of these men stand in need of advocates and judges, and others require surgeons and physicians, and the help which may be received from them.[29]

Surgeons and physicians are here quoted together, although the 'hostility' mentioned here might well have resulted in injuries needing surgical care. This is apparently why surgeons are cited first.

Surgery in the Talmud

We shall consider in this overview some surgical procedures, which may be compared with Graeco-Roman sources. While describing some of these operations, Preuss hinted at such comparative sources, without however going into detail. Regarding brain injuries, we read in the Babylonian Talmud, BT *Ḥullin* 45a:

> Rav and Samuel both said: [Even] if only the outer membrane [of the brain] was pierced [the animal is *taref*]. Others argued [that both Sages said] that it is not *taref* unless the inner membrane was [also] pierced. Samuel bar Naḥmani said: Think about the bag in which the brain lies.

This quote necessitates some explanations. First, the text speaks about animals, not human beings. In case an animal has a dangerous blemish, it is not allowed as food according to Jewish Law, it is *taref*. The outer membrane of the brain is called dura-mater, the inner one is called pia-mater. Today, we know that there is also a third membrane (arachnoid) between the two, but this was not known in ancient times. The mnemonic remark of Samuel bar Naḥmani refers to the fact the Aramaic term *teḥiyya* means both bag or pouch and revitalizing.[30] There is much to believe that Rav and Samuel, who both lived in the third century C.E., held the second opinion. Samuel is considered as the foremost Talmudic example of a trained physician and Rav had been studying for some time diseases of animals. Indeed, in a modern approach, a lesion of the inner membrane was fatal, whereas an injury of the outer membrane could eventually be cured.

Preuss correctly stated that both Aristotle and Pliny considered that a tear of the dura-mater was lethal, thus we learn that in both Greek and Roman literature the first version of our quote is preferred.[31]

The Disease of Titus

Titus destroyed the Second Temple in Jerusalem in 70 C.E. It says in the Talmud (*Gittin* 56b) that a gnat entered his nose and settled in his brain. The gnat then 'knocked' in his head for seven years. Titus once passed by a smith's shop and suddenly the knocking stopped. It began however again, after 30 days. When Titus died his skull was opened and they found something like a sparrow there inside, obviously a tumour.[32]

It is striking to note that a similar legend has been ascribed by al-Tabari to the Biblical ruler Nimrod, the initiator of the Tower of Babel.[33] When a host of 'flies' attacked his army Nimrod fled to Babylon, but a gnat entered his nose and penetrated his brain. He felt then constant hammering in his head. A blacksmith's hammer was brought, and noblemen struck Nimrod's head, which alleviated his pains. The gnat grew and finally, according to one version fifteen days after the gnat had entered his nose, his skull burst and Nimrod died.

There are in these legendary stories no surgical attempts at treatment, but another version can be found in *Midrash Rabba Genesis* 10, 8, where it says that they called the physicians, who opened Titus' skull and extracted a fledgling weighing two *litras* (around 350g). This was allegedly performed on Titus as he was still living but the text does not say that he died then and there. One rabbi even asserts that he saw this fledgling in Rome and that it weighed indeed two *litras*.

A similar story is told on the death of Nebuchadnezzar II (ca. 634-562 B.C.E.), the great King of Babylon, who conquered Judea and destroyed the First Temple of Jerusalem in 587 B.C.E. In Chapter 4 of the *Book of Daniel*, it says that the king suffered during seven years from a kind of insanity called 'boanthropy'.[34] However, the king recovered, and no treatment is mentioned. The prophet Jeremiah makes many statements on the Babylonian king, whom he calls Nebuchadrezzar, but nothing related to this ailment.

In two places in the Babylonian Talmud (*Ḥagigah* 13a and *Pesaḥim* 94 ab) the same Midrashic text presents Nebuchadnezzar on his death as an evil person, son of an evil one and grandson of Nimrod who enticed the whole world to rebel (Hebrew: *himrid*) against the Lord.[35] Preuss discusses the cases of Titus and of Nimrod in his *Biblical Talmudic Medicine* (p.205). Trepanning the skull was indeed practised in ancient times. The Talmud mentions, among other instruments a skull-borer (trepan) which could have been used by physicians or surgeons (*Oholot* 2, 3).

Referring again to the gnats, a colleague remembered having read many years ago a fable of Aesop entitled 'The Gnat and the Lion'. The gnat, perhaps rather a mosquito, challenged a lion, allegedly the king of all beasts. As the lion spurned it, the gnat placed itself on the lion's nose and struck it several times. The lion was unable to chase it and had to admit its inferiority. The fable however sees to it that the conceited gnat is condemned. It flies away, straight into a spider's web, where it is eaten up. But we have in this tale an illustration of the three mighty kings being trapped by gnats, which graze into their brains. Aesop died in 564 BCE in Delphi and his *Fables* were translated into Latin by Phaedrus in the first century CE. We have here a Graeco-Roman fable, which can be considered relevant to our topic.

Traumatic Evisceration

The following case is told in the Babylonian Talmud (BT *Ḥullin* 56b -57a):

> A Roman (or an Aramaean)[36] witnessed [an accident]: a man fell down from the roof to the ground; his belly burst open and his entrails protruded. [The Roman] called the son of the injured and made his father believe that he was going to slaughter the boy. The father fainted and sighed deeply, which drew his bowels inside. The Roman immediately stitched up his abdomen.

It implies the fact that the surgeon did not touch the bowels of the patient, which allowed better chances of recovering. The healer was not called a surgeon or physician but the fact that he closed the wound with stitches makes the designation likely. There is no author mentioned for this tale. Celsus (25 BCE-50 CE) writes in his *De Medicina* (Book VII, chap.16) on abdominal wounds that when intestines spill out, the bowels must be replaced *in situ* as soon as possible but does not mention the striking method described in the Talmud.

Operation for Obesity

It is told (BT *Baba Metsia* 83b) that Rabbi Eleazar was exceedingly obese. He was given a sleeping draught, taken to a room covered with marble stones, and then operated upon. His belly was opened, and the surgeon removed a number of baskets of fat. The outcome of this alleged operation is not documented.[37] The context of this striking story is not medical at all. It has to do with animal offerings and the question was, whether fat can be separated from flesh or not. Let us remark that the Talmud is describing an anaesthetic preparation which is not mentioned and is using a specially isolated room with marble walls. The word 'surgeon' does not even appear.

We find in the *Natural History* of Pliny (23-79 C.E.) a quite similar story. We read:

> It has been asserted that the fat was drawn from the body of a son of Lucius Apronius, a man of consular rank, and that he was thus relieved of a burden which precluded him from moving. (XI, 85)

Here also, the context is not medical – it is situated under the caption 'Animals who do not grow fat'! and Chapter XI deals with 'The various kinds of insects'.

Rabbi Eleazar ben Simeon (second century) had been hiding from the Roman authorities in a cave with his father for several years; his diet was then indeed minimal. Was this the reason for his (later?) metabolic problems? This question must be left open.

Splenectomy

The spleen had a special place in ancient physiology. According to the humoral theory accepted in Graeco-Roman medicine, the 'black humour' which causes melancholy was stored in the spleen. It says in the Talmud (*Berakhot* 61b) 'The spleen laughs', in other words, the spleen causes, or allows laughter, as it neutralizes the agent of sadness (melancholy).When Adoniyah, the son of King David, nominated himself king in place of his aged father, it says: 'Hagit, prepared chariots and horses and fifty men to run before him' (*I Kings* Adoniyah, son of 1: 5).

The Talmud (*Sanhedrin* 21a) affirms that these running men had their spleen and the flesh of the sole of their feet cut off.[38] The spleen is not a heavy organ; however, it was apparently thought that the spleen caused a sense of heaviness.[39] The Talmudists knew that animals and humans could live without a spleen. It says (*Mishnah Hullin* 3, 2):

> The following injuries do not render the animal *taref* […] In case the spleen is removed – it may thus be eaten, for it will not die from this injury.

This statement is discussed elsewhere in the Talmud (*Hullin*, 42b), where we read:

If the spleen is gone, the animal is permitted. Said Rabbi Avira in the name of Raba: But if the spleen is pierced, it (the animal) is *taref.*

There is moreover an addition to this, later in the same chapter (*Hullin* 55b):

It is *taref* only if it has been pierced in the thick part [of the spleen]; if in the flat part it is permitted.

We are impressed by the anatomical and physio-pathological expertise of these rabbinic authorities. Indeed, if the spleen is pierced, there is a clear vital danger from major bleeding. Preuss stated (p.215) that Pliny also noted that the spleen may be removed without impeding normal life

The spleen sometimes offers a peculiar impediment in running, for which reason the region of the spleen is cauterized in runners who are troubled with pains there [...]. There are some persons who think that with the spleen man loses the power of laughing, and that excessive laughter is caused by the overgrowth of it.(*Hist. Nat.* book 11, chap. 80).

Although writing on animals in this chapter, Pliny here notes that if the spleen is removed by an incision, the animal may survive. We do not infer from this that the rabbis had taken their information from Pliny as they might well have taken it from some earlier source.

Hypospadias

Hypospadias is an abnormality of the penis, in which there is an opening of the ventral side of the urethra. There is therefore an issue of urine and of semen before arriving at the meatus, at the end of the penis. We read:

If there is a hole underneath [the penis], the man is *passul* [invalid, or disqualified], because [the semen] is flowing out [through the hole]. If the hole has been closed, the man is valid [Heb. *Kasher*], for he may inseminate. (*Tosefta Yebamot* 10, 4)

The text of this *Tosefta,* which is parallel to the *Mishnah,* is under the caption 'severed membrum' (Hebrew: *kerut shofkhah*).[40] Indeed, when there is such a hole, it is as if the membrum had been cut off, for it usually causes sterility, and such an invalid is prohibited to marry. This Mishnaic saying is also mentioned in the Talmud (*Yebamot* 76a), but we find there a very special and original therapeutic procedure, advocated by Abbaye (278-338 CE). Abbaye was head of the Talmudic Academy in Pumbedita (Babylonia) and was well informed on medical items, many of them transmitted to him by his stepmother, who was most probably a midwife. In this case however, he does not say 'Mother told me'. (Hebrew: *amra lieim*).[41] We read:

> Abbaye said: The spot [i.e. the hole] is scratched with a grain of barley. Then tallow is rubbed on it. Then a big ant is procured, it will bite in, its head is then cut off. It must be a kernel of barley, for an iron [instrument] would cause inflammation. This is only fit for a small hole, for a large one would be peeled off. (*Yebamot* 76a)

This procedure requires some explanations. The scratching with barley kernel will cause some blood to ooze from around the hole, which will add to cicatrisation through the action of fibrin, which is rich in platelets.[42] This is obviously an anachronistic explanation, but it shows that they had observed, or heard about, this effect of scratching. Big ants have indeed been used in several parts of the world, particularly in Africa and South America, for suturing wounds. The Dorylus and the Eciton ants have particularly strong mandibles. Such kinds of ants have also been found in Bengal, at the North-Eastern part of India.[43] We think that there is much to presume that the Talmudists heard about this method of suturing from Hindu sources (cf. *Sushruta Samhita*), which may well have reached Babylonia.

Preuss (p. 219) noted that Abulcasis also used such a method for suturing intestinal wounds (*De Chirurgia* II, 85). Abulcasis lived in the tenth century in Andalusia. We did not find Graeco-Roman sources in this case but think that a Hindu source through Babylonian transmission could have been relevant.

Circumcision

In the Bible, we read:

> This is my covenant, which you shall keep between Me and you and your seed after you. Every man-child among you shall be circumcised [...] and it will be a token of the covenant between Me and you. Aged eight days every man-child among you shall be

circumcised [...] and my covenant will be in your flesh for an
everlasting covenant. (Genesis 17: 10-13)

The first circumcision performed at the age of eight days was that of Isaac,
the son of Abraham (*Genesis* 21: 4). We are told that Moses had left one of
his two boys uncircumcised, while living with his father-in-law Jethro.
When Moses was ordered to travel back to Egypt, he was threatened with
death and his wife Tzipora performed the circumcision herself in haste.[44]
We read:

Tzipora took a [sharp] stone and cut off the foreskin of her son and
cast it at his feet, and said: 'Surely a bloody bridegroom you are for
me'. (Ex. 4: 25)

When the Children of Israel were ready to cross the Jordan river, the Lord
commanded Joshua as follows: 'Make flint knives and circumcise again the
Children of Israel.' Those who had left Egypt on their way to freedom had
been circumcised, however those who were born during the wandering in
the wilderness were not.[45] All men were therefore circumcised, and
everyone waited there till they had recovered (*Exodus* 2-8). It is striking to
acknowledge that there is no detailed description of the operation of the
foreskin in the Bible, which was and remains so fundamental in Jewish law.

The procedure is detailed in the Mishnah (*Shabbat* 19, 2).We shall not
here describe in detail the operation. Let us however say that the three main
parts of the operation are firstly cutting the foreskin, then tearing the
membrane which covers the corona and finally suction of the blood that
covers the wound.[46] Then the corona is covered with a compress after
putting a suitable powder on the wound. In the time of the Mishnah this
was ground cumin. A few remarks cannot be omitted. First, all this must
be performed on the eighth day after birth, even if it is a Sabbath, unless
there is a medical contra-indication. Second, 'suction' may be performed
through a glass tube, since diseases may be transmitted orally. The official
who performs the operation is called *mohel*, who may or may not be a
physician. Topics such as the bandage, the aftercare as well as the possible
complications of the procedure are fully described by Julius Preuss.[47]

Conclusion

In this part of the chapter, we have tried to describe surgical data gathered
from ancient Jewish literature. In the Hebrew Bible, we noticed traumatic

injuries such as wounds and fractures, but mainly in an allegoric context. War injuries are mentioned quite often, but rarely discussed in detail; no military surgeon is ever called upon. One should of course remember that the Bible is a theological work in which the ultimate healer is the Lord.

In the Talmud, whose scope is very wide and encompasses all aspects of life, many more data can be selected, including surgical cases. We chose only a few of them, where comparative descriptions could be documented in Graeco-Roman sources. We hope to have thus contributed to the history of medicine in ancient Hebrew and Jewish literature.

Select Bibliography

Albright, W.F., 'The Chronology of the Divided Monarchy of Israel', *Bulletin of the American Schools of Oriental Research*, 100, 1945), p.29.

Gesenius, W., *Hebräisches und Aramäisches Handwörterbuch* (Leipzig: 1915), (16th edition), p.282.

Josephus in nine volumes, trans. Thackeray, H. St. J. and Marcus, R. (Cambridge: Harvard University Press [Loeb Classical Library], 1929-1962).

Kottek, S., 'La Bible, la santé et l'hygiène', Paris, Glyphe Ed., 2012 [See pp.248-289 on Surgery].

Kottek, S., 'The Surgeon as depicted in Talmudic Literature', *Proceedings of 37th International Congress of the History of Medicine*, Galveston, Texas, 2002, pp.280-284.

Lowin, S.L., *Narratives of Villainy: Titus, Nebuchadnezzar and Nimrod in the Ḥadith and Midrash, in The Lineaments of Islam* (Leiden: Brill, 2012), pp.261-293.

Morgenstern, L., 'A History of Splenectomy', in Hiatt, J.R., Phillips, E.H. and Morgenstern, L. (Eds), *Surgical Diseases of the Spleen* (Springer, 1997), pp.3-14.

The Works of Philo (C.D. Yonge trans.), Hendrickson Publ. [new updated edition], 2008. See 'On the Contemplative Life or Suppliants', pp.698-706.

Pliny the Elder, *The Natural History*, trans. John Bostock (London, 1855).

Preuss, J., *Biblical and Talmudic Medicine*, trans. Fred Rosner (New York/London: Sanhedrin Press, 1978).

Thorwald, J., *Science and Secrets of Early Medicine: Egypt, Mesopotamia, India, China, Mexico, Peru* (New York: Harcourt, Brace and World, 1963).

Notes

1. In fact, the Egyptian practitioners of embalming were not physicians. The physicians of Joseph attended the embalming operation in order to delete the magical and ritual customs appended to it.
2. The three Hebrew terms are in the singular form.
3. The term 'stripes' is not currently understood as meaning 'blow' or 'stroke', it is however used in the Bible for the forty blows inflicted by judges as punishment for evil actions (*Deuteronomy*, 25: 2-3).
4. This king is unknown; some commentators consider that it was King Aḥaz, who reigned on Judah from 743 to 727 BCE).

5. See also *Obadiah* 1, 7. Here *mazor* is translated as snare, viz. A trap in which you are caught.
6. *Makkot* is the plural form of *makkah*.
7. Cf. Mishnah, *Aboth* 5, 4; Tosefta *Sotah* 9, 4.
8. Calendula officinalis is a flower also known as Garden Marigold. Calendula oil has been used as well during the First World War and during the American Civil War for wounds.
9. Uzziah, King of Judah, reigned from 783 to 742 BCE according to Albright (cf. Bibliography). He was aged 16 when being enthroned. He was quite successful in the wars against his enemies.
10. Abimelekh was in fact the son of Gideon, who was also known under the name Yerubaal, living in the period of the Judges. He wanted to be King of Shekhem; he was however unsuccessful.
11. Rashi is the acronym of Rabbi Salomon ben Isaac, or Salomon Itshaqi (1040-1105), the foremost commentator of the Bible and Talmud.
12. *Metsudat David* is a commentary written by Rabbi David Altschuler, first published in 1753.
13. Hahaleiti means literally 'I have been made sick' but here we may choose the closely related term 'debilitated'.
14. Regarding this comment, see Rashi (ad loc.) and others after him.
15. Ahaziah, King of Israel (ca. 870-850 BCE), was the son of Ahab and Jezebel.
16. Jeroboam, son of Nebat, was the first king of the Kingdom of Israel, as opposed to the Kingdom of Judah.
17. See Gesenius, W., *Hebräisches und Aramäisches Hand wörterbuch*, Leipzig 1915 [(16. Ed.). p.282. Gesenius translates: Absterben (Atrophie oder Paralysis) der Hand.
18. The right eye is the 'eye of intelligence and wisdom'. Thus action (the arm) and intelligent judgment (the right eye) will be impaired.
19. See, for instance BT *Berakhot*61a.
20. Cf. manual, manufacture, manuscript.
21. See BT *Derekh Erets Zuta*, 10.
22. Minutor (Latin) But here the Hebrew term 'gara' is chosen; It means the one who diminishes the quantity of blood – hence the Latin minutor.
23. Rabbi Samuel Edeles (1555-1631) gave this widely accepted interpretation in his commentary on the Talmud.
24. Cf. *The Works of Flavius Josephus* (trans. Whiston, W.), Edinburgh, not dated, page 277 (with slight changes).
25. See Celsus, *De Medicina*, Book 7, 26. This operation remained afterwards in use, with minor change, throughout the Middle Ages. See Herr, H.W., *Cutting for the Stone: The Ancient Art of Lithotomy*, B.J.U., vol. 101, 10 (2008), pp.1214-1216.
26. In the translation of Whiston (cf. note 24, above), see p. 444.
27. Herod was made 'King of the Jews' by the Roman Senate, under Mark Anthony, in 37 BCE. He reigned till his death in 4 CE.
28. In this work, particularly appreciated by Christian Church Fathers, Philo describes the Jewish sect known under the name Therapeuts, who lived close to Lake Mareotis in Egypt. They had a kind of monastic life, comparable though not quite similar to the Essenes established around the Dead Sea. Eusebius considered the Therapeuts as early Christians.

29. In the translation of Yonge, C.D. (new updated edition, 2008), see *On the Contemplative Life*, pp. 698-706.

30. Samuel bar Naḥmani (or ben Naḥman) lived mainly in Palestine, later than the first mentioned Samuel, who lived in Babylonia.

31. See Preuss (1978), 'Brain Injuries' p.203, notes 222 and 223: Aristotle, *Hist. Animal.* 3: 13, and Pliny, *Natural History*, 11: 83.

32. This legend has been apparently widely circulated in Midrashic literature. See for instance *Midrash Tanḥuma, Ḥuqat,* 1; also *Leviticus Rabba* 22, 2 and in *Genesis Rabba* 10, 8.

33. Muhammad al-Tabari lived in the ninth-tenth centuries. His work comprises 40 volumes. Vol 1: 'From Creation to the Flood' was translated by Franz Rosenthal and published in 1989. The death of Nimrod was described several times in early Arabic literature.

34. Boanthropy means a psychic symptomatology where someone behaves like a bull. We read (Daniel 4: 22): 'You will be driven from men, and your dwelling will be with the beasts of the field; and you will be made to eat grass like oxen...' See also Ibid., 29-30.

35. In fact, there is no actual account, either in the Talmud, or in the Midrash, on King Nebuchadnezzar having experienced the same kind of death as his alleged forefather Nimrod. Both are however often seen as archetypic antagonists of the Jews.

36. Literally, 'an Aramaean'. However, on certain manuscripts it says 'A Roman'.

37. Even the stitching of the wound is not mentioned. Nowhere else in the Talmud or in the Midrash is such an operation recorded. The soporific draught is not detailed either.

38. We were unable to find a Graeco-Roman source for the alleged operation of the foot sole. It has been contended that ancient Greek runners ran barefoot. Indeed, running on the tip of toes (forefoot running) may well increase velocity. Foot fasciitis and pains in the arch of foot incur frequently in runners.

39. Some authors have argued that there might have been many cases of splenomegaly from malaria, or even from sickle-cell disease; this is uncertain

40. *Kerut shofkhah* is usually translated as 'castrated'; In fact, the literal translation is 'cut in the pipe' – that is the urethra. Such a type of castration as described here can therefore be cured by a successful operation.

41. See my paper (in French):'Amra li ém, La transmission de la médecine populaire par les femmes dans le Talmud'; *Revue des Etudes Juives,* 169, 3-4 (2010), pp.419-437.

42. The action of the fibroblasts may also reduce the size of the hole, however then one would have to wait a certain time before continuing the operation.

43. See Thorwald, J., *Science and Secrets of Early Medicine* (1962), p.212. We read that the big ants from Bengal were used for suturing the wounds following intestinal operations. And further: The formic acid secreted by these insects played the role of an antiseptic and would hinder any infection of the wound.

44. Moses had not performed the circumcision. He thought he could not delay his mission even for a few days, till the child was healed, as Joshua did later, when the children of Israel were circumcised, before crossing the river Jordan (see *Joshua* 5: 8).

45. They were not circumcised, because they did not know in advance when they would leave for the next station in the wanderings in the desert. They would have been obliged to wait till being healed.

46. Sucking the blood that covers the corona was considered important in order to allow healing, as it seems. Since the nineteenth century this sucking is performed, in a number of European Jewish communities, through a glass tube, with some gauze inside.

47. This is detailed in Preuss (1978), pp.244-247.

B. Medicine

Kenneth Collins

Jewish medicine is firmly based within the Jewish religious tradition. It utilises the canon of the *Tanach* (the Hebrew Scriptures) as understood in the voluminous commentaries and discourses of the rabbis as recorded in the *Mishna* and *Gemara*. Together, these works, known collectively as the Talmud have formed the basis for further rabbinic elaboration over the millennium and a half since the final redaction of the *Gemara*. Jewish traditional medicine also uses the rich symbolism inherent in Jewish ritual and the Hebrew language. Thus, the fragrant herbs used at the *Havdalah* ceremony at the end of the Sabbath could be used as an inhalation for colds, a treatment for diarrhoea, high blood pressure, hair loss and pestilence during the following week.[1]

The Land of Israel was strategically placed on the trade routes of antiquity and was especially open to the medical practices and traditions of its many neighbours. These included Egypt, where the Israelites lived for some centuries, to Mesopotamia, home of the Jewish patriarchs. In differing periods Egyptian and Mesopotamian medicine were highly esteemed even though many of the medications came with their own associated religious and cultural practices often inimical to that of Israel. Further, Israel enjoys a special climate located between sea and desert, with such remarkable land features as the Dead Sea and the River Jordan and is located at the conjunction of three continents with their varied plant and animal populations.

Medicine in the Bible

The Hebrew Bible records that the *Cohenim* (priests) supervised cases of contagious diseases but, unlike in other contemporary cultures, did not perform the functions of a physician. The Prophets, however, occasionally practised the art of healing. Elijah and his disciple Elisha both restored life to a child who appeared to have died (I Kings xvii. 17-22 and II Kings iv. 18-20, 34-35). Isaiah cured King Hezekiah, at the direction of God, of an inflammation by applying a plaster made of figs (II Kings xx. 7). Ben Sira wrote in the Apocrypha:

Honour a physician with the honour due unto him for the uses which ye may have of him, for the Lord hath created him…The Lord has created medicines out of the earth; and he that is wise will not abhor them…And He has given men skill that He might be honoured in His marvellous works…My son, in thy sickness be not negligent… give place to the physician…let him not go from thee, for thou hast need of him. (*Ecclesiasticus*, 38:1-12)

While the Bible is clearly not in any way a medical text, its voluminous account of the early history of the Jewish people and their constant religious struggles contains some references of a medical nature. However, it is difficult to find any reference of a medication to be taken internally though many of the products which are mentioned do have a medicinal component. There are indications of the understanding of quarantine, health protection and sanitary regulations concerning the eating of meat, the requirements for speedy burials and the rules for social hygiene. There were practising midwives as well as physicians. Treatments included bathing, anointing with oils, wine, balm and medical compresses and splinting for fractures.

The health benefits of music were already known in Biblical times. The minstrel's music enabled the prophet to be more receptive to the Divine Message while King David played on his harp to drive away the melancholy from King Saul.[2] The Book of *Proverbs* describes trust in God as 'potions, *sku'l*, for the bones'. *Ezekiel* 47:19 talks of waters flowing from Jerusalem as 'wherever the waters come they shall be healed, and everything lives wherever the river comes'.

The Bible also lists the traditional plants of the area. The *Book of Genesis* relates that when Joseph was sold into slavery in Egypt the Ishmaelite traders were carrying gum, balm and laudanum. These plant resins, including balsam, were used for a range of medical disorders, such as fevers, stomach problems and excessive sweating. When Jacob sent his sons to Egypt for the second time to buy food, they were to take some of the produce of Canaan, including balm, honey, gum, laudanum, nuts and almonds as a gift for Joseph.

The Book of Exodus records details of the special ointment used to consecrate the vessels of the Temple and anoint the *Cohenim* (priests). This ointment contained cassia, cinnamon, myrrh, calamus and olive oil. Calamus remains an essential ingredient in the manufacture of perfumes while it is also a psycho-active product being hallucinogenic at high doses. Cassia is closely related to cinnamon and was praised for its aroma while myrrh has analgesic properties and can stimulate the appetite. Hyssop, which has mild purgative properties, is mentioned in the Book of Psalms (51:9) as a cleanser from sin.

We have seen the reference to the healing of King Hezekiah. However, one of Hezekiah's acts, for which he was praised by the rabbis, was to conceal the legendary *Book of Remedies* which was said to have contained the cures for all diseases and whose authorship was attributed to King Solomon by the great mediaeval rabbi-physician Nachmanides, Ramban, (1194-c.1270). The Biblical commentator Rashi (1040-1105) believed that people were being healed so quickly by these remedies that they did not develop the humility that their illness should have produced and so they failed to see God as the true Healer.[3] Moses Maimonides (1138-1204), however, commented that the *Book of Remedies* contained treatments based on astrological phenomena and magical incantations which might lead people to use them for idolatrous purposes. Further, it contained details of the formulas for poisons and antidotes and this might have led unscrupulous people to use the poisons to kill their enemies.

Medicines in the Talmud

The nature of the Talmud, with its encyclopaedic view of the Jewish world spanning many centuries of Jewish life both in the Land of Israel and the Babylonian Diaspora, lent itself to coverage of a wide variety of traditional medical themes including folk remedies and health beliefs. The Talmud builds on the range of medicinal products and hygienic procedures in the Bible supplemented by oral traditions, some said to have been preserved from the time of Moses. In addition, the Talmud contains a large number of medical references dealing with the rights and duties of the physician. From Talmudic times it was recommended that no wise person should live in a town which did not have a doctor. It was required for a patient to seek help for healing even on the Sabbath when religious restrictions might be set aside if there is any possible danger to health.

Some of the popular medicine tradition recorded in the Talmud will naturally seem strange, even outlandish, to the modern mind but we should remember that in mediaeval Europe as late as the sixteenth century the apothecary was legally required to keep woodlice, ants, vipers, scorpions, crabs, sparrow brains and fox lungs in stock.[4] Leading rabbis of the Talmudic period, such as Abbaye and Raba, did have concerns about the use of magic and charms but, mindful of contemporary sentiment, accepted that whatever is done for therapeutic purposes is not to be regarded as superstitious.[5] Further, given the strictness of Jewish dietary laws and their proscription of certain animals and birds for food they record cases of permitted and forbidden treatments.[6] The use of forbidden animal products for medication remained a problem for observant Jews. While the theoretical lists of available Jewish traditional remedies and *materia medica* contain many products from such animals as the eagle, lion, frog, hyena and crocodile they feature much less in lists of Jewish practical pharmacy. This is thought to be less due to commercial availability than to halachic considerations.[7]

The medication mentioned in the Talmud is derived mainly from plants and trees. Often the trees are used in their entirety, while sometimes just the leaves and rarely the bark are used. Plant oils were popular and olive oil might be used as a gargle for sore throat. The most important animal product is honey 'with sweet a person heals the bitter'.[8] Drugs might be prepared in different ways. Mostly the drugs were cooked individually or together, such as the liquid remedy called *shikyana*. Sometimes drugs were pulverised and taken internally either as dry powder or suspended in water. *Samma de naftza,* an abortifacient remedy, was imbibed in this way.[9] Wax and base tallow were used as the base for salves. One such, collyria, was used for eye disease. Salves could also form the basis of poultices and plasters. Plaster, *retiya,* may be applied to a wound, or if the whole body is injured as in a fall then the whole body is covered with a plaster, one of ingredients of which is wheat. Theriac, a great compound medication with a variety of often potent ingredients, such as snake flesh, was widely employed in Talmudic times. The rabbis counsel against the use of theriac from heathen sources because of the risk of adulteration with poisons.[10]

Other products used for treatment include many common foodstuffs. Bread soaked in wine is recommended as an eye compress and green leaves may be applied on inflamed eyes.[11] Ripe or unripe gourds can be placed on the forehead to relieve fever.[12] Mar Samuel (c.165-c.257), a leading scholar and physician of the Talmudic period, considered that cool water for eye compresses is the best collyrium in the world and children were bathed in wine for healing purposes.[13] (*Tosefta Shabbat* 12,13) The use of natural springs and waters was also well known – and the springs of Tiberias, on the shore of the Sea of Galilee, were particularly prized for their healing properties. Rabbi Yochanan explains that the absence of *tsaraat,* leprosy, in Babylon was because of their bathing in the Euphrates.[14]

In addition to the use of specific medications the Talmudic records additional details which would seem to add a magical dimension to the treatment. The use of garland, or knotted plants, is said to be especially efficacious – three knots arrest the illness, five heal it and seven help even against magic.[15] A particularly efficacious medication was said to be *samtar.* If this is placed on a wound caused by an arrow or spear wound this would help the victim survive.[16] If someone is bitten by a rabid dog, they would be given liver from that animal to eat.[17]

There is little in the way of so-called *filth pharmacy* in the Talmud which appears extensively in Greek and Roman sources. In the Talmud Rabbi Chanina records the use of a measure of forty day old urine for a wasp sting or scorpion bite – presumably this was to be applied externally.[18] In the Jerusalem Talmud, a shorter and less complete compendium produced in the Land of Israel rather than in Babylonia, Rabbi Yochanan records that he learned from a Roman woman that the faeces of children were a cure for scurvy.[19]

Many non-medicinal remedies are also recorded in the Talmud. These include the application of heat, for example by the use of warm cloths on the abdomen and hot cups on the navel.[20] The beneficial effects of sunshine on health were also known from Biblical times and recommended by the rabbis.[21] Dietary considerations relative to health were also recorded in detail in the rabbinic literature. The rabbis took care that while patients might be given advice about diet, for incurable patients some are of the opinion that such patients be allowed to eat what they want.[22]

Physicians were advised that they should handle such situations with delicacy – not giving specific difficult orders but saying the same, 'don't sleep in a damp place or drink anything cold', adding 'lest you die like so and so' – as this will make a better impression.[23] Sick people were advised to avoid eating gourds but could eat the more delicate food known as *hatriyot.* A physician came to heal Rav Yirmiyahu and saw gourds present and exclaimed, 'How can I heal him – the Angel of Death is in this house!'[24] Eating beef, fat meat, poultry, roasted eggs, cress, milk and cheese could make illness worse while beneficial foods, which could heal sickness, included: cabbage, mangold, camomile and small fish.[25] Specific foods for the sick would include the gruel-like tisane or *arsan*, which is made from old peeled barley from the bottom of the sieve, or fine barley flour. *Schathitha*, dried baked corn flour mixed with honey, was prepared in thick and thin forms. The thick version was used as nourishing food and the thin form as medication. A similar product, made from lentil flour mixed with vinegar was used as a remedy for fever.[26]

The commonest forms of surgical treatments to be considered within the framework of traditional medicine include bleeding and cupping. Bleeding, by performing phlebotomy, is often mentioned in the Talmud, sometimes accompanied by a special blessing, and was widely performed as a medical treatment until as late as the nineteenth century. Sanhedrin 129b gives direction for cupping and bleeding. Mar Samuel, greatest of Talmudic physicians advised that a patient should fast before bloodletting and take their time before resuming normal activities after the procedure.[27] The rabbis were concerned about the risks of bleeding and constructed a calendar of propitious days for the procedure.

There is a voluminous literature in the Talmud and in the New Testament (Matthew 10:1) about demons and their role in the causation of illness and the Rabbis believed that magic and the evil eye operate through them. The demon aetiology is even susceptible of a theory of contagion. One shouldn't drink liquid left by another or the spirit that comes out of the other, if he has a disease, can pose a mortal danger. Demons inhabit marshy places, damp and deserted houses, latrines, squalid lanes and foetid atmospheres which obviously became associated with disease and ill-health.[28]

Notes

1. Matras H., 1995. *Jewish Folk Medicine*, p.122.
2. 2 *Kings*, 3, 15; 1; *Samuel* 16, 16.
3. Epstein, I. (Ed. and trans.) *The (Babylonian) Talmud* (London: Soncino Press, 1981). Commentary on Tractate Pesachim, Babylonian Talmud, 56a.
4. Rosner, F. (Ed. and trans.) *Julius Preuss' Biblical and Talmudic Medicine* (New York: Sanhedrin Press, 1978), p.433.
5. Epstein, I., *The Talmud*. Shabbat 67a and Hullin 77b.
6. Tosefta Shabbat, VII, VIII (Hebrew).
7. Lev, E. and Amar, Z., *Practical Materia Medica of the Eastern Mediterranean According to the Cairo Genizah* (Leiden: Brill, 2008), p.511.
8. Rosner, F., *Julius Preuss*, p.435.
9. Epstein, I., *The Talmud*, Niddah 30b.
10. Epstein, I., *The Talmud*, Shabbat 109b.
11. Epstein, I., *The Talmud*, Shabbat 108b,
12. *Epstein, I., The Talmud, Yoma 78a,*
13. Tosefta Shabbat 12, 13 (Hebrew).
14. Epstein, I., *The Talmud*, Ketubot 77b.
15. Epstein, I., *The Talmud*, Shabbat 66b.
16. Epstein, I., *The Talmud*, Baba Batra 74b.
17. Epstein, I., *The Talmud*, Yoma 8b.
18. Epstein, I., The Talmud, Shabbat 109b.
19. Shabbat 14:14d, Jerusalem Talmud (Hebrew).
20. Epstein, I., *The Talmud*, Shabbat 40b.
21. Epstein, I., *The Talmud*, Nedarim 108b; Malachi 3:20.

22. Freedman, H. and Simon, M. (Eds and trans.), *The Midrash* (London: Soncino Press, 1977), Exodus Rabbah 30:22; Ecclesiastes Rabbah 5:6.
23. *Sifra* on Leviticus, 16:1 (Hebrew).
24. Epstein, I., *The Talmud*, Nedarim 49a.
25. Rosner, F., *Julius Preuss*, p.441.
26. Epstein, I., *The Talmud*, Avodah Zarah 38b; Gittin 70a.
27. Epstein, I., *The Talmud*, Shabbat 128a/b.
28. Trachtenberg, J., *Jewish Magic and Superstition: A Study in Folk Religion* (New York: Atheneum Press, 1970), p.198.

3

Islamic and Jewish Traditional Medicine

A. Islamic: Aspects of Amulets, Charms and Evil Eye

Aref Abu-Rabia

Introduction

The Arabs in the pre-Islamic period practised traditional medicine that some learned from neighbours and nations with whom they came in contact. Some ancient Arab medical practices depended on amulets, charms, sorcery and witchcraft. Among the methods of treatment was divination (*sihr*), magic (*sha'wadha*), talismans (*talsim*), and astrology (*tanjim*).[1] The aim of traditional medicine is to deter the causes of illness by hanging amulets or talismans on a person, making vows, visiting the tombs of saints or using stratagems to mislead the sources of the disease, such as the evil eye. The influence of the evil eye is counter-acted by devices designed to distract its attention and annul its power through the practice of magic. The concept of the evil eye appears to be a psychological idiom for the fear of misfortune. It may relate to fear of outsiders and their envy. Adhering to the rules of social ethics, religion and hygiene can also help to prevent illness.[2]

The healer in traditional society could be a shaman, herbalist, bonesetter or a medium. In western society they could be a family physician, cardiologist, oncologist or a psychiatrist.[3] Both the Palestinians and the Israelis have western medical systems in addition to traditional medicine, yet there is more of a coexistence of patterns of medical pluralism among the Palestinians than the Israelis.

According to Popper-Giveon and Kiev,[4] traditional healing embodies the methodology, theology and cosmology of the community and protects it and its children from the forces of evil. The role of the healer as an intermediary and mediating agent between members of the community and the 'World Beyond', grants the healer esteemed status. The healer is viewed as an important figure from a religious and even a political perspective, and is perceived as a guardian of the community's cultural heritage, responsible for preservation of the social order and the spiritual equilibrium within it, and at times owner of a monopoly on the ability to heal. At the same time, the traditional healer is described as a marginal and exceptional figure who engenders awe in others due to the healer's powers and proximity to the spirit world. He often appears as one who can recruit the spirits to do his bidding, and even through them to do harm to members of the community.[5]

Popper-Giveon's research deals with traditional Arab female healers in Israel, and the women who turn to them for treatment. The Arab society in Israel is influenced by deep change processes, such as urbanisation, acculturation and modernisation. These processes impact on the circumstances and social setting of Arab women in Israel in general, and on the form taken by traditional healing in particular. It also effects the role of the healers, their work methods and the context within which they operate. Therefore, one can assume that the character and the actions of the traditional Arab female healers living in mixed cities in the centre of Israel where the Arab population is influenced by accelerated acculturation, would be different from those of traditional female healers living in Bedouin communities in the Negev, who even today still maintain a high level of cultural uniqueness.

Traditional medicine is practised by Jewish Israelis. The research conducted by Lieberman-Avital examines the image and practices of Jewish female traditional healers of Maghreb origin (north and north-western Africa between the Atlantic Ocean and Egypt, from Morocco to Libya) currently working in Israel.[6] Lieberman-Avital has observed how these traditional female healers have adopted the narrative of 'ancestral merit' (of one's forefathers). This is a dominant element in the authority of a blessed saintly-righteous figure in Israel since the 1970s and the healers have gendered this element with a narrative of 'maternal ancestral merit'. This narrative contains their personal story and through their narratives they raise spiritual and cultural capital that grants them authority to operate as female healers and as persons endowed with divine qualities in the modern and post-modern Israeli domain. In a broader sense, in regard to the intersection of traditional medicine with Israeli identity, field research suggests that support for traditional medicine in the modern world emanates from the perseverance of traditional cosmology. This outlook includes belief in the existence of harmful forces: the evil eye, witchcraft and even demons. While the belief in demon-possession has weakened in the Israeli domain, it has not disappeared entirely. Rather it has been 'melted' together with the evil eye into one broader category of harmful spiritual powers. It is worthy of note that in regard to the use of incense (*bakhur*), this practice has actually become more widespread in the Israeli context under the influence of New Age discourse and alternative medicine. This development has been made possible due to the similarity that exists between traditional religions and New Age spirituality, and the similarity between alternative medicine and traditional medicine. Thus, traditional medicine enjoys renewed cultural capital, and the intersection of traditional medicine with New Age currents has aroused renewed interest in traditional medicine. For example, as part of this process, the practice of burning incense has become widespread, prevalent and accessible not just to those of North African (Maghreb) origins, but for many other Jews too.[7]

Treatment

Traditional healers among Palestinians-Arabs in Israel, as described by Massalha and Baron, have claimed that, for generations, the Arab woman has learned to use plants growing in her vicinity for medicinal purposes, knowledge passed down from mother to daughter.[8] For example, the bark of the eucalyptus tree constitutes a medicine for the flu. The bark of the tree is ground to a powder and brewed as a tea. In cases of a serious cold or backache, one seeks out an expert in cupping. The healer heats the cups using a piece of burning paper and places the hot cups on the patient's back. After a time, he removes the cups, which leave red puffy circles on the skin where they were applied. Afterward, the healer makes a series of shallow incisions on the swollen areas with a razor blade or straight razor. The blood that oozes out of the lacerations is considered the source of the malady. After the body rids itself of the source of the illness, it is restored to equilibrium and the patient is cured.

Other treatment regimens include burns on the painful spot, limb or organ. It should be noted, however, that modern medicine offers more effective solutions, and the need for popular or folk medicine for essentially physical problems is declining. Yet, when modern medicine fails to offer a solution to a problem, there is a tendency to turn to healers in the hopes that they can succeed where modern medicine has failed. In cases of psychological/mental health problems, it is customary to turn to recognized/prominent healers, who demand a fee for their services, but such healers are willing to treat only mild mental disorders. The folk healers themselves recognize the advantages of modern mental health care and in serious cases they will refer to psychiatric hospitals. Folk healers, male and female, treat fertility problems among couples, infertility among women and impotence among men, break spells and curses of the evil eye. They also deal with anxieties tied to making a livelihood or finding a marital match, and they intervene to ameliorate marital disputes, and so forth.[9] The rise in the status of alternative medicine in Western society in general and Israeli society in particular has contributed to the expansion of the work of healers. The populations who seek out folk healers are very diverse, and all levels of Arab society are represented: villagers and urbanites, housewives and working women, educated and uneducated persons, rich and poor. Yet, it has been found that simple folk and those with low education turn to folk medicine more frequently than educated segments of the population. It is important to note that simple folk and educated individuals turn to healers for similar problems. The primary difference is that simple folk turn to healers routinely as a matter of course, while educated persons seek the help of a healer as a last resort, particularly for diseases diagnosed as incurable by modern medicine, such as terminal cancer.[10]

I have shown that traditional Arab healers use a range of techniques and medications in their work.[11] Illnesses are cured by means of remedies taken from vegetables, minerals and animals. Various plant parts are used, including flowers, fruits, leaves, juices, roots, seeds, bulbs, tubers and pulps. One of the most famous medicines in use among the Arab in the Middle East is the *arba'yn*, which consists of a mixture of 40 different types of plants and is considered to be a cure for all aches and pains. In traditional and folk medicine, the Bedouin appeal not only to the herbalist, but also to the dervish (a member of a Muslim, specifically Sufi, religious order who has taken vows of poverty and austerity, often noted for their ecstatic rituals), the amulet writer (*khatib*), the cauteriser, the setter of broken or fractured bones (*mujabbir*), midwives and the local pharmacologist and vendor of medicinal spices (*'attar*). They may also have recourse to visit the holy tombs of ancestors or prophets, the sea, rivers, and holy springs and other places. In addition, healers use techniques that stimulate physiological processes, including bathing, sweat-bathing, massage, cupping, emetics, burning or cauterizing, incision and bloodletting.

There are traditional healers who cooperate with modern medicine by sending patients to a particular physician who, they assure him, will bring them relief. In many cases, this is a good combination, since the patient has complete faith in it, takes his medicine and the advice given with absolute seriousness, and often quickly recovers. Many traditional healers insist that the patient's desire to recover is as important as the healer's desire to cure him. Treatment by traditional healers has established a relationship of psychological-therapeutic dependence on the part of the patient with regard

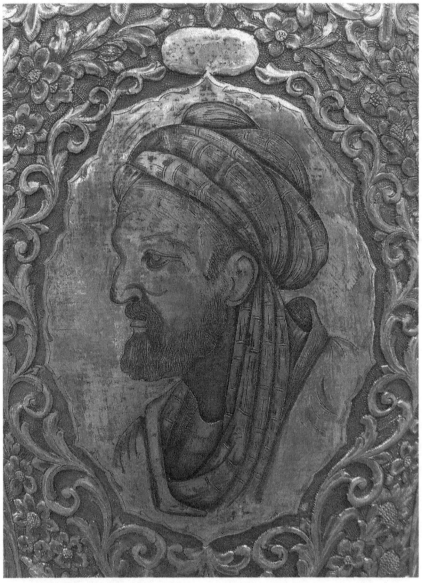

3. Avicenna Portrait on Silver Vase, Museum at Avicenna Mausoleum, Hamadan, Iran.

to the healers. This dependence is deeply rooted in their psyches and is reinforced and legitimised by their culture.

Pinczuk found that Bedouin women in the Negev eat or swallow several roasted coffee beans or seeds of Ricinus Communis (*khirwia'*) after delivery or after menstruation. They put cotton wool in indigo dye powder (*nilih*) and insert it in the vagina taking it out just before sexual intercourse. They drink tea with anise or with Coriandrum sativum (*kuzbarah*). She reported that Negev Bedouin women treated babies with *ktur* as mentioned above, or with incense (*bakhkhur*) on Mondays and Thursdays and allowed children who were thought to be afflicted with the evil eye to inhale the smoke.[12] She found that among the Bedouin women of the Negev, in order to encourage uterine contractions following delivery, mothers drink several cups a day of an infusion of the following plants for two to three weeks: Teucrium (*ja'adih*), Salvia triloba (*marmariyih*), Artemisia judaica (*b'aythiran*), Tamarixaphylla (*tarfa*), Matricaria chamomilla (*rabil*), and Trigonella foenum-graecum *(hilbih)*. They also eat a dish of dates with olive oil called *makhtum*, Portulaca oleracea (*farfahina*) cooked with rice, or dried leaves of eminium spiculatum (*irgita*) cooked with egg.

Gorkin and Othman observed that many Palestinians, when in need of psychotherapeutic intervention, prefer to go to traditional healers within their community both in Israel and the West Bank.[13] All the healers emphasized that they did not choose the healer's role, but were chosen for it, by spiritual dreams or visions. Usually their parent or grandparent were healers and some of the healers had ties to Sufism or had trained with a mentor associated with Islamic mysticism. The healers treated patients with different illnesses and health disorders. These included infertility, impotence, marital problems, dizziness, fainting, digestive problems, psychotic and neurotic disorders, heart disease and cancer. They also deal with the effects of sorcery, the evil eye or spirits known as *jinn*. The healers used different methods for treatments: herbal medicine (zaatar-wild thyme; Miramiya-wild sage (*marmariyih*); Baboonag-camomile). Also employed are some forms of massage with olive oil, rose water or a herb and water mixture used as a lubricant. Some of the healers used diets advising patients to eat, or abstain from, certain foods. Some of the healing process included reading phrases from the Quran as a religious healing ritual.

The use of traditional medicine, particularly herbal medicine, was widespread throughout the Middle East in the twentieth century.[14] The philosophy of traditional medicine draws its strength from the belief in fate, the conviction that all things that happen to man, both good and evil, are the will of Allah. Allah acts through the mediation of man, and therefore cures illness by means of a doctor or folk healer. In some cases the patient may appeal to both simultaneously.[15] Patients used to refer first to home remedies and traditional medicine, but now they often rely upon Western medicine initially or first after home medicine. If these fail, they finally resort to traditional healers, including religious healers. Healers use a range of techniques and medications in their work. Illnesses are cured by means of remedies taken from vegetables, minerals and animals. Various plant parts are used. In addition, healers use techniques that stimulate physiological processes, including bathing, sweat-bathing, massage, cupping, emetics, burning/cauterizing, incision and bloodletting.[16]

Most Arab healers learn from their fathers or mothers during their practice of a healing trade. There is no time limit for acquiring the skills, but it is not uncommon for famous healers to have apprenticed for ten years or more. In the Middle East, the healer's role is perceived as a religious skill related to proximity to saints, which enables the healer to fight the forces of evil that cause illness. Proximity to saints can be more easily attained within a family blessed with many religious healers, dervishes, who treat mental and physical illnesses using a variety of religious and cultural rituals. Men and women usually become dervishes by virtue of having received a *baraka*, a blessed gift from God or by virtue of a birth-right, from father or mother, through family members renowned as wise or righteous people or purported to have special visionary powers, and so forth. Illness is said to be ultimately determined by the will of Allah.[17] Illness is defined holistically as a deviation from states of normal health, manifested by changes in social, psychological and physical states. Traditional therapies are not only the means for curing sickness, but also means by which specified types of illness are defined and made culturally recognisable. When healing fails, a patient remains with his disease until he discovers the correct cure from another healer. Healers and patients explain that this is the will of Allah. Healers examine the facial expression and the eye colour of the patient as part of their attempt to diagnose the disease and prescribe treatment. Their reputations as good healers result from their attitudes toward patients. Healers are always warm, friendly and supportive, and offer good hospitality to those that they treat. Usually their treatments are successful, and patients recover from a majority of their illnesses.[18] The influence of the evil eye is counteracted by devices designed to distract its attention and annul its power through the practice of magic. The concept of the evil eye appears to be a psychological idiom for the fear of misfortune. It may relate to fear of outsiders and their envy.[19]

When a person is ill, or wants to take protective measures for himself, his children or his property, he beseeches Allah to help him through His saints. Among the Bedouin of the southern Sinai, such a pilgrimage can foster any of three kinds of rites: those between members of the tribe, those between the tribes of southern Sinai, and those between members of all the tribes and Islam.[20] Notably, the Bedouin of Jabaliya near St. Catherine's Monastery in Sinai have developed a unique form of folk medicine, designed to overcome the diseases and mishaps that typify their desert environment.[21]

Background

The earliest known beads, made of mollusc shells and associated with early modern humans, Homo sapiens, were discovered at Middle Palaeolithic sites in Asia and Africa. In the Near East, beads containing green minerals were found for the first time in significant numbers in the context of archaeological sites associated with the beginning of cultivation around 12,000 years ago. The onset of agricultural practices brings with it a special interest in fertility, both of plants and animals and of humans.[22]

The use of beads for ritual purposes has been found in many settings. Among the Native-American Iroquois, wampum shell beads had both practical and magical meanings.[23] In various societies, the shells were symbols of eternal life and gifts from the gods to help the dead during their voyage toward the afterlife.[24]

Humans have utilised cowries throughout the world since the dawn of history for decorative and monetary purposes. Most cowries are found in tropical waters, although several species do exist in the Mediterranean. Large cowries symbolized sex among peoples bordering the Indian Ocean and the Red Sea, because of the resemblance of the underside of the shells to female genitalia.[25]

The role of beads in Islamic belief seems to have begun as early as the eighth century when Muslims established hospitals and hospices for old people and the mentally ill.[26] These were free of charge regardless of the gender, social status, or age of the patient.[27] Beads, gemstones and corals are mentioned in descriptions of Islamic mental healing treatments in the Middle Ages.[28] Places of worship of all religions were and are still adorned with stones and linked with stones. An example of this is the Black Stone of *al-Ka'bah* in Mecca.[29] The Prophet embraced the stone and his companions were advised to do the same. The advice to Muslims is to salute the Black Stone as they pass by, as the sacred stone will register the salutation and bear witness on the Final Day.

There is a theory that gemstones have vibrational rates. Placing these vibrations of fields of energy within the human energy system is believed to improve its vibrational rate. The vibrational qualities of the gemstones can further help achieve balance and awareness at the physical, emotional, mental and spiritual levels. Different stones have been reported to have different effects on people who wear them and people nearby.[30] Stones are most popularly used in magical cures.[31] A glance in a round mirror of polished jet is said to protect against cataract.[32]

Islamic Attitudes to Wearing Beads, Gemstones and Metals

According to the consensus of Muslim scholars, it is forbidden for a man to wear golden rings because of the authentic prophetic narrations on the prohibition of gold for men.[33] Therefore, it is permissible to wear a carnelian ring, but better to remove it and wear a silver ring as 'the Prophet had a ring made of silver'.[34]

Coral (*marjan, murjan, mardjan*) is used in jewellery and is supposed to possess curative powers. It comes in many colours, from white to light pink, orange, red, and brown. Black and white coral are also mentioned in the Quran. In Islam, coral belongs to organic products along with the pearl (*lu'lu'*) and amber (*kahruba*), which are associated with precious stones (*jawahir*).[35] Coral and pearls are mentioned together as symbols of the mercy and benefits of God.[36] Beads and corals are used in certain societies as preventive and curative medicine as well as spiritual medicine.[37] Arabic sources recommend hanging coral on epileptic patients as a treatment. Coral is also used to treat gout (*niqris*), cure scurvy, strengthen the gums, treat eye diseases and inflammations, palpitations, the coughing up of blood (haemoptysis), abrasions, urine retention, stomach diseases, and bleeding and whiten teeth.[38] Beyond these specific indications, they are intended to prevent and treat harms caused by the evil eye, bad souls/spirits, and *jinni*. Prayer beads (*sibha*) made of coral have been popular among devotees of Islam since its early days.[39] Arab mothers place coral on their children's necks to protect them. Wearing coral is believed to send out vibrations of harmony, friendship, beauty, and unity. A ring of coral is thought to protect against heat stroke, improve vision, and promote success.[40] According to Popper-Giveon et al., beads and corals are used by the Bedouin in the Negev and Sinai as adornment and for medical purposes; healing powers, as well as the power to exorcise evil spirits.[41]

Some psychiatrists trace bead adornment to feelings of security connected with the eye and sight.[42]

In Bethlehem, the headdress for married women, the *shatweh*, is embroidered and adorned with gold coins and pieces of coral.[43] The triangle of coins (*shbeika*) on the forehead signifies a girl's status as *bint*, young and unmarried.[44] Two medical coins and a metal ring are sewn to a piece of cloth, which is tied to the aching part of the body, are used among the Bedouin women of southern Sinai. A *wuqaa* from Ramallah has a stiff, horseshoe-shaped brim decorated with silver coins, and on the back, a silver amulet with a light blue stone and coins. Children's caps among the Bedouin of the Negev are covered with coins, cowries, corals, blue beads and charms against the evil eye.[45] Medicinal properties are assigned to the *iznaq*, the costly silver chain descending from either side of the *burqa'* and fastened under the chin.[46] Elderly Bedouin women wear a heavy cap that fits tightly on their heads. Its weight is supposedly a potent means of driving away headaches.[47] At festive occasions among the Negev Bedouin, women wear a robe embroidered in different shades of red, with a long waist belt (*hizam*). The lower part of the belt is wider than the upper part and plaited with brown and white stripes. The upper, narrower section features a repeating arrowhead pattern plaited in shades of red, blue, and black, as well as buttons, coins and four-petalled flowers made of cowries. Bedouin women are usually modestly shrouded from head to foot, but the red embroidery on their black dresses, their woven ornaments and their coin decorations make them conspicuous.

When they walk, the decorative panels attached to their costumes flutter, and the coins produce a jingling sound.[48] Beyond its important social and economic symbolism and healing properties, Bedouin women's attire also carries other significant meanings. It attests to the wearer's sexual virtue and fertility and indicates her marital status and group origins. By declaring her own fertility through symbolic attire, the Bedouin woman also announces her husband's virility and boasts of his contribution to the expansion of his agnatic group, that is sharing the same male line, which makes him worthy of a higher social status. The married woman's attire is more conspicuously ornamented. Her *wuqaa* is decorated with shells which are symbols of sexuality and fertility. Coins and stones are added to its back part, so that the *wuqaa* rests more securely on the head.[49] In the nineteenth and early twentieth centuries, women wore headdresses decorated at the front with gold, silver coins, metal ornaments, and coral, cowry shells, buttons, stones, and glass beads.[50] Bead necklaces worn by Palestinians, both Bedouins and villagers, include a variety of beads, cloves, coral, imitation coral, amber, glass and silver, blue beads, tortoise-shell, and triangular cloth amulets, small hands that represent the hand of Fatimah (the daughter of the Prophet Muhammad), and 'eyes' ('*owaynah*).[51]

As a young girl gets older, the amount of jewellery she wears increases. These pieces of jewellery are made of cheap metal, chains of shells, stone, plastic, coral and simple coins. A special head ornament is worn by girls in the full flower of youth as they go to pasture with their herds, to signal that they were still available. The strings of beads that adorn the neck have protective value and are also used as amulets. They are made of gemstones, glass, coral, shells and plastic. A small number of the glass beads are saved and used in new strings of beads, especially because they are thought to have special healing properties. The women save them because of their scarcity and high market price.[52]

In Jordan and the Negev, headstalls (*rasan*) for camels are made of multi-coloured wool in twined weave, and decorated with blue beads, cowries, and shells, buttons and coins.[53] Women wear multicoloured woollen girdles decorated with tassels and beads of bone, blue or brown glass, and cowry shells.[54] They use as amulets and charms many stones and beads thought to have particular powers. Women also wear the *gladeh* or *giladeh*, a choker of various kinds and colours of beads, with a pendant of three multiple strings of cloves (*qrunful*) interspersed with beads, coral, and mother-of-pearl spacers, blue, maroon and orange silk tassels and tiny glass beads. Other necklaces ('*uqdmirjan*) are made of coral with amber and mother-of- pearl spacers.[55]

The Relation between Ornaments and Islamic Religion

Religion has influenced jewellery design significantly in all periods and regions. Islam is an all-encompassing religion and its principles guide all aspects of life, including art and design. In order to prevent idolatry, Islamic art has remained primarily abstract and symbolic, consistently avoiding pictorial representation of the divine. Four basic patterns are used: geometrical, floral, calligraphic designs, and stylised animal and human figures. This language of decoration provided a unified framework of imagery within which Islamic craftsmen have had considerable freedom of expression. Islam created a unity in the diversity: differences exist from region to region, yet a strong, underlying, iconographic concept unified much of the artistic output.[56] Even in the pre-Islamic period, Arabs used gems, crystals, beads and stones as medicine. They believed that precious stones were useful to wear as ring-stones. Corals and cowries were believed to have magical powers of healing, preventing diseases and bringing omens.[57] Certain beads and coins were also assigned magic, symbolic and healing qualities.[58] In ancient Arabia, mothers plaited their daughters' hair, put rings in the side-locks (*jadayil*), and strung them with sea-shells, in addition to adorning them with chains of cowries and necklaces of dried date stones.[59]

The Symbolism of Beads

Arab-Bedouin women adorn their hair with strings of cowry (*couri*) shells called wada'. From the side, with its opening facing outwards, the cowry resembles a woman's vagina, while the colour of the cowry is white, like a man's sperm, symbolizing fertility. When a woman is seen wearing the

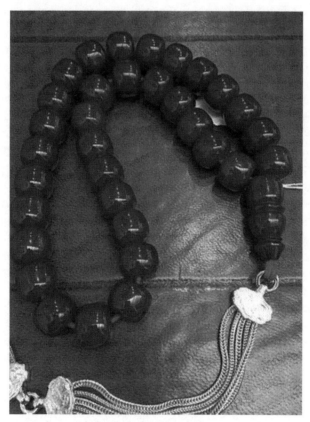

4. Ottoman-era Muslim prayer beads (*subḥa* or *tasbīḥ*).

cowry string, it means she is at the peak of her fertility. If a Bedouin woman does not have access to such shells, she will collect the bulbs of crocus (Colchicum sp.: *wada'*) as she herds her livestock. The bulbs of the wada' are used as a medicine to treat sexual diseases (in both men and women), mainly among the pastoral nomadic Bedouin in the Middle East.[60] According to Shinar, the shapes of cowry and certain other seashells are also claimed to have magical significance.[61]

Among Arabs, beads are also connected with mourning and burial rituals. Amulets described by Latin writers, shells, coral, amber, glass beads, flints, horns and animal teeth, have been found in graves all around the Arabian Peninsula and the Mediterranean area, from both pre-Roman and Roman times.[62] Interestingly, the very same amulets described by the Romans were used for magical purposes until modern times, both in Italy and other European/Mediterranean countries.[63] In the twentieth century, a male Bedouin child was buried with his toys, his small water jug, alum (*shabbeh*) and a blue bead (*kharazahzarga*) that had been intended to ward off the evil eye ('*ayn al-hasad*) during his life. A girl was buried with her bracelets and necklaces that included corals and coins. Both young and old men and women were buried with coins or pieces of gold as a sign of respect.[64]

Beads of necklaces, in addition to their material and aesthetic value, have acquired a wide set of attributed magical-medical properties. Some of these beads are amulets that work with the power inherent in the material or in the shape of the object itself. Cowrie shells, which are attached to necklaces, are used to ward off the evil eye, and in addition symbolize fertility among the Arabs in Jordan and Palestine.[65] Reddish plastic beads are designated as *kahrab*, a local variant of *kahraman*, designating amber, and referring to its electro-magnetic properties. Red glass cylinders that imitate coral are called *murjan*, like real coral. The use of corals in amulets is widespread. In Jordan, their magical power is related to the symbolism, as its red colour is believed to give the coral a positive effect on the blood.

The Bedouin mother hangs two corals on her breast. One of these is called *khrazat al-dirrih*, and is for her, while the other, the *murjan*, is for her new-born.[66] Bedouin healers, men as well as women, relate that when a mother's breast or nipple is painful, infected or swollen, preventing her from feeding her infant, she will wear a white coral necklace called 'breast beads' (*kharazat al-dioud*) on her cleavage.[67] According to folk wisdom, this will cure her. Arab-Bedouin women will sprinkle ground coral on their breasts to ensure plentiful milk and to cure any swelling or infection. This coral is white and perforated, as are her nipples.[68] The colour of the bead is white, like milk, and the bead originates in the sea, signifying fluids, so the wish is that the breast will supply plenty of milk. These practices are based on a belief in the logic of reciprocal action in sympathetic magic, that of 'like cures like'.[69] Some of these practices are also evident in other cultures.[70]

Forty days after delivering the baby, the mother washes (*ghassalat*) her body with water in which she has put an 'impurity bead' (*kharazatkbass*) and a gold coin (*dhahab*) to symbolize the end of her impurity. She is then considered pure (*rab'anat*) and allowed to have conjugal relations with her husband, as well as to carry out her household duties.[71] It should be noted that in Pre-Islamic Arabia, if someone is bitten by a snake, he must hold women's jewellery in his hands and rattle it all night.[72]

Beads, as well as seashells, human bones, and *mushaharat* necklaces are usually obtained during the holy Islamic pilgrimage to the Saudi Arabia

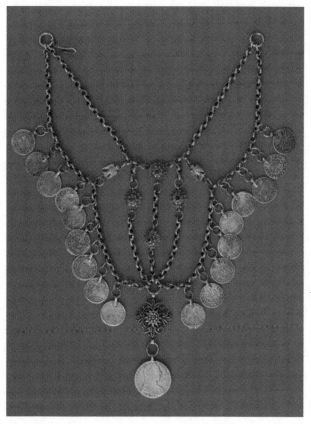

5. The *iznaq*, a silver chain descending from either side of the *burqa'* and fastened under the chin is believed to have medicinal properties.

cities of Mecca and Medina and are therefore considered to be 'of the Prophet Muhammad' and hence especially sacred. Most *mushaharat* necklaces of this type contain seven relatively large beads, often of different sizes and shapes. The beads are considered to be symbols of the various causal categories of *kabsa*, a condition which is thought to be caused by an encounter with a menstruating woman. For example, *mushaharat* necklaces usually contain a red, 'bloody' bead and a white, 'milky' one. Likewise, a black bead symbolizes death, and several beads in the yellow-amber-orange-brown spectrum represent both gold and human bodily secretions, especially urine. Traditional midwives and other healers who own these necklaces are often expert at explaining the symbolic meanings of these beads.[73]

Married Bedouin women wear a plaited woollen girdle (*sufiyih*) decorated with cowrie shells. The girdle has two parts: a broad striped grey and black under-girdle, and, worn over it, a narrower black sash with coloured chevron patterns and fringed and tasselled ends.[74]

The Bedouin of Southern Sinai,[75] appeal to the *hawi* (dervish, folk healer) to treat snake bites and scorpion stings. The *hawi* places a cowrie bead (*kharazat al-hwaia*) that has a solid black on its back or, alternatively, a mixture of flour, onion, sugar and olive oil on the sting. The Bedouin believe that the cowry bead draws the venom from the afflicted person and relieves pain.[76] Among the Rwala nomadic Bedouin, small sea shells with red, white, and green spots, called *kharazat al-nafs*, or a pair of marbles are recommended for protection against the evil eye.[77] Among the Bedouin of the Negev and Sinai, ear-shaped seashells called *idhynih*, diminutive for *idhyn*, ear, are hung on the child's cap to treat ear-ache. A special seashell worn as a necklace treats dental pains.[78] Using clamshells (*sadafah*) and cowries (*wada'*) and coral from the sea in ritual bathing ensures that the impurity of the *qarina* is washed away, since clamshells and cowries bear a strong resemblance to the female genitalia, as mentioned above.[79] Blue beads, coins, cowries, shells and amulets may also be hung on the baby's head covering to protect the baby from the evil eye and the *qarina*.[80]

Conclusion

The role of the traditional healer as an intermediary and mediating agent between members of the community and the World Beyond grants the healer esteemed status. The healer is viewed as an important figure from a religious and even a political perspective, and is perceived as a guardian of the community's cultural heritage, responsible for preserving the social order and the spiritual equilibrium within it; at times the healer holds a monopoly on the ability to heal. At the same time the traditional healer is described as a marginal and exceptional figure who engenders awe in others due to the healer's powers and proximity to the spirit world. He often appears as one who can recruit the spirits to do his bidding and even through them, to do harm to members of the community.

When serious illness strikes, particularly in the case of incurable diseases, even educated people turn to traditional medicine for a remedy. Overlapping realms between traditional medicine and modern medicine have morphed in the form of alternative medicine as a legitimate aspect of western healthcare. One observes more and more physicians and paramedics including psychologists and social workers taking an interest in alternative medicine which has slowly been introduced as a welcome adjunct to modern medical services.

It is not my intention to claim traditional medicine should *replace* modern medicine, yet I would like to re-examine and refresh current thinking and argue in favour of a synthesis between the two for their reciprocal enrichment, and to suggest there is an advantage to adopting a comprehensive therapy where the two are fully integrated, a step I believe can only benefit those who seek relief from diseases and other medical conditions.

Notes

1. Abu-Rabia, A., *Indigenous Medicine among the Bedouin in the Middle East* (New York and Oxford: Berghahn Books, 2015), pp.6-25; Amin, A., Fajr al-Islam (Islamic Dawn). (Beirut: Dal al-Kitab al-'Arabi (Arabic); 1969, pp.1-35); al-Najjar, A., *Fi tarikh al-tib fi al-Dawlah al-Islamiya* (History of Medicine in the Islamic Empire) (Cairo: Dar al-Ma'arif (Arabic), 1994), pp.2-53; al-Shatti, A., *al-'Arab wal-tibb* (The Arabs and Medicine).(Damascus: Manshurat Wazarat al-Thaqafa (Arabic), 1970), pp.5-100. For more details about uses of beads among the Arabs in different periods, see Tifashi, 1977.
2. Abu-Rabia, A., *Indigenous Medicine among the Bedouin*, pp.6-25.
3. Baer, H., Singer, M. and Susser, I.., *Medical Anthropology and the World System: A Critical Perspective* (Westport, CT, and London: Bergin & Garvey, 1997), p.9.
4. Popper-Giveon, A., *A Tale of an Amulet: Traditional Arab Women Healers in Israel* (Haifa University Press, 2012), pp.15-21; Kiev, A., *Magic, Faith, and Healing: Studies in Primitive Psychiatry Today* (New York: Free Press, 1964).
5. Popper-Giveon, A., *A Tale of an Amulet*, pp.15-21; Kiev, A., *Magic, Faith, and Healing.*
6. Lieberman-Avital, L., *In the Name of the Mother: Traditional Women Healers of Maghreb Origin in Israel Narratives, Models & Types*, Ph.D. thesis, Ben Gurion University of the Negev, 2015.
7. Lieberman-Avital, L., *In the Name of the Mother.*

8. Massalha, K. and Baron, B., *Souls in Narrow Lanes: Popular Healers among Israeli Arabs* (Hebrew). (Beit-Berl: The Institute for Israeli Arab Studies, 1994), pp.10-23.

9. Ibid.

10. Ibid.

11. Abu-Rabia, A., *Indigenous Medicine among the Bedouin in the Middle East*, pp.6-25.

12. Pinczuk, S., *Pregnancy and Delivery among the Negev Traditional Society*. Paper submitted to the Environmental High School at Sde Boqer, 1994.

13. Gorkin, M. and Othman, R., 'Traditional Psychotherapeutic Healing and Healers in the Palestinian Community', *Israel Journal of Psychiatry*, 1994, 31(3), pp.221-231.

14. Ali-Shtayeh, M.S., Yaniv, Z. and Mahajna, J., 'Ethnobotanical survey in the Palestinian area: a classification of the healing potential of medicinal plants'. *J Ethnopharmacol 2000*, 73 (1–2), pp.221–232; Krispil, N., *Medicinal Plants in Israel and Throughout the World: the complete guide* (Or Yehuda: Hed Arzi Publishing House, 2000); Palevitch, D. and Zohara, Y., *Medicinal Plants of the Holy Land* (Tel Aviv: Modan Publishing House, 2000).

15. Ben-Assa, B., 'The Bedouin as a Patient', *Harefuah*, 1974, 87 (2), pp.73–76 (Hebrew)

16. Abu-Rabia, A., *Indigenous Medicine among the Bedouin*, pp.6-25.

17. al-Krenawi, A. and Graham, J., 'Spirit Possession and Exorcism in the Treatment of a Bedouin Psychiatric Patient', *Clinical Social Work Journal*, 1997, 25 (2), pp.211–22.

18. Abu-Rabia, A., *Indigenous Medicine among the Bedouin*, pp.6-25; Ben-Assa, B., 'The Bedouin as a Patient', *Harefuah*, 1974, 87 (2), pp.73–76 (Hebrew)

19. Abu-Rabia, A., 'Evil Eye and Cultural beliefs among the Bedouin tribes of the Negev', *Folklore*, 2005, vol. 116, no. (3), pp.241–254.

20. Marx, E., 'Bedouin Pilgrimages to Holy Tombs in Southern Sinai', *Notes on the Bedouin*, 1977, 8, pp.14–22. See also 'Tribal Pilgrimages to Saints' Tombs in South Sinai' in Gellner, E. (Ed.), *Islamic Dilemmas: Reformers, Nationalists and Industrialization* (New York: Mouton Publishers, 1985), pp.104-131.

21. Ben-David, J., *Jabaliya, a Bedouin Tribe under a Monastery's Patronage* (Jerusalem: Kanna, 1981).

22. Bar-Yosef, M., and Porat, D. and N., 'Green stone beads at the dawn of agriculture', *PNAS*, 2008, 105 (25), pp.8548–8551.

23. Snyder, G., 'Wampum: A Material Symbol of Cultural Value to the Iroquois Peoples of Northeastern North America' in Robb, J.E. (Ed.), *Material Symbols: Culture and Economy in Prehistory* (Carbondale: Center for Archaeological Investigations, Southern Illinois University, 1999), pp.362–381.

24. Perego, E., 'Magic and Ritual in Iron Age Veneto, Italy', *Papers from the Institute of Archaeology*. 2010 (20), pp.67–96.

25. Abu-Rabia, A., *Indigenous Medicine among the Bedouin*, pp. 6-25; Jackson, J.W., *Shells as Evidence of the Migration of Early Culture* (London: Longmans Green, 1917).

26. Melling, J. and Forsythe, B. (Eds), *Insanity, Institution, and Society, 1800–1914: A Social History of Madness in Comparative Perspective* (London and New York: Routledge, 1999); Dols, M., 'The Origins of the Islamic Hospitals: Myth and Reality', *Bulletin of the History of Medicine*, 1987 (62), pp.367–390.

27. The first hospitals were established during the reign of al-Walid ibn 'Abd al-Malik (R. 705-15) in Damascus (al-Shatti, 1970).

28. Dols, M., *Majnun: The Madman in Medieval Islamic Society* (Oxford: Clarendon Press. 1992). It was also customary to invite groups of dancers, singers and entertainers to perform for the patients.

29. Lazarus-Yafeh, H., 'The Religious Dialectics of the Hajj', in: Lazarus-Yafeh, H. (Ed.), *Some Religious Aspects of Islam: a Collection of Articles* (Leiden: Brill; 2006), pp.168-189.

30. https://www.facebook.com/notes/ali-gems-and-jewellery/gemstones-and-birthstones-in-islam/423058561101218

31. Ullmann, M., *Islamic Medicine* (Edinburgh: Edinburgh University Press, 1978).

32. al-Tamimi, M.A., *The Guide to the Fundamentals of Foodstuffs and the Powers of Simple Drugs*. N.P.

33. An-Nawawi I., Sharh of Sahih Muslim (14/65). See also Fatwa No: 90906, Islamweb, 'Wearing a ring made of gold and silver for men'. Accessed at http://www. islamweb.net/emainpage/index.php?page=showfatwa&Option=FatwaId&Id=90906

34. Islamweb, Fatwa No. 147235
http://www.islamweb.net/emainpage/index.php?page=showfatwa&Option=FatwaId&Id=147235

35. *Encyclopaedia of Islam*, second edition.
http://referenceworks.brillonline.com/entries/encyclopaedia-of-the-quran/coral-EQSIM_00094
http://referenceworks.brillonline.com/search?s.q=coral&s.f.s2_parent=&search-go=Search

36. 'He released the two seas, meeting [side by side]; between them is a barrier [so] neither of them transgresses. So which of the favours of your Lord would you deny? From both of them emerge pearl and coral' (*Quran*, 55:19–22); 'So which of the favors of your Lord would you deny? As if they were rubies and coral' (*Quran*, 55:57–58). See also (*Quran*, 35:12).

37. Abu-Rabia, A., *Indigenous Medicine among the Bedouin*, pp.6-25; Erikson, J.M., *The Universal Bead* (New York: W.W. Norton, 1969); Abu-Rabia, A., *Evil Eye and Cultural Belief*.

38. Tifashi, A., *Azhar al-afkar fi jawahir al-ahjar (Arab roots of Gemology: the best of stones)* (Cairo: al-Hay'ah al-Misriyal al-'Ammah lil-kitab, 1977).

39. sibha subha, misbaha: a strand of 33 or 99 prayer beads corresponding to the 99 'beautiful names of Allah', The Quran refers to stars as 'beads of the sky' (*Quran*, 24:35); Stars, like beads, are bright and shining 'heavenly eyes' that offer protection by lighting up the darkened skies (Erikson, *The Universal Bead*, pp.164-176; *Quran*, 6:97; 67:5).

40. Borhany, Qazi Dr. Shaikh Abbas, 'Gems Science in Islam: its Medicinal and Mystical Value', *Daily News*, Pakistan, March 2010.

41. Popper-Giveon, A., Abu-Rabia, A. and Venture, J., 'From White Stone to Blue Bead: Materialized beliefs and sacred beads among the Bedouin in Israel', *Material Religion*, 2014, 10 (2), pp.132–153.

42. Erikson, J.M., *The Universal Bead.*

43. Saca, I., *Embroidering Identities: A Century of Palestinian Clothing* (Chicago: The Oriental Institute Museum of the University of Chicago, 2007).

44. Meir, C., *Crown of Coins: Traditional Headdresses of Arab and Bedouin Women* (Tel Aviv: Eretz Israel Museum, 2002).

45. Meir, C., *Crown of Coins;* Abu-Rabia, A., *Indigenous Medicine among the Bedouin*, pp.6-25.

46. 'Palestinian/Bedouin women wear burqas, face ornaments, coral and bead pendants', Weir, *Palestine Costume* (London: British Museum Publications, 1994), p.190.

47.   Meir, C., Crown of Coins.

48.   Saca I., 'Embroidering Identities'; Vogel, T., 'Negev Bedouin Women and their Clothes', in Meir, C. (Ed.), *Crown of Coins*.

49.   Vogel, T., *Negev Bedouin Women and their Clothes*.

50.   Weir, S., *Palestine Costume*.

51.   Ibid.

52.   Goren, O., 'The Jewelry of Bedouin women in the Negev and Sinai', in Zeevy, R. (Ed.), *Israel People and Land* (Tel Aviv: Eretz Israel Museum, 1994).

53.   This is also true regarding headstalls for horses. Weir, S., *The Bedouin* (London: British Museum Publications, 1990).

54.   Weir, S., *Palestine Costume*; Weir, S., *The Bedouin*.

55.   Weir, S., *The Bedouin*.

56.   Meyerhans, A., 'A Bejeweled Journey', *Signature Magazine*, 2011: http://www. acmeyerhans.com/publications/andre_c_meyerhans_acmeyerhans_signature_ 1112. pdf

57.   Abu-Rabia, A., *Indigenous Medicine among the Bedouin*, pp.6-25; Amin, A., *Fajr al-Islam (Islamic Dawn)* (Beirut: Dal al-Kitab al-'Arabi (Arabic), 1969), pp.1-35. al-Shatti, A., *al-'Arab wal-tibb (The Arabs and Medicine)*(Damascus: Manshurat Wazarat al-Thaqafa (Arabic), 1970), pp.5-100. For more details about uses of beads among the Arabs in different periods, see Tifashi, 1977; Bailey, C., *Bedouin Religious Practices in Sinai and the Negev*.

58.   Abu-Rabia, A., *Indigenous Medicine among the Bedouin*, pp. 6-25; Meir, C., *Crown of Coins*.

59.   Bailey, C., 'Bedouin Religious Practices in Sinai and the Negev', *Anthropos*, 1982, 72 (1-2), pp.65-88.

60.   Abu-Rabia, A., 'The Significance of Colours in Pastoral Nomadic Society', in Hertzog, E. and Hazan, H. (Eds), *Serendipity in Anthropological Research: The Nomadic Turn* (Surrey: Ashgate Publishing Ltd., 2012), pp.247–256.

61.   Shinar, P., 'Elements of Magic in Modern North African Jewelry, Yesodot magiyim ba takhshitanut ha-Maghribit ba-'et ha-hadashah', *Pe'amim*,1982 (11), pp.29-42.

62.   Perego, E., 'Magic and Ritual in Iron Age Veneto, Italy', *Papers from the Institute of Archaeology*, 2010 (20), pp.67–96.

63.   Paine, S., *Amulets: A World of Secret Powers, Charms and Magic* (London: Thames and Hudson, 2004).

64.   Abu-Rabia, A. and Khalil, N., 'Mourning Palestine: Death and Grief Rituals', *Anthropology of the Middle East*, 2012, 7 (2), pp.1–18.

65.   Mershen, B., 'Amulets and Jewelry from Jordan: A Study on the Function and Meaning of Recent Bead Necklaces', *TRIBUS*, 1989, (38), pp.43-58.

66.   Dirrih means 'mother's breast' or 'cattle/livestock udder'. This coral's shape resembles that of the breast and the udder. Coral (marajan, murjan) is found and used in North Africa as a charm against the evil eye and other afflictions. It is strung by mothers into necklaces for their infants to wear (Shinar, 1982). For more on the uses of coral in Morocco, see also Westermarck, E., *Ritual and Belief in Morocco*, 2 vols. (London: Macmillan, 1926), pp.1:439, 2:98, 2:381–383, 2:419, 2:421.

67.   Abu-Rabia, A., 'Breastfeeding Practices among Pastoral Tribes', *Anthropology of the Middle East*, 2007, 2 (2), pp.38–54.

68.   Bailey, C., *Bedouin Religious Practices in Sinai and the Negev*.

69.   Abu-Rabia, A., 'Breastfeeding Practices among Pastoral Tribes'.

70. Turner, V., *The Forest of Symbols: Aspects of Ndembu Ritual* (Ithaca: Cornell University Press, 1967); Frazer, J., *The Golden Bough: A Study in Magic and Religion* (London: Macmillan, 1950).

71. Abu-Rabia, A., 'Childbirth in Traditional Arab-Bedouin Society', in Abuhav, O., Hertzog, E. and Marx, E. (Eds), *Perspectives on Israeli Anthropology* (Wayne State University Press, 2010), pp.453-464.

72. Ullmann, M., *Islamic Medicine.*

73. Inhorn, M., 'Kabsa and Threatened Fertility in Egypt', *Social Science and Medicine*, 1994, 39 (4), pp.487-505.

74. Weir, S., *The Bedouin.*

75. Levi, S., 'refu'ah, higyenah ve-beri'ut etsel ha-Bedvim be-drum Sinai. Bayt sefer sadeh, marumi Sinai', 1978; Levi, S., *The Bedouin in the Sinai Desert* (ha-Bedvim be-Midbar Sinai) (Tel Aviv: Schocken, 1987) (Hebrew)

76. Bailey, C., 'Bedouin Religious Practices in Sinai and the Negev'; Abu-Rabia, A., *Indigenous Medicine among the Bedouin in the Middle East.*

77. Musil, A., *The Manners and Customs of the Rwala Bedouins* (New York: American Geographical Society, 1928).

78. Abu-Rabia, A., *Indigenous Medicine among the Bedouin in the Middle East.*

79. A female demon (qarina) can cause madness, postpartum depression, in a new mother, or the instant death of her newborn baby. See Abu-Rabia, *Childbirth in Traditional Arab-Bedouin Society*, pp.453-464.

80. Abu-Rabia, A., *Childbirth in Traditional Arab-Bedouin Society.*

B. Traditional Jewish Medicine

Kenneth Collins

Introduction

The Jewish people have always seen medicine and faith as inextricably linked.[1] There has been continuing Jewish fascination with medicine from earliest times usually associated with reverence for the healer with an understanding that treatment and cure carries with it something of the divine. Traditional medicine, sometimes also referred to as popular or folk-medicine, occupies the ground between the use of natural medicinal substances and the traditional religious quest for the victory of the forces of good in an uncertain world. Though the pharmacology of Biblical and Talmudic medicine, as well as that of medieval Jewish practitioners, may seem strange to the modern health consumer Jewish folk practices have remained remarkably persistent surviving to the present day.

Jewish popular medicine has often been seen as the superstitious legacy of the encounter between Jews and their neighbours, especially in the medieval Christian and Arab worlds, over millennia of dispersion. Thus, at times this tradition has been seen as primitive, the product of an era best forgotten, while others, less disparagingly, see elements of a rich historical tradition in these practices. In recent years, especially following the movement of the previously marginalised Jews from eastern communities into the political mainstream in Israel, there have been serious attempts to understand this folk medicine culture in its proper context.[2]

Medieval Jewish Medicine

In the Middle Ages there was often a narrow line delineating the role of traditional healers and practising physicians. The physician was often seen as a powerful exponent of science and religion while the rationale of superstition and magic in medicine had become part and parcel of the Jewish cultural heritage.[3] Magical cure and incantations were occasionally permitted by the rabbis – not because of their likely efficacy but to set at ease the minds of the superstitious. Thus, it was not really necessary for the patient to resort to the magician for treatment as the ordinary remedies used by doctor and layman used the full range of magical devices. Many of these treatments follow theories of aetiology and pathology which we can readily see today as being wrong but from medieval beliefs about cause and effect the treatments follow a logical pattern.[4] The traditional Jewish healer required knowledge of the Jewish lore surrounding his practice besides an expertise in medicinal plants and an ability to exorcise the evil eye.[5]

Jews and Christians shared much of this popular medicine. Rabbi Menahem of Speyer was quoted as saying that as sound effects a cure so a Christian may be permitted to heal a Jew by incantation even if he invokes the aid of Jesus and the saints in his spell.[6] However, religious views differed on the attitude to healing. Important rabbinic authorities, such as

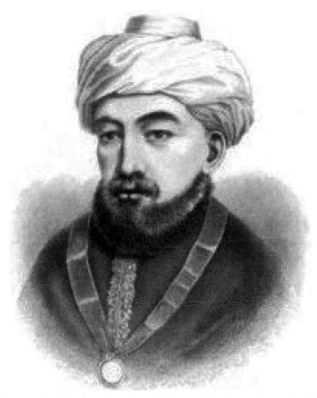

6. Moses Maimonides (Rambam), 1138-1204, practised in Fostat (Cairo) and his medical texts were written in Arabic. (image from the eighteenth century)

Nachmanides, *Ramban,* considered that the righteous should be protected by God's blessing while Moses Maimonides, *Rambam* (1138-1204), the greatest of Jewish medieval rabbis and himself a physician, believed that the Divine mandate to heal derives from the Torah. In short, true healing is a gift from God who has given the doctor what is required to heal by natural means.

Medieval medicine had inherited from late antiquity the conviction that there was a close correlation between the universe, the macrocosm, and man, the microcosm. Both were said to be formed of the four elements: air, fire, earth and water and endowed with the same four qualities: heat, cold, dryness and humidity. The four humours: blood, yellow and black bile and phlegm had to be kept in balance by, for example blood-letting, and doctors had special zodiacal calendars to identify the best times for bleeding.[7] The Talmud gives clear evidence of the widespread practice of blood-letting and while Maimonides himself counselled against it as a reliable treatment it retained its popularity down to modern times.

The rabbinic *Responsa* literature of the Middle Ages, where the medieval rabbis respond to questions by their followers, contains much of medical interest. Here, we see the attitudes of people distressed by illness, to healing practices and what they had recourse to in the hope of returning to full health. Some treatments seem benign. There was an association between sanctified wine for the ceremonies of Kiddush and Havdalah and the strengthening of weak eyes as medieval Jews saw the drinking of the wine or merely bathing the eyes with it as a remedy in itself.[8] Other treatments posed religious problems. Patients would ask the rabbi for permission to undergo procedures which might be in conflict with the laws of Shabbat and many of the medications would have required the taking of foodstuffs forbidden by a kosher diet. In general permission seems to have been given for the consumption of the most outlandish products if it would benefit health although some rabbis indicated that they would withhold consent 'to all remedies which are biblically forbidden'.[9]

Zimmels records what he calls medicines in their natural state such as goat's milk, fish oil, warm animal blood, human milk and urine. More commonly, medicines contained a number of ingredients. One celebrated ingredient was the Egyptian mummy, the embalmed flesh of which was taken internally or more often applied as a plaster. Given the scarcity of mummies from Egypt eventually the bones and flesh of ordinary corpses were ground up and sold as mummies. Some rabbis had problems about using 'the flesh of corpses' which the mummy represented but usually permitted it considering that the product no longer resembled its original matter. Using the principle of sympathy, it was the upper half of the mummy, containing as it does the heart, lungs and stomach which was considered most likely to be effective.

Some treatments were considered to have specific effects. A modest Jewish herbal of the fifteenth century copied and illustrated in Italy preserves a sense of plants and their properties. Here St John's Wort (*Hypericum perforatum*) is considered to be a diuretic and expectorant.[10] These included fish oil for coughs, drinking urine for jaundice and ass milk for asthma and haemoptysis. Epileptics could be given such products as broth from a reptile or a mole, while people with mental illness could be given the flesh of a fowl which had died a natural death. Topical treatments, including ointments and bathing and the application of plasters and poultices, such as oats or barley, were also used. One plaster that was 'proved by experience' had sheep fat, butter, olive oil, wax, egg yolk, almonds, alum and herbs all fried together.[11]

Medieval Herbal Therapy

Herbs often have natural healing properties which have been accepted by medical science and the search for active ingredients in traditional medicines has intensified in modern times. Substances of medicinal plants played a major part in the lives of medieval Jews. They served as foodstuffs, herbs, cosmetics, condiments and incense as well as in home industries like tanning, dyeing and ink production.[12] The medieval mind often associated the healing herbs with magic qualities and it is usually impossible to divorce the purely therapeutic from the magical and superstitious in such prescriptions. Thus, herbs gathered in a cemetery were considered of high medicinal value because of their association with the spirits and their occult potency.[13]

In the Roman period medicine sellers had their own professional and social organisation and in the Middle Ages, during periods of both Moslem and Christian rule, herbalists and purveyors of medication had proper supervision and were educated in medicine and pharmacy. In the Arab world many of these practitioners inherited their skills through numerous generations of the same family. It should not be thought that these medications were without effect. Indeed, the efficacy of many plant medicines has long been understood for simple symptom control and some products could be used for more specific conditions. To this day there are many plant-based remedies in official national pharmacopoeias which have stood the test of time and have met the criteria of randomised control trials.[14] The Jewish community in Cairo relied on the trade in medicinal remedies for much of its commercial success with Jewish traders in port cities around the extensive medieval diaspora.[15]

Hebrew sources record use of fennel for abdominal disorders and threatened miscarriage, celandine sap for cataracts and columbine taken internally for bad eyes.[16] A decoction of sage was employed as a cure for paralysis and to aid digestion. The mixture included saltpetre, sage, bay and cinnamon, which was beaten thoroughly with honey. After drinking the decoction the disturbance should leave and the patient is then recommended to drink some wine.

In the *Materia Medica* of Maimonides there are a number of plant medications with an identifiable psycho-active effect and given his custom of tailoring his prescriptions to individual patients we have a clear idea of his clinical practice. Maimonides, practising in Cairo and personal physician to the Sultan of Egypt, was well aware of psycho-somatic factors in disease considering that 'the skilled physician should place nothing ahead of rectifying the state of the psyche by removing these passions'. There has been considerable concern in recent years to understand the nature of the placebo response as it is conceded that one of the reasons for the popularity of alternative complementary medicine is the time, support and empathy provided by its practitioners. Indeed, it is concluded that a good doctor-patient relationship can tangibly improve patients' responses to treatment, placebo or otherwise.[17]

Paavilainen records more than a hundred different drugs used by Maimonides in the treatment of melancholy with about two dozen of them used most frequently.[18] Most commonly prescribed were *Rosa canina, citrus, ox tongue (helminthia echioides)* and *pistacia* (mastic and pistachio) along with jacinth, a mineral and castporeum, a secretion from beaver glands used today in the manufacture of perfumes. She considers that almost two thirds of Maimonides' treatment for melancholy would have had some level of efficacy either as a mood enhancer or as a tranquilliser. Basil is anti-depressant and sedative while citrus may be a mood enhancer, neuro-protective and anti-amnesiac. The pepper genus has numerous psycho-active properties while raisins and grapes are also neuro-protective and wine, of course, can relieve stress and improve the mood if taken in appropriate quantities. Maimonides also liked to prescribe spikenard (*Nardostachys jatamansi*) also called nard, which is a flowering plant of the valerian family. It can be crushed and distilled into an intensely aromatic amber-coloured essential oil, which is used as a perfume as well as a sedative and hypnotic.

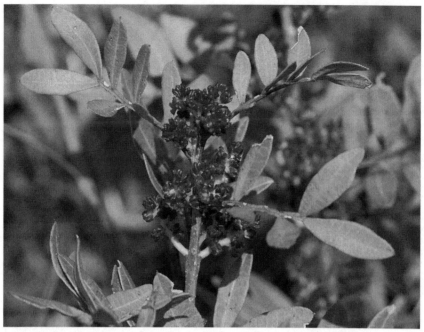

7. Pistacia lentiscus: (mastic) a favourite remedy of Maimonides for melancholy.

Ibn Ezra (1092-1167) was a poet, astronomer and Bible commentator whose writings detail his own medical knowledge as well as that of contemporary physicians usually accompanied with the formula 'and this has been verified with testing'.[19] He divided active medication into those which purge the body whether by vomiting or diarrhoea, those which are beneficial for diseased organs when hung on the arm or neck or by ablution or by drinking, in a poultice or by fumigation and others which counteracts the poison of creeping animals or deadly poison of beverages.[20] He wrote that when drugs are acting through their whole essence it is impossible to define their action by logical judgement but when people examine them by testing the truth of their efficacy will come to light.[21]

Among the hundreds of his treatments are extract of absinth together with ashes, commonly used in his time in place of soap. The patient wraps it tightly round the head in a bandage then rinses the ashes from the head. This is done two or three times a week to cure headaches of every kind.[22] The juice of a sempervivum plant which has been buried for a year underground if instilled into the ear is said to cure any deafness even if it is from childhood.[23] A further treatment for a headache involves taking the peganum herb with marjoram and pennyroyal and putting them in a bag on the sufferers head. The pain, throbbing and swelling of haemorrhoids will be relieved by finely ground leek, cooked with butter.[24] However, he also recorded that excrement of a bear when hung on the thigh of one who has colic pain makes him healthy and soothes his pain. Amongst his recordings of spells and incantations is that if you write the following three names on the patient's forehead – *kita, zvi* and *lekh* – while blood comes out of his nostrils it will stop immediately.[25]

Alternative Therapies

Some traditional remedies did not require ingestion of medication but rather relied on *segulot*, which originally referred to charms but came to be attached to the concept of an 'occult virtue' which was inherent in a particular object. Nachmanides believed that King Solomon had gained all the appropriate knowledge in this area from the Torah 'even the potency of herbs and their *segulot*'. Rabbi Bayha ben Asher (d.1340) believed that God had taught Moses the nature and occult virtue of plants and herbs which had the power to heal but could also 'sweeten the bitter and make the bitter sweet'.

The principles of 'sympathy', where the effect resembles the cause and 'contact', where objects which have been in contact continue to act on each other after the contact has ended, can also be found in the Jewish sources. Accordingly, we find such remedies as rubbing a stillborn baby with its placenta or eating the liver of a mad dog as a cure for the dog's bite. Sympathy was even extended to looking at specific colours to influence the red or black humours or trying to destroy an enemy by destroying his image. As for contact, it was believed that anyone who got possession of someone's cut hair or nail clippings could assume power over them. The name given to a person gives them some of the character of its original owner. Rabbi Jacob Emden (1697-1776) referred to a drug which heals sword wounds when the drug is in contact with the blood on the sword even if the wounded person is now some distance away. The noted physician and Padua graduate Tobias Hacohen (1652-1729) reported cases of family illness where brothers, even those living in different countries, developed the same illness or died at the same time.

The principle of antipathy was the basis for the use of amulets. Thus, the supposed antipathy between deer and snakes led to people wearing the tooth of a deer to keep snakes away. Maimonides was careful to avoid magical treatments unless there was evidence as to their efficacy and claims for benefit for them could be proved or if withholding them would cause psychological distress to the patient. Rabbi Samson Morpurgo (d.1740) noted the principle of sympathy as well as the working of specific remedies. He also noted that other 'remedies', whether of vegetable or animal origin, were hung on the neck or arm of the patient who had fever, jaundice, epilepsy or dysentery, and these were to be considered *segulot* as doctors were aware that they were not conventional treatment. However, Morpurgo made a specific case for the use of snake products, found in the medication known as theriac, as doctors had indicated that it could be prescribed for disorders of the white humour and thus did not work by occult virtue alone. In general though, the consumption of many of the noxious medicaments was not recommended for Jewish patients and there was a particular revulsion to the use of blood and products of vermin and reptiles.[26]

There is a wide variety of treatments recorded within the rabbinic *Responsa*. Among the popular prescriptions are many items that owe their place to tradition and long-established associations such as cutting the beard as a cure for sore eyes or washing being harmful to aching teeth. As a treatment for toothache salt, pepper and a little garlic were mixed, and the mixture was left on the pulse overnight.

Some years ago the actress Gwyneth Paltrow made headlines when wearing a backless dress showing the marks from having cupping during an acupuncture treatment. Today cupping is most commonly used to treat coughs, asthma and muscle aches and pain, especially back pain, but it has been used in cultures across the world for centuries and was especially popular in Eastern European Jewish traditional medicine, where it was known as *bahnkes*. Cupping was especially popular as a treatment especially for weak and obese patients and pregnant women. Despite the enduring popularity of the procedure, the old Yiddish proverb, *Es vet helfen vi a toiten bahnkes,* 'it will help like applying cups to a dead person', indicates a more sceptical view of its efficacy. Cupping techniques vary but *bahnkes* involves the use of small cups containing a small amount of alcohol which is heated, and a vacuum is produced by the absence of oxygen. The cup is then pressed tightly against the skin. This suction is thought to draw out noxious substances from the body thus restoring the balances of bodily humours.

Numbers also played an important part in healing. The numbers 3, 7 and 9 were particularly efficacious and invocations used were similar for Jew and Christians with the wording adapted to the sensitivities of the patient. *Sefer Hasidim,* a book of medieval pietistic literature, records that a person who has been harmed by a demon needs to have the charm repeated nine times, as they do in Germany, for a cure.[27] The principle of transference was also employed in treatment. For a severe headache a thread was wound three times around the patient's head and hung in a tree. When a bird flew through the loop it took the headache with it.[28] The placing of the patient's excrement on a growing plant to which the illness will be transferred, is recorded by Tobias HaCohen (1651-1729) who indicates that its value is greatly exaggerated.[29] The principle could even be used to gauge the progress of the illness. The patient's belt was stretched over the length and width of his body. The belt was then hung on a nail with the appropriate incantation and measured: any change in length was interpreted as being prognostic of the course of the illness. Circling round the patient, initially seen as preventing the action of demons, could also be used as a remedy against various diseases.[30]

The mere repetition of a magic name may effect a cure, or the magic name may be written on the person or inscribed on an amulet. Having the name written on the forehead was said to be very effective in stopping bleeding. A magic name written on an apple and consumed on three separate occasions was used to heal fevers.[31] To ease a confinement Psalm 20 was to be recited nine times. This might be repeated or combined with a call on the angel Armisael, who governs the womb, to help the woman and baby to life and peace.[32] The variety of spells available for treatment was infinite and often did not need to be accompanied by medication or blood-letting. Many German magical cures, which would otherwise have been lost, have been preserved in Hebrew manuscripts.

A person's name is considered as playing a role in deciding his fate; it is given to him when he enters the Jewish world and has been described as serving as a social and cosmological identity card.[33] The Talmud records that a change of name can cause a change of fortune.[34] To confuse the Angel of Death it may be necessary, *in extremis*, to change the name and thus the fate of the patient. In the Middle Ages the name might be chosen by lot or by randomly finding a name in the Bible while in more modern times the change of name was usually to one associated with life, health or old age, such as Chaim (life) or Alter (old one).[35] Change of name was also used for childless couples wishing to have children and for those parents whose previous children had died. The ritual for such a name change can still be found in many contemporary Jewish prayer books. The angelic name Refael, shares the same Hebrew root as *refua*, medicine, and is thus an auspicious name for health or for inscription on an amulet. Many of these amulets carry the numerical equivalents of holy words because of what is seen as the intrinsic holiness of the Hebrew letters.

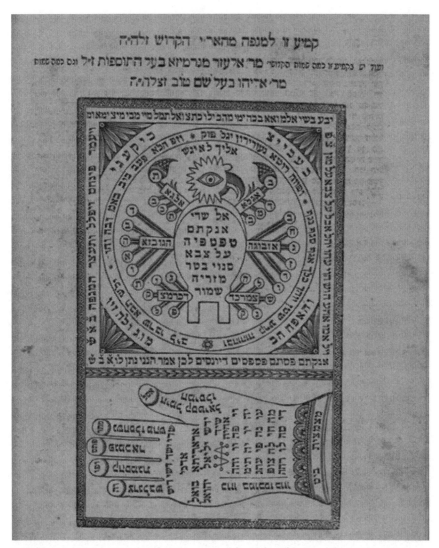

8. Hebrew Amulet against the plague to protect the Holy Rabbi Isaac Luria (Ha-Ari). From *Shaar HaYichudim* (The Gate of Unifications) by the Safed Kabbalist Hayyim ben Joseph Vital.

There are passages in the Torah the recitation or inscription of which can be efficacious in treating illness. Particularly popular are talismans from the Book of Psalms. The entire Book of Psalms was considered as a potent protection against danger while Psalm 121 is used especially for protecting women after childbirth and Psalm 91, using either the first or last letters of each verse, is for general protection.[36] Charms and incantations remained popular in Jewish traditional medicine especially for the treatment of eye disease, headache and epilepsy.[37]

The Early Modern Period

The migration of Jewish physicians during the sixteenth to eighteenth centuries, many with an Iberian background and trained in Italian medical schools such as Padua and Pisa, brought modern medicine into the Ottoman Empire. These Jewish doctors filled an important gap in the numbers of physicians in the area and records indicate that they formed a larger proportion of the population than the number of Jewish inhabitants might have indicated.[38]

During this period there was a wide variety of medication available, whether of animal, vegetable or mineral material, mostly based on locally available products. One such, a potion made from almond milk, honey and roses, was popular amongst Jerusalem's Jews. Rabbi Refael Mordekhai Malkhi, who arrived in Jerusalem from Italy in 1676, mentions many items in his writings.[39] He noted that the potion of almond milk, honey and roses could cause diarrhoea and suggested the use of sweet wine with sugar. However, he expressed his concern about the poor quality of medication on offer and noted that much of what was available to the Jewish population was based on superstition.[40] A poultice for the eyes was made from dried plums and seedless raisins cooked with some spices like cinnamon, ginger or rose water. Malkhi's grandson, Rabbi David de Silva, describes some compounds in a chapter entitled Pri Megaddim, choice fruit, in his work *Pri Hadas*. De Silva includes about two hundred items in his pharmacopeia which Amar notes shows similarities with works from Hippocrates, the early modern period as well as contemporary popular medicines.[41] At the same time the baths and hot springs at Tiberias were restored during the sixteenth century and thousands of Jewish, Muslim and Christian pilgrims came to enjoy the curative power of the waters.[42]

While modern medicine developed rapidly especially in Western countries during the eighteenth and nineteenth centuries much of the new knowledge remained out of the reach of the majority of the population usually because of cost. At the same time there was little popular understanding of the pathology or physiology of disease and many could easily be fooled by exaggerated claims of effectiveness. Consequently, a market grew from the seventeenth and eighteenth centuries in Britain and North America for commercial medications supplied by apothecaries, as well as by untrained and unlicensed providers of patent medicine.

Patent medicines were marketed effectively, and their popularity can be gauged by the existence of over a thousand of such products by 1830. British products dominated the international market until well into the nineteenth century. Many of the suppliers of these products were known as quacks or charlatans, usually meaning that they pretended to have qualifications they did not possess. In the late eighteenth century two such Jewish charlatans, William Brodum and Samuel Solomon, tested the boundaries of orthodox medicine in Britain by supplying patent medicines and obtaining genuine medical qualifications by subterfuge.[43]

Contemporary Jewish Popular Medicine

Judaism's approach to healing is illuminated in the traditional centuries old *Mi Sheberach* prayer for healing which is said when someone is ill. The prayer calls for a 'complete healing' (*r'fuah shleimah*) which includes a 'healing of body' (*r'fuat ha-guf*) and a 'healing of spirit' (*r'fuat ha-nefesh*). It is understood that this is no guarantee of a cure but gives patient, family and community to give voice to their belief that the course of the illness will reach a favourable outcome. Prayer is naturally a familiar source for achieving a cure and even in modern times, despite studies of prayer effectiveness producing negative results, it retains its popularity as evidenced by the existence of websites like www.jewishinghealing.com Many believe that prayer can aid in recovery, not just due to divine influence but due to the psychological and physical benefits to a person who knows that he or she is being prayed for. The increase in morale may thus aid recovery. Many studies have suggested that prayer can reduce physical stress and that 'the psychological benefits of prayer may help reduce stress and anxiety, promote a more positive outlook, and strengthen the will to live'. The rise of the pietistic Hasidic movement in Eastern Europe in the eighteenth century with its veneration of leaders, known as *Zaddikim*, led to a belief in the power of the *Zaddik* to cure the sick.

It should not be thought that traditional Jewish medicine has disappeared in the modern period with its emphasis on scientific progress and evidence-based procedures. Customs that were common in Eastern Europe a century ago, such as placing pigeons on the abdomen of a jaundiced patient, have become common practice in Israel among all sectors of the population.[44] Popular adherence to the use of amulets and charms has persisted even among contemporary Jews. These amulets are often made of stone or metal to be worn by the patient and over the past few years it has been observed that there has been an increasing tendency for the use of amulets in Israeli hospitals. A study of parents of children admitted to a paediatric intensive care unit in Zerifin (Sarafand), Israel, showed that around a third of Jewish families used such amulets claiming that it reduced parental anxiety and warned medical staff to respect the emotional and psychological value they present.[45] Such persons find the contact with the healer to be of value even if he fails to bring a cure. Moslem patients in Israel also made use of healing charms, many of Jewish origin with Hebrew lettering, reflecting a tradition dating back to medieval times. Amulets have persisted despite almost universal opposition through the ages by rabbis and Jewish physicians who consistently described their use as irrational and superstitious.

Of course, religious Jews have long regarded positively the value of prayer, whether by the reciting of Psalms or the direct blessing of the patient and as we have seen there remained a strand within the rabbinic leadership which preferred to see healing in divine hands without negating the value of medical interventions. In extreme cases, which I have witnessed myself on a couple of occasions, the name of a seriously sick person was changed in an attempt to thwart the evil designs of the Angel of Death.

Given the survival of these customs, and an increasingly pervasive concern about the direction of modern medicine, it is not surprising to record the continuing use of traditional practices. In recent years studies have indicated the use of medicinal plants amongst the rural population of Israel and within the country's ethnic groups, especially those from such countries as Iraq, Iran and Yemen. These substances, usually obtained from local rather than imported products, are considered to be based on the Galenic tradition and adapted to an Arabic and Moslem form during the Middle Ages. The contemporary emphasis on modern therapeutics has modified this tradition but not eliminated it.

Lev and Amar have identified animal, mineral and especially plant products used in the modern Israeli popular medicine market.[46] They found well over two hundred plant products in common usage. While enumeration of all the products is beyond the scope of this chapter many will be familiar to those who would keep a supply of simple herbal home remedies for minor ailments not thought sufficiently important to call on the services of a physician. Thus, there are such common vegetables as onion, cauliflower and garlic, cereals such as oats, herbs and spices such as tarragon, wormwood, cumin, cloves and dill. Hyssop oil is used for backache, clove oil for toothache and rosemary remains a popular remedy for kidney stones while the use of the seed of the emetic nut *Strychnos nux vomica,* substantially having the properties of the poison strychnine, is used for its stimulant action on the gastro-intestinal tract, for itch and for inflammations of the external ear. In chronic constipation it is often combined with cascara and other laxatives with good effects. The list of products only includes cultivated plants. Wild plants are still gathered by healers and patients, but they are not commonly sold in the traditional shops.

The twenty animal products include such substances as beeswax and honey used for burns, eye inflammation and coughs but also deer horn employed as a general tonic and for drug addiction. Musk oil and grain is used for high blood sugar while snail operculum, from the shell lid, deals with the evil eye. There were less than twenty mineral products available many, like clay, earth, sulphur and ferrous citrate, known also as green vitriol, used to treat skin problems. Galena, otherwise known as lead sulphide but often containing silver admixtures, antimony and zinc products are used for eye problems. Apart from sulphur the most frequent mineral prescribed was alum, long known to have anti-bacterial properties and used in modern deodorants, is not only used as a disinfectant but also to reduce liver size and as a general tonic. Nevertheless, Lev and Amar relate that the commercial field for the sale of traditional medicines in Israel is declining and businesses have closed, and the inventory of medicines has diminished.[47] Their work in documenting the decline of this sector is a window into the medieval world, using philology, comparisons across Levantine cultures and comparisons with Biblical and Talmudic medicine.

If commercial popular medicine is fighting for survival against the current fads for modern alternative medicines one Jewish folk remedy still seems to hold sway. From Talmudic times rabbis such as R. Abba used chicken soup as a remedy.[48] Maimonides stated that chicken soup is an excellent food suitable for those convalescing from illness and fattening those who have lost weight due to illness, finding it beneficial for those with asthma while noting that it helps the chronic fevers that develop from white bile.[49] Chicken soup is not without its risks: hypernatraemia and anaphylaxis have been recorded and one child has been recorded as choking on a chicken bone being which lodged in his bronchus while drinking unstrained chicken soup.[50] Nevertheless, Ohry, Tsafrir and Rosner all conclude that the medical uses of chicken soup is part of the armamentarium of successful traditional remedies.[51]

Conclusion

The subject of Jewish medicine has a long history described in literature stretching back to the Biblical period. The practice reflects the Biblical and Talmudic period with additions reflecting the encounter between Jews and their Christian and Moslem neighbours over fifteen hundred years of Diaspora. The resurgence of interest in medical botany and herbalism in recent years has encouraged further study of the content and practice of popular medicine in its widest context and has emphasised its cross-cultural nature. Even the spells, charms and incantations of an earlier era still find their echo today and might claim a place in the search for cure as long as patients are given recourse to the evidence-based medicine that they require for recovery.

Notes

1. Bermant, C., *The Jews* (London: Sphere Books, 1978), p.138.
2. Matras, H., *Jewish Folk Medicine in the 19th and 20th Centuries* (Tel Aviv: Bet HaTfutsot, 1995), pp.113-135.
3. *Jewish Encyclopaedia* (New York: Funk and Wagnalls, 1925, vol.8, p.417. Available online at www.jewishencyclopedia.com (Accessed 23 January 2019); Zimmels, H.J., *Magicians, Theologians and Doctors: Studies in Folk-medicine and Folk-lore as reflected in the Rabbinic Responsa (12th to 19th Centuries)* (London: Edward Goldston & Son, 1952), pp.193-194.
4. Rivers, W.H.R., *Medicine, Magic and Religion: Fitzpatrick Lectures, Royal College of Physicians, London 1915-6* (London International Library of Psychology, Philosophy and Scientific Method, 1924), pp.7,51; *Jewish Encyclopaedia*, vol. 5, pp.426-427; Trachtenberg, J., *Jewish Magic and Superstition* (University of Pennsylvania, 2004), p197.
5. Matras, H., *Jewish Folk Medicine*, p.123.
6. Trachtenberg, J., *Jewish Magic and Superstition*, p.200.
7. Metzger, T. and Metzger, M., *Jewish Life in the Middle Ages: Illuminated Hebrew Manuscripts of the Thirteenth to Sixteenth Centuries* (Fribourg (Switzerland): Chartwell Books, 1982), p.174.
8. Metzger, T. and Metzger, M., *Jewish Life in the Middle Ages*, p.195.
9. Zimmels, H.J., *Magicians, Theologians and Doctors*, p.124.
10. Metzger, T. and Metzger, M., *Jewish Life in the Middle Ages*, p.173.
11. Zimmels, H.J., *Magicians, Theologians and Doctors*, p.132.
12. Lev, E. and Amar, Z., *Practical materia medica of the medieval eastern Mediterranean according to the Cairo Genizah*, Sir Henry Wellcome Asian Series, vol.7 (Leiden and Boston: Brill, 2008), p.511.
13. Trachtenberg, J., *Jewish Magic and Superstition*, p.207.
14. There is an extensive contemporary literature relating botanical species and modern pharmacological research. See, for example, Lansky, E.P., Paavilainen, H.M., Pawlus, A.D. and Newman, R.A., Ficus spp. (fig): Ethnobotany and potential as

anticancer and anti-inflammatory agents', *Journal of Ethnopharmacology*, 2008, 119, pp.195-213.

15. Lev, E. and Amar Z., *Practical Materia Medica*, p.510.
16. Ibid., p.207.
17. Spiegel, D., and Harrington, A., 'What is the placebo worth?' *BMJ*, 2008, 336, pp.967-8.
18. Paavilainen, H., 'Psychoactive plants in Maimonides' Regimen Sanitatis and de Causis Accidentium', *Korot, Israel Journal of the History of Medicine and Science*, 2007, 18, pp.25-54.
19. Leibowitz, J.O. and Marcus, S. (Ed. and trans.), *Sefer Hanisyonot: The Book of Medical Experiences, Attributed to Ibn Ezra, Medical Theory, Rational and Magical Therapy: A Study in Medievalism* (Jerusalem: Magnes Press, 1984).
20. Ibid., p.137.
21. Ibid., p.147.
22. Ibid., p.171.
23. Ibid., p.181.
24. Ibid., p.213.
25. Ibid., pp.148, 183.
26. Trachtenberg, J., *Jewish Magic and Superstition*, p.204.
27. Ibid., p.201.
28. Ibid., p.204.
29. Zimmels,H. J., *Magicians, Theologians and Doctors*, p.141.
30. Ibid., p.147.
31. Trachtenberg, J., *Jewish Magic and Superstition*, p.201.
32. Ibid., p.202.
33. Matras, H., *Jewish Folk Medicine*, pp.118-119.
34. Epstein, I., *The Talmud*, 16b, Babylonian Talmud.
35. Trachtenberg, J., *Jewish Magic and Superstition*, p.205.
36. Matras, H., *Jewish Folk Medicine*, p.120.
37. Zimmels,H.J., *Magicians, Theologians and Doctors*, p. 140.
38. Amar, Z., *The History of Medicine in Jerusalem* (Oxford: Archaeopress, BAR International Series 1032, 2002), pp.116-119.
39. Benayahu, M., *Medical Works of Rabbi Refael Mordekhai Malkhi* (Jerusalem: 1985), (Hebrew)
40. Singer, A., 'Ottoman Palestine 1516-1800: Health, Disease and Historical Sources', in Waserman, M., and Kottek, S.S. (Eds), *Health and Disease in the Holy Land: Studies in the History and Sociology of Medicine from Ancient Times to the Present* (Lampeter (UK): Edward Mellens Press, 1996), p.200.
41. Amar, Z., *The History of Medicine in Jerusalem*, p.117
42. Singer, A., 'Ottoman Palestine 1516-1800', p.202.
43. Collins, K., *Go and Learn: the International story of Jews and Medicine in Scotland 1739-1945* (Aberdeen University Press, 1987), pp.37-41. The degrees were obtained in absentia on the recommendation of bona fide physicians. One later physician who tested the boundaries was Samuel Levenston (1821-1914) who had begun his practice as an unqualified practitioner, gained the MD in Glasgow in 1859 but was removed from the medical list in 1880 for irregular medical practices. See *Minutes of the General Council of Medical Education and Registration of the United Kingdom* (London: W. J.

Goldbourn, 1877), pp.37, 106, 231; *Medical Times and Gazette* (London: J. & A. Churchill, 1881), II: pp.478-480.

44. Matras, H., *Jewish Folk Medicine*, p.129.

45. Barr, J., Berkovitch, M., Matras, H., Greenberg, R., and Eshel, G., 'Talismans and Amulets in the Pediatric Intensive Care Unit: Legendary Powers in Contemporary Medicine', *Israel Medical Association Journal*, 2000, 2, pp.278-281.

46. Lev, E. and Amar, Z., 'Ethnopharmacological Survey of Traditional Drugs Sold in Israel at the end of the 20ᵗʰ Century', *J Ethnopharmaco.*,2000, 72, pp.191-205.

47. Lev, E. and Amar, Z., *Practical Materia Medica*.

48. Epstein, I., *The Talmud*, Shabbat 145b.

49. Rosner, F. (trans.), *The Medical Aphorisms of Moses Maimonides* (Maimonides Research Unit, Haifa, 1989), pp.293-312; Rosner, F. (trans.), *Moses Maimonides Treatise on Asthma* (Maimonides Research Unit,1994), p.176; Rosner, F., *Encyclopaedia of Medicine in the Bible and Talmud* (Northvale, NJ: Jason Aronson, 2000), pp.74-75.

50. Ohry, A. and Tsafrir, J., 'Is chicken soup an essential drug?', *Canadian Medical Association Journal*, 1999, 161, 12, pp.1532-3; Leiberman, A. and Bar-Ziv, J., 'Unstrained chicken soup [letter]', *Chest*, 1980, 77, p.128.

51. Rosner, F., 'Therapeutic Efficacy of Chicken Soup', *Chest*, 1980, 78, pp.672-674; Rosner, F., 'Its uncanny (letter)', *Canadian Medical Association Journal*, 1980, 162, p.973.

4

Islamic Medicine from the Eighth to Eighteenth Centuries

Aref Abu-Rabia

Introduction

To understand the development of Islam and Islamic civilization, we must recognize that the Middle East region into which Islam expanded was a rich repository of centuries of accumulated intellectual exchanges, religious experiences and administrative practices. Islamic society built upon these existing foundations and was shaped by them.[1]

Ancient Near Eastern civilizations began to develop in Iraq around 3500 BCE. These settled communities developed written alphabets, governing institutions, and religious rituals, improvements in agricultural and military technology. This process reaches its first culmination in Egypt's Nile Valley, where an advanced civilization took shape under the rule of the Pharaohs (3200-332 BCE). A similar unifying effect was achieved by the Iranian-based Acheminid Empire (550-331 BCE), which brought all the lands of the Middle East from Egypt to the Oxus River into a single imperial framework. In the wake of the conquests of Alexander the Great in the fourth century BCE, the lands of the Middle East lying between Iran and the Mediterranean Sea absorbed yet another layer of tradition as Greek was implanted as the language of administration and high culture.[2]

The Arabian Peninsula is the home of the Arabs, an ancient Semitic people. Tribes were the largest units of social and political organization to which an individual's loyalties were given. Mecca was a religious site of major significance. The city's shrine – the Ka'ba – became the centre of an animistic cult that attracted worshipers throughout western Arabia. By the time of Muhammad's birth in 570 the Ka'ba had become the site of an annual pilgrimage during which warfare was suspended, and Mecca's sanctuary became a kind of neutral ground where tribal disputes could be resolved.[3] The city celebrated a special style of Arabic poetry known as a *qasidah*.[4]

Islam must be understood as a product of the societies into which it spread as well as of the society in which it originated. Muhammad was born into the clan of Quraysh. He is the Prophet of Islam; his prophethood can be divided into two phases, the period at Mecca (610-622), and the years in al-Madina (622-632). The Quran was transmitted from God to Muhammad by the angel Gabriel. Muslim scholars agreed that since God had chosen Muhammad to receive final revelation, he must have possessed exemplary human qualities. Therefore, the words and actions of Muhammad in his daily life were taken as divinely approved guides for human conduct. This source of law became codified as scholars sifted through the many stories – *hadith* – about Muhammad that were in general circulation. When the Muslim jurists collectively agreed that certain practices were forbidden or permitted, their decisions became part of the *shari'a* (the sacred law of the Islamic community).[5]

Ancient Arab Medicine

In order to understand Islamic medicine, one must first gain an understanding of ancient Arab medicine in the pre-Islamic and early Islamic periods. The Arabs in the pre-Islamic period were influenced by many cultures and civilizations, among them their neighbours and kin-the Nabateans, the Palmyrens, the Ghassanids, the Lakhmids and the Byzantine and Persian cultures. Areas of contact between the Arabs and other civilizations included commerce and trade as well as political, military, religious (Judaism and Christianity), and intellectual fields.[6] Beyond these realms, the influence of neighbouring cultures was felt in the practice of medicine, health and hygiene.[7]

Ancient Arab medicine was also influenced by Greece and Rome. The Greco-Roman system of medicine developed based primarily on the writing of Hippocrates (460–360 BCE), Dioscorides (c. 54 to 68), and Galen (130–201). Alexandria, Rome, Constantinople, Antioch, Edessa, Amida and Gundishapur flourished as centres of scientific and medical activity.[8] A combination of political and religious events caused many Greek and Syriac-speaking scholars to move eastward to Persia and establish a centre of learning, including a medical school, in the city of Gundishapur in the sixth century. In the year 489, the Roman emperor closed the school at Edessa, and the learned men, mostly Christians of the heretical sect of Nestorians, took refuge in Nisibis in Persia, taking with them Greek texts and Syriac translations and epitomes. The city of Gundishapur in southwest Iran also became a centre of learning, blending many languages and cultures – Greek, Syriac, Persian and Hindu. The medical school of Gundishapur supported the translation of Greek and possibly Sanskrit texts into Middle Persian and Syriac; Greco-Roman medicine was practiced and there was a forum where medical texts could be read. A college remained in Alexandria where philosophy and medicine were taught. Several physicians taught there in the Greek language however, their works survived only in Arabic translations.[9]

The Arab medical system grew out of the works of physicians who were contemporaries of the Prophet Muhammad (570–632), including al-Harith b. Kalada (d. 634), and Ibn Abi Rimtha.[10] The sayings (*hadith*) of the Prophet Muhammad on health and illness were systemized and became known as *Medicine of the Prophet (al-Tibb al-Nabawi)*.[11] In the early period of Islam, a number of physicians or traditional healers practised, among them al-Nader b. al-Harith (the son of al-Harith b. Kalada), Zaynab al-Awadiya from Bani Awd, al-Shamardal b. Qibab al-Ka'bi al-Najrani, Ibn Hudhaym from Tim al-Ribab, Hammad b. Tha'labah al-Azadi, Abd al-Malik Abjar al-Kinani and Um 'Attyya al-Ansariyya.[12] Rufaida bint Sa'ad of the Bani Aslam tribe in al-Madinais was recognized as the first Muslim nurse. Her father was a physician and she worked as his assistant and went out into the community and tried to solve the social problems that lead to disease. She was, in essence, both a public health nurse and a social worker.[13]

Umayyads and Abbasids

During the period of Umayyad rule (661–750 in the East) based in Damascus, translations of ancient medical works began. The first Umayyad caliph, Mu'awiya b. Abi Sufyan (reg. 661-680), employed the physician Ibn Uthal, a Christian from Damascus. The grandson of Mu'awiya, Prince Khalid b. Yazid (d.704) had a passion for medicine and instructed a group of Greek scholars in Egypt to translate Greco-Egyptian medical literature into Arabic. The physician of Caliph 'Umar b. 'Abd al-'Aziz (reg. 717-720) was 'Abd al-Malik b. Abjar al-Kinani, a convert to Islam who had studied at the surviving medical school in Alexandria.[14]

Over the course of the following five centuries (750–1258), the Abbasids dominated the socio-political life of the greater part of the Muslim world. The ten caliphs of the period were generous in their promotion of knowledge and medicine, and medical translations and writings flourished under the Abbasids. Particularly notable in this regard were al-Mansur

(754–775), Harun al-Rashid (786–802), and al-Ma'mun (813–833). A hospital was built and became the cradle of the Baghdad School of Medicine. Countless manuscripts, particularly those written in Greek, were collected and stored in the Bayt al-Hikmah (the House of Wisdom) established in Baghdad in 830 by Caliph al-Ma'mun, where scholars laboured at translating such manuscripts into Arabic.[15] One of the early translators was the Nestorian Christian Yuhanna b. Masawayh (d. 857), a pupil of Jibril b. Bakhtishu' and a teacher of Hunayn b. Ishaq. Al-Ma'mun appointed him superintendent of his library/academy and he was responsible for all scientific translation into Arabic.[16]

Hunayn b.Ishaq (810-877) a Nestorian Christian originally from al-Hira in southern Iraq, was the physician of the caliph al-Mutawakkil. His treatise 'Questions on Medicine for Students' (*al-Masa'il fi al-tibb li-lmuta'allimin*) was extremely influential, as were his 'Ten Treatises on the Eye' (*Kitab al-'AshrMaqalat fi al-'Ayn*). Another translator was Thabit b. Qurra (d.901), a member of the Sabian sect of Harran in northern Mesopotamia. 'Ali b. Sahl Rabban al-Tabari from Marw, south of the Caspian Sea, was the son of a Christian scholar who later converted from Christianity to Islam. He was a physician, translator and author and dedicated his book *Paradise of Wisdom* (*Firdaws al-Hikma*) to the caliph al-Mutawakkil in 850. Qusta b. Luqa al-Ba'albaki (d. 912) a physician and translator, wrote on various topics including blood, phlegm, yellow bile and black bile.[17]

It was during this period, too, that the philosopher Ya'qub b.Ishaq al-Kindi (d. 873) authored several works on medicine. His *Formulary of Compound Medicines* (*Agrabadhin*) has been translated from Arabic to English.[18] Another scholar, Abu 'Abd Allah b Sa'id Al-Tamimi (d. 980) from Jerusalem, went to Egypt to work as physician for the Vizier Ya'qub ibn Killis. He wrote *The Guide to the Fundamentals of Foodstuffs* and the *Powers of Simple Drugs* (*Kitab al-Murshid ila Jawahir al-Aghdhiyawa Quwa al-Mufradatminal-Adwiya*), and a book about plague: *The Extension of Life by Purifying the Air of Corruption and Guarding against the Evil Effects of Pestilences [Plagues]* (*Maddat al-Baqa' bi-Islah Fasad al-Hawa' w-al-taharruz min Ḍarar-il-Awbā*).His other important medical works include: *Treatise on the Nature of Ophthalmology and its Types, Causes and Treatment* (*Maqalah fi Mahiyat-ul-Ramadwa Anwauhuwa Asbabuhuwa 'Ilajuh*), *Dear is the Bride, but the Souls are Fragrant Basil* (*Habib al-'arus, wa-rayhan al-nufus*), *The Key to Pleasure in all Worries* (*Miftah al-Surur fi kul al-Humum*).

Ishaq ibn Sulayman al-Isra'ili (855-950), Isaac Judaeus or Israeli, was both a physician and a philosopher. He first worked as an oculist was in

Cairo and later he emigrated to Qayrawan (Kairouan) in Tunisia, where he studied medicine under Ishaq b. 'Imran and became court physician to Ziyadat Allah III (reg.903-909), the last Emir of the Aghlabid dynasty. His finest works were the *Book of Fever* (*Kitab al-Hummayat*) and the *Book of Urine (Kitab-al Bawl)*[19]. One of the most highly-regarded ophthalmological manuals was *The Oculist's Notebook* (*Kitab Tadhkirat al-Kahhalin*), by Sharaf al-Din 'Ali b. 'Isa al-Kahhal (d.1010), who practised as an oculist and physician in Baghdad. The text covered 130 eye ailments.

Abu Hanifah Ahmad ibn Dawudd al-Dinawari (d. 894) the herbalist (*al-'Ashshab*) an Arab scholar of Iranian origin, was an Islamic Golden Age polymath, astronomer, agriculturist, botanist, metallurgist, geographer, mathematician and historian. He is the author of *The Plants* (*al-Nabat*), six volumes that describe 1,120 plants, giving their different names and meanings in Arabic while preserving others in their Persian or Latin names.[20]

Within a century of the birth of Islam, Muslim physicians and scientists were making original contributions to medical and botanical knowledge. One of the greatest and most well-known Islamic doctors was Ibn Sina (Avicenna, 980–1037), who compiled the *Canon of Medicine* (*Kitab al-Qanun fi al-Tibb*).[21] The *Canon* distilled Greek and Islamic medical knowledge, which included medicine, anatomy, physiology, pathology and pharmacology with many descriptions of uses for medicinal plants. It is the epitome of Islamic medicine, and the culmination and masterpiece of Arab systematization. Another leading Arabic philosopher/physician was al-Razi (Rhazes, 865-923), who was born in Rayy, Persia. He studied in Baghdad where he lectured, practised medicine and compiled the *Comprehensive Book on Medicine* (*Kitab al-Hawi fi al-Tibb*).[22] The works of Ibn Sina and al-Razi were later translated into Latin. The *Canon* was taught for centuries in Western universities and was one of the most frequently printed scientific texts in the Renaissance. Thus, from their Latin translations, Ibn Sina and al-Razi continued to influence medical practice until as late as the nineteenth century.[23]

Islamic Spain

In the western end of the Islamic empire, the Umayyads of Andalus (Islamic Spain from 711 to 1492) established themselves after the downfall of the Umayyads of Damascus in 750 and made their capital at Cordoba. Science, arts and medicine flourished under the Umayyads of Cordoba. Areas of Cordoba and Granada became centres of learning. The period of the Caliphate is seen as the golden age of al-Andalus. Under the Caliphate of

Cordoba, al-Andalus was a beacon of learning, and the city of Cordoba became one of the leading cultural, economic, scientific and technological centres in both the Mediterranean Basin and the Islamic world.[24] Cordoba, Seville and Madinat al-Zahra were one of the greatest centres of art and culture in the tenth century. In fact, Madinat al-Zahra, the caliphate residence, was regarded as one of the 'wonders of the age' until it was destroyed in the eleventh century.[25]

From the earliest days, the Umayyads wanted to be seen as intellectual rivals to the Abbasids, and aspired that Cordoba have libraries and educational institutions that could rival Baghdad's. Although there was a clear rivalry between the two powers, freedom to travel between the two Caliphates was allowed, which helped spread new ideas and innovations over time.[26]

The rich diverse flora of Spain was a contributing factor to the development of medical botany. *The Compendium of Simple Drugs and Food* (*al-Jami' li-Mufradat al-Adwiyawa'l-Aghdhiya*), by Ibn al-Baytar [al-bitar] (1197–1248), describes more than 1,400 medicinal drugs, including 300 not previously described. This is probably the best known of all Arabic herbal books.[27] The medicinal use of plants was a popular topic in Arab medical writings. Among the well-known physicians who wrote on the uses of plants was Sulayman b. al-Hasan b. Juljul (d. 994), who worked at the court of 'Abd al-Rahman III and assisted in the translation of Dioscorides' herbal into Arabic. He was the author of *History of Medicine and Physicians* (*Tabaqat al-Atibba' wa-l-Hukama'*).[28] Hamid Ibn Samajun (d.1010) compiled a large volume on herbs, *The Comprehensive Book of Sayings of Ancient and Modern Physicians and Philosophers Concerning Simple Drugs* (*al-Kitab al-Jami' li-Aqwal al-Qudama' wa'l-Mutahaddithinmin al-Atibba' wa'l-Mutafalsifinfi'l-Adwiya al-Mufrada*).[29] Abu Ja'far Ahmad b. Muhammad al-Ghafiqi (d. 1135), originally from Ghafiq, near Cordoba, compiled a large text on herbs and drugs, *Book of Simple Drugs* (*Kitab al-Adwiya al-Mufrada*).[30]

Among the well-known physicians who wrote on the uses of plants was 'Abd al-Malik b. Zuhr (Avenzoar 1113–1162), the first of a five-generation family of prominent Andalusian physicians. A native of Seville, he achieved widespread fame as a physician in Spain and North Africa. He wrote *The Nutrition Book/Book on Foodstuffs* (*Kitab al-Aghdhiya*), but his best-known book was *Facilitation of Treatment in Therapy and Diet* (*Kitab al-Taysirfi'l Mudawatwa'l-Tadbir*).[31] Abu-Bakr Muhammad Ibn-Bajjah (Avempace d. 1139) authored the *Kitab al-Nabat* (The Book of Plants), a popular work on botany, which defined the sex of plants.

Significant contributions to medical science were also made by Al-Zahrawi [Abu al-Qasim Khalaf b. 'Abbas al-Zahrawi] (Abulcasis or Albucasis 936-1013),[32] born in Zahra, near Cordoba, who laid the foundations of modern surgery. He authored three books that remained standard textbooks for nearly a thousand years. The most famous of these was his*Manual for Medical Practitioners (Kitabal-Tasrif li-man 'Ajiza 'an al-Ta'lif)*. Its primary contribution to the field of medicine is that it contained 278 illustrations of equipment used for surgery.

Ibn al-Jazzar and his Era

During this fruitful period of medical writing, Ibn al-Jazzar (d.980), an Arab physician, a student of Ishaq ibn Sulayman al-Izraili and member of a distinguished medical family in Qayrawan, (Kairouan) the medieval capital of Tunisia, authored several works that added much to the medical knowledge of the time. His writing earned him renown in medieval Western Europe. Some of his books were translated into Greek, Latin and Hebrew: *Treatise on Simple Drugs (Kitab al-Adwiya), Medicine for the Poor (Tibb al-Fuqara' wa-al-Masakin); On Forgetfulness and Its Treatment (Risala fi al-Nisyanwa 'ilajihi); On the Education and Regimen of Children (Kitab Siyasat al-Sibyanwa-Tadbirihim)* and *On the Stomach, Its Diseases, and Treatment (Kitab fi al-Ma'idahwa-Amradihawa-Mudawatiha)*. His *Provision for the Traveller and Nourishment for the Sedentary (Zad al-Musafirwa-qut al-Hadir)* is, contrary to what its title suggests, an excellent medical text on sexual diseases and their treatment. This one of the seven books written by Ibn al-Jazzar, provides a concise presentation of sex-related ailments, providing an illuminating snapshot of the development of medical science in the tenth century. It also provides insights for anyone interested in the view of sex and sexuality in Arab society in that period. It constitutes a great advance in the understanding of the history of Islamic and Western medicine. The work was translated into Greek, Latin and Hebrew, and stood among the standard texts for medical instruction at Salerno, Montpellier, Bologna, Paris and Oxford.[33] Another significant contributor to medical sciences was Muhammad b. Ahmad Ibn Rushd (Averroes 1126–1198). Born in Cordoba, his main medical work is *Colliget* (Latin) (*Kitab al-Kulliyyat*). Ibn Rushd had a major influence on the intellectual life of medieval Europe. He is considered the founder of the Averroism School of philosophy, and his works and commentaries had an impact on the rise of secular thought in Western Europe. He also developed the concept of 'existence precedes essence'.[34] It is worth mentioning that the Scotsman

Michael Scot (1175-1235) travelled to Paris, Bologna, Palermo and Toledo where he learned Arabic to study the Arabic versions of Aristotle and the many commentaries of the Arabs upon these, as well as the original works of Avicenna and Averroes which he took to Italy where it would have a significant impact on the formation of the European Renaissance.[35]

The influence of Arab medicine, which is so closely interwoven with the Greco-Latin legacy, has proved to be of critical importance for Western medicine.[36] The Arabic texts became available mainly through two successive waves of translations into Latin. The first of these became available in southern Italy in the second half of the eleventh century, while the second became available in Spain about a hundred years later. In the middle of the thirteenth century, the three great medical faculties of Paris, Montpellier and Bologna gradually integrated the fundamental works of Ibn Sina and al-Razi and the surgical section of the *al-Tasrif* of al-Zahrawi into their curricula.[37]

During the Fatimid rule (909-1160) and Ayyubic rule (in 1164) in Egypt, Cairo became a centre of learning, attracting physicians such as Musa ibn Maymon, Moses ben Maimon or Maimonides,(1138-1204). Maimonides was born in Cordoba and achieved fame not just as one of the outstanding physicians of his era but also as the leader of the Jewish community in Egypt writing many works on codifying Jewish law and on philosophy with an Aristotelian influence. He served as a personal physician to Salah ad-Din's son al-Malik al-Afdal Nur ad-Din 'Ali in Egypt and some of his medical works are addressed to him. His books were all written in Arabic and one of the most famous is his *Aphorisms* (*Kitab al-Fusul fi al-tibb*).[38]

Other famous physicians included Abd al-Latif al-Baghdadi (1162-1231) and Muhadhdhab al-Din 'Abd al-Rahim ibn 'Ali, known as al-Dakhwar (1170-1230), who was the leading influence on the development of learned medical care in Syria and Egypt in the thirteenth century. Al Dakhwar was born and raised in Damascus where his father and brother were oculists. He was appointed 'Chief of the Physicians in all of Egypt and Syria' and was the personal physician to Ayyubid ruler al-Malik al-'Adil Sayf al-Din, the brother of Salah ad-Din. Two famous pupils of al-Dakhwar were Ibn Abi Usaybi'a and Ibn al-Nafis. Ibn Abi Usaybi'a (d. 1270) born in Damascus of family physicians was a noted oculist practising at the Nuri hospital in Damascus. He authored *Information on the Classes of Physicians* (*Kitab 'Uyun al-anba' fi tabaqat al-atibba'*), in which he presents the biographies of over 380 physicians. Ibn al-Nafis (Ali abi al-Hazm al-Qurashi, d. 1288), born in Damascus, was a physician-surgeon and an authority on religious law, logic and theology, as well as a prolific writer of medical tracts. Among his writings was *The Perfected Book on Ophthalmology* (*Kitab al-Muhadhdhabfi 'l-kuhl*), a summary of ophthalmological practices, which is a commentary on *Questions on Medicine for Students* by Hunayn ibn Ishaq. His most famous writings are the *Concise Manual* (*Kitab al-Mujaz*), on Ibn Sina's *Canon of Medicine*, and a large commentary on the *Canon* in which he developed his theory of pulmonary circulation, the first to accurately explain the circulation of the blood hundreds of years before the Spaniard Michael Servetus (Miguel Servede, 1509–1553).[39] It is worth noting that al-Razi, Ibn-Sina, Al-Zahrawi and Ibn al-Nafis described in detail specific cancer and tumour types, which were known at this time, and suggested several treatments.[40] Dawud ibn Omar al-Antaki (d. 1599) was born in Antioch and lived in Egypt. Before settling in Egypt, he travelled to many countries collecting information about the uses of medicinal plants. He wrote more than twenty-five books on pharmacology and medicine, including the *Treatise of Dawud* (*Tadhkira ulu' al-Albab*) known simply as *Tadhkirat Dawud*.[41]

Among Arab physicians, music was a prominent mode of healing. Music is a means of communication and can be a powerful therapeutic tool. Here the basic objective of the healer is to establish communication with the spirits through music. One of the well-known Arab doctors who employed music for healing was Abu-Nasr al-Farabi (d. 950) (Alpharabius Avenassar) who invented a musical instrument on which he played melodies that strongly affected patients, causing them to laugh or cry, wake up or fall asleep.[42]

Hospitals in the Islamic Lands

The hospital as a medical institution was one of the great achievements of medieval Islamic society as hospitals were built throughout Islamic lands, with hospitals for the elderly and the mentally ill beginning at the dawn of Islam.[43] All these hospitals were financed from the revenues of charitable trusts (*waqfs*) and were open to males and females, rich and poor, and to Muslims and non-Muslims. In the early eighth century, Muslims established hospitals and hospices that were free of charge regardless of the gender, social status or age of the patient.

Islamic hospitals provided patients with systematic treatments based upon humoral medicine (*al-akhlat*) including exercises, baths, dietary regimens and a comprehensive *materia medica*, in addition to bone-setting, cauterizing, venesection and eye surgery.[44] Caretakers would wash patients, dress them in clean clothes, help them pray, and have special chanters with pleasant voices read them verses from the Qur'an. Sometimes the *Mu'adhdhin* (who calls the faithful to prayer from the minaret of the mosque) would recite prayers and supplications (*ibtihalat*) before sunrise to relieve patients of their insomnia and pain. In addition to the daily provision of song and instrumental music in the hospital, it was also customary to invite groups of dancers, singers and entertainers to perform for the patients. The burning of incense (*bakhkhur*) further enhanced the healing milieu. Sometimes the floors of the hospital were strewn with branches of pomegranate (*rumman*), mastic tree (*mustaka*), balsam of Mecca (*balsam Makka*), henna (*hinna*) and pleasant-smelling spice trees.[45]

The general health of the Islamic community was influenced by many factors, including: the climatic conditions of the desert, the different living conditions of nomadic, rural, and urban populations; and the incidence of plague and other epidemics as well as the occurrence of endemic conditions such as trachoma and other eye diseases. Medical care is always multi-faceted with the needs of the society being served by various local traditional practices as well as the formal learned medicine. In early Islam, the general histories and chronologies of a realm or dynasty were written in comprehensive encyclopaedias, containing sections on medical topics and travel literature. Both belles-lettres and a genre of literature termed *adab*, which addressed specifically manners and ethics of society, on occasion discussed physicians.[46] Philosophical writing frequently dealt with medical topics and theological and juridical opinions regarding medicine and the practice of physicians were of great importance.[47]

Prophetic Medicine

The records of the Prophet Muhammad's reputed saying and deeds, compiled mostly in the ninth century in a body of literature called *hadiths*, contain many statements on health and illness. It is a combination of religious and medical information, providing advice and guidance on the two goals of medicine – the preservation and restoration of health, in careful conformity with the teachings of Islam as enshrined in the *Qur'an* and the *hadith*. It includes customs and sayings of the Prophet, as well as on herbal and medical practices. It is a concise summary of how the Prophet's guidance and teaching can be followed, as well as how health, sickness and cures were viewed by Muslims. The original Arabic text offers an authoritative compendium of Islamic medicine and still enjoys much popularity in the Muslim world. *Medicine of the Prophet* will appeal not only to those interested in alternative systems of health and medicine, but also to people wishing to acquaint themselves with, or increase their knowledge of, the *hadith* and the religion and culture of Islam.[48]

An understanding of the conceptual aspects of Islamic medicine requires an understanding of Islam itself. Islam has its own concepts of maintenance of health and the alleviation of disease, that entwine Islam's conceptions of the nature of creation, the status of humankind, the path of wellbeing along with almost every aspect of life. The welfare of mothers and children is well regulated in the *Qur'an*, and the *hadith* in regard to hygiene and sanitation; in short, the Prophet provided the foundation for a medical tradition that considered a human being in his totality.[49] In a later development, these medical traditions were termed Prophetic Medicine (*al-tibb al-nabawi*). It should be noted that by the tenth century *al-tib al-nabawi* developed parallel to that based upon the Hellenistic and Byzantine systems of medicine. During the thirteenth and fourteenth centuries, this topic attracted particular attention. Such writings were fuelled by aspirations to both attest to the religious value of medicine, arguing that medicine represents the highest service to God, and to appropriate medicine for Islam rather than allowing it to be dominated by Greco-Roman traditions. In other words, the final authority for medicine is Prophetic revelation, not Galen or Hippocrates.[50] For all writers on Prophetic medicine, prevention was always viewed as better than a cure (echoed in similar sentiments expressed in the old Western saying that 'an ounce of prevention is worth a pound of cure').[51]

Well-known authors in the field of Prophetic medicine included prominent Muslim religious scholars, especially those specializing in *hadith*.[52] Interest in Prophetic medicine has not died out in modern times as both contemporary religious scholars and physicians still make intriguing contributions to the field of Prophetic medicine. Further, the number of Prophetic traditions varied widely from one book to another.[53] Up to the fourteenth century, when this genre witnessed its golden age, books just listed the relevant traditions without further analysis of their medical content. Commentaries on the medical content of these traditions were introduced to consider Prophetic medicine when practising physicians such as al-Baghdadi and Ibn Tarkhan became interested in this topic. Subsequent works such as that by al-Dhahabi dedicated whole chapters to theoretical issues widely discussed in the Greco-Islamic medical tradition, such as the theory of humours, elements, temperaments and general causes of illnesses and contagion and preventive medicine. Books on Prophetic medicine also addressed religious-ethical and medico-legal issues, such as the traits of an ideal physician, the education of the physician and the assigned punishments for malpractice. Some of these books touched on gender issues, such as the practice of medicine by females and whether medical treatment and care provided by women for men and vice versa is permissible.[54] Excessive emotions such as passionate love (*'ishq*) were treated by spiritual cures and Islamic rituals such as prayer, fasting, remembrance of Allah and Qur'anic recitation.[55]

Conclusion

The authors of the prophetic traditions claim that the Prophet of Islam had already discovered recent western medical findings many centuries ago. Contemporary authors try to stress that prophetic medicine should not at any rate replace Western medicine as an academic discipline and a highly developed profession.[56] The objective here is to provide food for thought and suggest new thinking about a synthesis between the two systems and their reciprocal enrichment, on behalf of more comprehensive therapy that can only benefit those who seek relief from diseases and other medical conditions.

The main achievements of medieval Arabic-Islamic medicine were in five areas: systematisation, hospitals, pharmacology, surgery and ophthalmology.[57] The development of Arabic medical literature can be described as a constant reshaping and rearranging of the Greek heritage by shortening, expanding, commenting on and systematising ancient source material.

Ibn-Sina combined the legacy of Greek medical knowledge with the Arab contribution in his massive *Canon of Medicine* which is the greatest masterpiece of Arab systematisation. Numerous Arab authors, who added some 500 names of simple and compound drugs to the ancient stock, thus broadened the basis of pharmacology Dioscorides' *Materia Medica*.[58]

The Islamic medical tradition, established by *al-tibb al-nabawi* in the seventh century, was systemised in the tenth century, developed in the eleventh and twelfth centuries and reached its peak in the thirteenth to sixteenth centuries, but later declined in the seventeenth to nineteenth centuries. Medical literature and healing methods that had been the focus of traditional medicine for over a thousand years were marginalised in the nineteenth and twentieth centuries by the advent of Western medicine, becoming the exclusive domain of traditional medicine and folk healers. Folk healers continued to consult medical texts originally written in the

Middle Ages, but we should not conclude that they marked the decline of the Islamic civilisation.

Notes

1. Cleveland, W., *A History of the Modern Middle East* (Boulder, Colorado: Westview Press, 2004), pp.1-35; Lapidus, I.M., *A History of Islamic Societies* 3rd edn (New York: Cambridge University Press, 2014); Hitti, P., *History of the Arabs* 10th edn (London: Macmillan, 1951), pp.1-25.
2. Cleveland, *History of the Modern Middle East*, pp.1-35; Hitti, *History of the Arabs*, pp.1-25.
3. Lazarus-Yafeh, H., 'The Religious Dialectics of the Hajj', in Lazarus-Yafeh, H. (ed.), *Some Religious Aspects of Islam:A Collection of Articles* (Leiden: Brill, 1981).
4. Cleveland, *History of the Modern Middle East*, pp.1-35; Hitti, *History of the Arabs*, pp.1-25; Arberry, A.J., *The Seven Odes* (London: George Allen & Unwin, 1957).
5. Cleveland, *A History of the Modern Middle East*, pp.1-35; Schacht, J., *An Introduction to Islamic Law* (Oxford: Clarendon Press, 1964); Amin, A., *Fajr al-Islam* (Beirut: Dal al-Kitab al-'Arabic (Arabic), 1969), pp.1-35; Zaidan, A.K., *Al-madkhal li-dirasat al-shari'a al-islamiya* (Baghdad: maktabat al-quds. (Arabic), 1981), p.47.
6. Amin, *Fajr al-Islam*, pp.1-35. al-Najjar, A., *Fi tarikh al-tib fi al-Dawlah al-Islamiya* (History of Medicine in the Islamic Empire) (al-Qahira: Dar al-Ma'arif (Arabic), 1994), pp.2-53; Elgood, C., *A Medical History of Persia and the Eastern Caliphate from the Earliest Times to the Year A.D. 1932* (London: Cambridge University Press, 1951).
7. Abu-Rabia, A., *Indigenous Medicine among the Bedouin in the Middle East* (New York and Oxford: Berghahn Books, 2015).
8. Mursi, A., *Dirasattfi'l-Shi'ūn al-tibbiyah al-'arabiyah* (Studies on Arab Medical Affairs) (al-Iskandariya: al-ma'arif. (Arabic), 1966); Savage-Smith, E., 'Medicine', in Rashid, R., and Morelon, R. (eds.) *Encyclopedia of the History of Arabic Science*, vol. 3 (London and New York: Routledge, 1996), pp.903-962.
9. Savage-Smith, 'Medicine', pp.903-962; Murad, A.S., *Lamhat min tarikh al-tibb al-qadim* (Glimpses from the History of Early Medicine) (al-Qahira: Maktabat al-nashr al-haditha (Arabic), 1966); al-Said, M.S., 'Medicine in Islam', in: Selin, H. (ed.) *Encyclopedia of the History of Science, Technology, and Medicine in Non-Western Cultures* (Dordrecht, Boston and London: Kluwer Academic, 1997), pp.695-98; al-Shatti, A.S., *al-'Arab wal-tibb* (The Arabs and Medicine) (Dimashq: ManshuratWazarat al-Thaqafa (Arabic), 1970), pp.5-10; Ullmann, M., *Islamic Surveys: Islamic Medicine* (Edinburgh: Edinburgh University Press, 1978), pp.1-40.
10. Al-Harith b. Kalada (Kilda) (d. 634) travelled to Jundishapur in Persia and studied medicine prior to the advent of Islam. He returned to Ta'if (in Arabia), where his medicine became renowned among the Arabs. He is said to have been a relative of the Prophet Muhammad. The Prophet would send sick people to consult al-Harith. One of these was Sa'd b. Abi Waqqss. See Hawting, G.R., 'The Development of the Biography of al-Harith ibn Kalada and the Relationship between Medicine and Islam', in Bosworth, C.E., Issawi, C., Savory, R. and Udovitch, A.L. (eds.), *The Islamic World, from Classical to Modern Times* (Princeton, NJ: Darwin Press, 1989), pp.127-137. Al-

Harith was very familiar with the doctrine of the four humours (al-Akhlat) Ibn Abi Usaybi'ah, *Kitab 'uyun al-anba' fi tabaqat al-tibbā'* (Baiyrut: ManshuratdarMaktabatal-hayat (Arabic), 1965), pp.13-17.

11.   Hawting, 'The Development of the Biography', pp.127-137. Ibn Abi Usaybi'ah, *Kitab 'uyun al-anba' fi tabaqat al-tibbā'*, pp.13-17.

12.   al-Labadi, 'A.A., *Tarikh al-Jiraha 'ind al-'Arab*. (Amman: Dar al-Karmel (Arabic), 1992), pp.80-81.

13.   Kasule, O.H., *Islamic Medical Education Resources: Historical Roots of the Nursing Profession in Islam*. Paper presented at the 3rd International Nursing Conference: 'Empowerment and Health: An Agenda for Nurses in the 21st Century', held in Brunei Dar as Salam 1-4 November 1998.

14.   al-Najjar, A., *Fi tarikh al-tib fi al-Dawlah al-Islamiya* (History of Medicine in the Islamic Empire) (al-Qahira: Dar al-Ma'arif. (Arabic), 1994), pp. 2-53; Savage-Smith, 'Medicine', pp.903-962; Haddad, S., *History of Arab Medicine* (Beirut, Lebanon: 1975).

15.   Many physicians were brought to Baghdad. One of these was Jurjis b. Jibra'il b. Bakhtishu'. For eight generations, well into the second half of the eleventh century, twelve members of the Bakhtishu' family of Nestorian Christians would serve the caliphs as physicians and advisors, sponsor the translation of texts and compose their own original treatises. See Al-Najjar, *Fi tarikh al-tib fi al-Dawlah al-Islamiya*, 1994, pp.2-53; Hitti, *History of the Arabs*, 1951, pp.311-312; Savage-Smith, 'Medicine', 1996, p. 910.

16.   Hitti, *History of the Arabs*, pp.1-25.

17.   Thus, by the end of the ninth century, the humoral system of pathology as outlined by the Greco-Roman physician Galen in the second century had been completely accepted and integrated into the learned medical thinking of the day (see Hitti, *History of the Arabs*, 1951, pp.311-312; Savage-Smith, 'Medicine', 1996, p.912; Ullmann, 1978, pp.7-40). This system was based upon the notion of four humours: blood, phlegm, yellow bile and black bile, derived from the earlier Hippocratic writings. Parallels were drawn with the four elements (air, water, fire and earth), while the four qualities were aligned in pairs with the humours in the following manner: blood is hot and moist, phlegm is cold and moist, yellow bile is hot and dry, black bile is cold and dry. The four seasons of the year were important and climatic and geographical conditions were also considered significant (see al-Azraq, 1948, pp. 2-7; Khan, 1986, pp.37-50; Ullmann, 1978, pp.55-62). Hippocrates, Galen and the Arab physicians, particularly Avicenna, were the principal authorities for medical theory and practice at the time. See Foster, G. and Anderson, B., *Medical Anthropology* (New York: John Wiley, 1978), p.59.

18.   Levey, M., *The Medical Formulary (Agrabadhin) of Al-Kindi* (Madison: University of Wisconsin Press, 1966).

19.   Kottek, S., Paavilainen, H. and Collins, K., *Isaac Israeli: the Philosopher Physician* (Hebrew University of Jerusalem Medical Library, 2013).

20.   Abū Ḥanīfa al-Dīnawarī, in Bearman, P., Bianquis, T., Bosworth, C.E., van Donzel, E. and Heinrichs, W.P. (Eds), *The Encyclopaedia of Islam*, 2nd edn, first published online: 2012. Accessed online on 15 January 2018.

21.   Ibn Sina, A.A. (980-1037). One of the greatest and most famous Islamic doctors was Ibn Sīnā (Avicenna) born near Bukhārā in Central Asia, of a family devoted to learning. Known as the 'Prince of Physicians', he combined the legacy of Greek medical

knowledge with the Arab contribution in his *Canon of Medicine* in Arabic, which is the epitome of Islamic medicine, and the culmination and masterpiece of Arab systematization and includes many descriptions of uses for medicinal plants. It was translated into Latin and taught for centuries in Western universities, being one of the most frequently printed scientific texts in the Renaissance and in some medical faculties employed as a textbook until 1650. Al-Canon concentrated Greek and Islamic medical knowledge, which included medicine, anatomy, physiology, pathology and pharmacopoeia (Al-Said, 1997, pp.695-698).

22. al-Razi's (Rhazes) most celebrated work was *Kitab fi al-Jadariwa al-Hasba, On Smallpox and Measles*, which was translated into Latin and later into other languages, including English. Another famous book is the *Kitab al-Tibb al-Mansuri, Book of Medicine*, a short general textbook of medicine of considerable influence, dedicated by al-Razi in 903 to the Samanid prince Abu Salih al-Mansur b. Ishaq, governor of Rayy. The material in al-Hawi is arranged under the headings of different diseases, with separate sections on pharmacological topics. This work, in 24 volumes, was one of only nine books used in the Medical Faculty of the University of Paris.

23. Murad, A.S., *Lamhat min tarikh al-tibb al-qadim*, 1966; al-Said, *Medicine in Islam*, 1997, pp.695-98;

24. Jayyusi, S.K., *The Legacy of Muslim Spain* (Leiden and New York: E.J. Brill, 1994); Said, H.M., 'Muslim Contribution to Medicine', International Symposium on Islam, Philosophy and Science (Paris: UNESCO, 1981); Al-Hassan, A., *Transfer of Islamic Science to the West* (Foundation for Science, Technology and Civilization, FSTC, Manchester: UK, 2006).

25. Maryam. N.B., accessed at http://www.hispanicmuslims.com/andalusia/andalusia.html

26. *Al-Andalus*, a document.

27. Johnstone, P., *Ibn Qayyim al-Jawziyya, Medicine of the Prophet*, trans. and Ed. by Penelope Johnstone (Cambridge: Islamic Texts Society, 1998).

28. Ibid.

29. Ibid.

30. Ibid.

31. Savage-Smith, 'Medicine', pp.903-962; al-Said, *Medicine in Islam*, 1997, pp.695-98; Johnstone, *Ibn Qayyim al-Jawziyya, Medicine of the Prophet*.

32. Albucasis, *Albucasis on Surgery and Instruments*, trans. and commentary by Spink, M.S. and Lewis, G.L. (Berkeley: University of California Press, 1973).

33. Abu-Rabia, A., 'Review of Zad al-Musafi r wa-qut al-hadir' (On Sexual Diseases and Their Treatment by Ibn al-Jazzar), *Middle Eastern Studies*, 2000, 36 (2), pp.224–29; Bos. G., *Ibn al-Jazzar on Sexual Diseases and their Treatment* (Zad al-Musafirwa-qut al-Hadir) (London and New York: Kegan Paul International, 1997), pp.1-18; Jacquart, D., 'The Influence of Arabic Medicine in the Medieval West' in: Rashed, R. (Ed.), *Encyclopedia of the History of Arab Science* (London: Routledge, 1996), pp.963-71.

34. Fakhry, M., *Averroes: His Life, Works and Influence* (Oneworld Publications, 2001); Irwin, J., 'Averroes' Reason: A Medieval Tale of Christianity and Islam', *The Philosopher*, 2002; LXXXX (2).

35. Scott, T.C., Marketos, P. and Michael Scott (1175-1235) accessed at http://mathshistory.st-andrews.ac.uk/Biographies/Scot.html

36. For more details see Campell, D., *Arabian Medicine and its Influence on the Middle Ages* (London: Kegan Paul, 1926); Browne, E.G., *Arabia Medicine* (London: Cambridge

University Press, 1983); Watt, W.M., *The Influence of Islam upon Medieval Europe* (Edinburgh: Edinburgh University Press, 1973).

37.	Jacquart, 'The Influence of Arabic Medicine', pp.963-971.

38.	Hourani, A., *A History of the Arab Peoples* (Cambridge, MA: The Belknap Press of Harvard University Press, 1991). Salah ad-Din was said to have had no less than eighteen physicians in his service including Muslims, Jews and Christians. See also Davidson, H., *Moses Maimonides: the Man and His Works* (Oxford: Oxford University Press, 2005); Collins, K., Kottek, S. and Rosner, F., *Moses Maimonides and his Practice of Medicine* (Haifa: Maimonides Research Institute, 2013).

39.	al-Najjar, A., *Fi tarikh al-tib fi al-Dawlah al-Islamiya*, 1994, pp.2-53; Ullmann, M., *Die Medizinim Islam* (Leiden: Brill, 1970); Khan, M.S., *Islamic Medicine* (London: Routledge & Kegan Paul, 1986), p.19; Nasr, S.H., *Science and Civilization in Islam* (Cambridge, MA: Harvard University Press, 1968), p.213.

40.	Zaid, H., Rayan, A., Said, O. and Saad, B., 'Cancer Treatment by Greco-Arab and Islamic Herbal Medicine', *The Open Nutraceuticals Journal*, 2010, (3), pp.203-212.

41.	al-Said, M.S., 'Medicine in Islam' in Selin, H. (Ed.), *Encyclopedia of the History of Science, Technology, and Medicine in Non-Western Cultures* (Dordrecht, Boston and London: Kluwer Academic, 1997), pp.695-98.

42.	al-Farabi, A.N., *Kitab al-Musiqi al-Kabir*. al-Qahira: MaktabatAnjlo al-Misriya (Arabic 1967); al-Shatti, a⊠Arab wal-tibb, 1970, pp.5-10; Shiloah, A., *Music in the World of Islam* (Jerusalem: Institute for Israeli Arab Studies; 2001), pp.81–95.

43.	The first hospitals were established during the reign of al-Walid ibn 'Abd al-Malik (705-715) in Damascus (al-Shatti, 1970). See also Dols, M.W., 'The Origins of the Islamic Hospitals: Myth and Reality', *Bulletin of the History of Medicine*, 1987 (62), pp.367-390; Melling, J. and Forsythe, B. (Eds), *Insanity, Institutions and Society, 1800–1914: A Social History of Madness in Comparative Perspective* (London and New York: Routledge, 1999).

44.	Reynolds, V. and Tanner, R., *The Social Ecology of Religion* (New York: Oxford University Press, 1995), pp.249–50.

45.	Abu-Rabia, *Indigenous Medicine among the Bedouin in the Middle East*, 2015; al-Shatti, al-'Arab wal-tibb, 1970, pp.5-10

46.	For more details see Rispler-Chaim, V., *Islamic Medical Ethics in the Twentieth Century* (Leiden: Brill, 1993); *Islamic Medical Ethics*: The IMANA Perspective (IMANA= Islamic medical association of North America), 2005, pp.1-12; Gareeboo, H., 1981, 'An Islamic Code of Medical Ethics', *Bulletin of the Islamic Medicine*, vol.1 (Proceeding of the First International Conference on Islamic Medicine. Kuwait: Ministry of Public Health; 1981), pp.625-630; Farooqi, M.Q., 'An Ethical Code for Islamic Medical Practice', *Bulletin of the Islamic Medicine*, vol.1 (Proceeding of the First International Conference on Islamic Medicine. Kuwait: Ministry of Public Health; 1981), pp.665-671.

47.	al-Najjar, *Fi tarikh al-tib fi al-Dawlah al-Islamiya*, pp.2-53; Savage-Smith, 'Medicine', 1996, pp.903-962; Haddad, S., *History of Arab Medicine* (Beirut: Lebanon,1975).

48.	Meyerhof, M., 'Science and Medicine', in Arnold, T. and Guillaume, A. (Eds), *The Legacy of Islam* (Oxford: Oxford University Press. 1931), pp.311–55; al-Jawziyya, I.Q., *al-Tib al-Nabawi* (Medicine of the Prophet) (al-Qahira: Dar Ihya' al-kutub al-'Arabiyya (Arabic), 1957).

49.	Abu-Rabia, A., 'Breastfeeding Practices among Pastoral Tribes in the Middle East', *Anthropology of the Middle East*, 2007, (2), 2, pp.38–54; Coulson, N.J., *Succession in the Muslim Family* (Cambridge: Cambridge University Press, 1971), pp.238-242; al-Sarakhsi, M.A., *Kitab al-Mabsut li-Shams al-Din al-Sarakhsi* (Beirut: Dar el-Ma'refah (Arabic), 1993); Abu-Rabia, 'Breastfeeding Practices among Pastoral Tribes in the Middle East', pp. 38–54; al-Said, *Medicine in Islam*, 1997, pp.695-98.

50. Ghaly, M., 'Prophetic Medicine: Muhammad in History, Thought and Culture' in *An Encyclopedia of the Prophet of God* (San Francisco, CA: , Academia.edu, 2016), pp.502-506; Rispler-Chaim, V., 'Egyptian Fatwas on Medical Matters: A Dialogue between Religion and Science', in Ilan, N. (Ed.), *The Intertwined Worlds of Islam* (Jerusalem: Ben Zvi, 2002), pp.493-512.

51. Abu-Rabia, A., 'Key Plants in Fighting Cancer in the Middle East', *Chinese Medicine*, 2015b 6, pp.124-135.

52. Ghaly, 'Prophetic Medicine: Muhammad in History, Thoughts, and Culture', pp.502-506.

53. Ibid., pp.502-506.

54. Levey, M., *Medical Ethics of Medieval Islam, with Special Reference to al-Ruhāwī's Practical Ethics of the Physician* (Philadelphia: The American Philosophical Society, 1967); Al-Ruhawi, I.A., *Adab al-tabib* (Ethics of the Physician) (Arabic), 1992); Abd al-Hamid, M., *al-Adab al-Tibbi wa-Adab al-Tabib* (Cairo: Najib Metri, (Arabic), 1927).

55. For more detail about treating by spirituality in Western medicine, see Koenig, H., *Spirituality in Patient Care, Why, how, When and What* (Philadelphia and London: Templeton Foundation Press, 2002); Koenig, H., McCullough, M. and Larson, D., *Handbook of Religion and Health* (New York: Oxford University Press, 2001).

56. Ghaly, *Prophetic Medicine; Muhammad in History, Thoughts, and Culture*, pp.502-506; Basha, H.S., *Al-Tibb al-Nabawi Bayna al-'Ilm wa al-'Ijaz* (Damascus: Dar al-Qalam (Arabic), 2008).

57. See Levey, M., *Early Arabic Pharmacology: An Introduction Based on Ancient and Medieval Sources* (Leiden: Brill, 1973).

58. al-Shatti, *al-'Arab wal-tibb*, 1970, pp.5-10; Burgel, C., 'Secular and Religious Features of Medical Arabic Medicine' in: Leslie, C. (Ed.), *Asian Medical Systems* (Berkeley: University of California Press, 1976), pp.44–62; Meyerhof, M., 'Science and Medicine' in Arnold, T. and Guillaume, A. (Eds), *The Legacy of Islam* (Oxford: Oxford University Press, 1931), pp.311–55.

5

The History of Military Medicine in the Holy Land

Eran Dolev

Introduction

Battles and wars have been an essential part of human history from the earliest time. For various national groups, battles have been the origin of myths and the source of pride, while for others the interpretation of the same events has been the origin of a sense of failure. Battles may be classified according to arenas, goals, magnitude, weaponry, tactics, etc. Yet one thing has been common to all military conflicts: they have always been the source of pain, injuries, crippling and death. In order to deal with this inevitable problem, as well as for the morale of the troops, medical services were introduced into military organisations as early as during antiquity.[1]

Military medicine is a unique discipline of the medical profession. While most other fields of medicine include diagnosis and treatment, integrated in basic sciences, military medicine also includes aspects of preventative medicine and organisation, mainly echeloning and medical evacuation. Military medicine is also involved in the research of effort physiology. It should be remembered that while doctors in general are committed only to their patients, military doctors are also committed to the organisation and to its missions.[2] This commitment, both to the patient and to the military organisation, defines the doctor as a 'medical officer'.

Military medicine is practised by doctors who are expected to be aware of any recent professional developments, in order to be able to prevent diseases among the troops and to save lives at the battlefield. On the other hand, due to harsh conditions in which military units have been functioning, medical officers have been those who contributed to the advancement of various aspects of preventative medicine.[3]

This introduction serves to provide a background for the contents of this chapter. It seeks to explain the difference between treating sporadic trauma casualties in the field and having an organised medical service which practises military medicine. Another factor should also be considered: the geographical setting of the Holy Land, located between Asia and Africa, between a Southern Empire and a Northern Empire, situated at the Western edge of the 'Fertile Crescent' and adjacent to the Mediterranean Sea. The Holy Land has been an arena for countless battles. Thus, the development of military medicine can be learned through the performance of the medical services of various military organisations through the ages.

On the other hand, it should also be remembered that in most armies which fought in the Holy Land, military medicine, as has been defined above, did not exist. This review intends to discuss only those cases where military medicine did exist and has left its mark on history.[4]

Biblical Period

There is no indication whatsoever that there was a military medical organisation in any army during the Biblical period. Practising physicians were very seldom mentioned in the Bible and it was not usually in a military context.[5] Injuries inflicted unto warriors on the battlefield were seldom described in the Bible, unless they were a part of the biography or the untimely death of a king or a leader.[6] Although treatments to various injuries were described in Ancient Egypt and Mesopotamia at that period of time and most probably these practices were known in the area,[7] no medical or surgical treatment was mentioned in the Bible in the military context.[8] Also, the laws and directives established in order to maintain health and prevent diseases are dictated generally and not in a military context.[9]

HellenisticPeriod: Fourth Century BCE – First Century CE

According to the *Iliad* of Homer, written most probably during Biblical times, military physicians were already treating wounded soldiers during the Trojan War. However, there was no military medical organisation during the whole Hellenistic period.[10] Alexander the Great, when he conquered the Near East, including the Holy Land, was accompanied by physicians; but they did not form any organised service and most probably were accompanying the King himself for his needs and not for the sake of the troops.

Hippocrates (460-377 BCE) has been credited for saying 'He who would become a surgeon should join an army and follow it.'[11] However, this aphorism should not be interpreted in the context of military medicine, but rather in the context of advice to a young physician who seeks a reliable source for acquiring experience in treating trauma.

Roman Period: 70 CE – Fourth century CE

The Romans' contribution to military medicine was, for the first time, the organisation of military medical support for their army. When, during the 1st century BCE, the Romans organised their army into legions, a military medical service was also established and physicians and surgeons became an essential part of every combat unit.[12] With the expansion of the Roman Empire and the necessity to care for sick and wounded soldiers far away from Rome, military hospitals, *valetudinaria*, were constructed as a component of this system and have been excavated in various locations throughout the Roman Empire.[13]

It is very interesting to note that no such hospital has yet been found in the Holy Land. Flavius Josephus, who described in detail the structure and the organisation of the Roman Legions that fought against the Jews during the First century CE, did not mention any medical elements. Also, no surgical instruments have been found in this area.[14]

Byzantine Period: Fourth century CE – Seventh Century CE

The Byzantine Empire, the Eastern successor of the Roman Empire, ruled parts of the Near East, including the Holy Land, for a long period of time. Thus, its influence on various facets of life in this area was significant. Roman legacy was kept very strictly by the Byzantines and the military organisation was one of the fields which remained unchanged for a long time. However, developments in both military science, and especially Nestorian and Islamic medicine, could not be ignored and penetrated even the rigid Byzantine tradition. One of the outcomes was that the Byzantine army had the best medical service during the Middle Ages.[15]

The Christian Byzantine Empire was surrounded by several Muslim territories which were always superior to it in manpower and did not miss any opportunity to capture territories from the Empire. This permanent threat forced the Byzantines to find some creative solutions in order to maintain its manpower and to use it in the most efficient way. First of all, it influenced the rulers' attitude towards their troops and Emperor Leo's (886-912) treatise on military science may serve as an example:

> Give all the care you possibly can to your wounded, for if you neglect them, you will make your soldiers timorous and cowardly before a battle, and, not only that, but your personnel whom you might preserve and retain by proper consideration for their health and welfare, will be otherwise lost to you through your own negligence.[16]

Another solution found by the Byzantines was the establishment of military hospitals in various parts of the Empire, including in the Holy Land. These hospitals were founded as early as the Fourth century CE and served both military and civilian populations.[17] These military hospitals did not serve the legions in the field as the Roman *valetudinaria* had before. The noteworthy fact about Byzantine military hospitals is that they served as a prototype for the hospitals of the Crusaders' Kingdom of Jerusalem. These, in turn, served as a template for the hospitals established in Europe from the thirteenth century onwards.

Muslim Period (634 – 1099)

We are not aware of any information considering medical support to Muslim forces during the conquest of the Middle East. However, one episode during the campaign in the Holy Land deserves a special mention: it was during 639 CE, after the Rashidun army, under the command of Abu Ubaidah Ibn al Jarrah, captured Jerusalem and camped at Emmaus. During April, the army was struck by outbreaks of plague and many soldiers died. The Caliph Umar was worried about Abu Ubaidah, whom he considered as his future successor, and wanted to save him from the disease. Thus, the Caliph wrote him a letter in which he told him that he needed him urgently. In his letter the Caliph told Abu Ubaidah to leave his command immediately and to join him. When Abu Ubaidah received the Caliph's letter, he immediately understood his aim and responded:

> I know that you need me; but I am in an army of Muslims and I have no desire to save myself from what is afflicting them. I do not want to separate from them until God wills. Please release me from your command and permit me to stay on with my troops.

He ended his letter to the Caliph by saying:

> If you hear the news of an outbreak of an epidemic at a certain place, do not enter that place, and if the epidemic falls in a place while you present in it, do not leave that place to escape from the epidemic.[18]

This story of the total commitment of a commander to his troops, might be key to understanding the future attitude of Islam towards the obligation of leaders to their communities during epidemics.

Crusader Period (1099 - 1291)

The Crusades are among the most exciting adventures in Western history, although they encouraged sometimes devastating violence against Jewish communities as the Crusaders crossed Europe. Inspired by Pope Urban II at the Council of Clermont on 27 November 1095, thousands of Europeans made their way to the East to liberate the Holy Land from the reign of Islam. Jerusalem was captured by the Crusaders on 15 July 1099. A short time later they established the Crusaders' Kingdom of Jerusalem in the Holy Land. It ruled the country, or parts of it, for almost two centuries until the fall of Acre in 1291. During this epoch, the Europeans who lived 'beyond the sea' or as they were called 'the Latins' or 'the Franks', created a new culture which was influenced to a large extent by local traditions, customs and science.[19]

The Latins were always a minority in their own kingdom and the conquest of the Holy Land and other territories in the Middle East by the Crusaders resulted in a continuous encounter with the local heterogenous population. Considering themselves as representatives of European culture, in many instances the Latins had to accept the fact that the level of science, of culture and of knowledge was higher in the Orient than in their homeland.[20] These encounters, in peacetime as well as on various battlefields, left their mark on both societies: the European and the native. Medicine was probably the sphere in which the Latins benefited most from their contacts with the local population.[21]

The Crusaders were cautious in warfare and preferred to defend fortified positions rather than engage in open battle. Thus, siege warfare was the principal method of fighting. Yet in many military engagements they were forced to fight in the open, relying on the knights' charge and their overall war-fighting ability. Most of the castles and strongholds were well prepared for siege. Several major castles were also organised for taking care of battle casualties.[22]

The unique innovation of the Crusaders' Kingdom was the creation of the military orders. While previous monastic orders had dedicated themselves to the Church, the Knights who belonged to the military orders were ready to fight but they also took the vow 'to be a serf and a slave to our lords the sick'. This meant to care for the sick and poor regardless of race, religion or language. The first order to be founded was the Order of the Knights of St. John of Jerusalem, known later as the Hospitallers. The order was officially recognized by Pope Pascal II in 1113.[23]

The greatest achievement of the order was the establishment of a hospital in Jerusalem, where knights from the aristocracy treated any person in need with great devotion and at considerable expense. The concept of the hospital was mainly based on the Byzantine hospitals, which had been located in various places in the empire, including in the Holy Land.[24] Diagnoses were established, mainly according to the school of Salerno. Yet, medicine practised at the Crusaders' Kingdom was also influenced by Muslim and Byzantine practices.[25] European pilgrims and travellers who visited Jerusalem during the twelfth century, were amazed by the hospital of the Knights of St. John, its capacity and the professional skills of its personnel, as they had never seen such an institution anywhere in Europe.[26]

There is a lack of information pertaining to the medical support given to the Crusaders at the battlefield. It is not known if there were designated medical orderlies among the troops.[27] The extraction of arrows at the battlefield was practised, most probably, by every soldier as a part of his training for war.[28] However, a lot of information may be obtained from one of the main primary sources of this epoch, William, the Bishop of Tyre. According to William, smoke was used by the Muslims as a tactical tool, but he also noted its use as a weapon causing suffocation. William described various injuries which were inflicted by different weapons. According to William, stretchers were used for evacuation of battle casualties.[29] One also may learn quite a lot about the function of the hospital in Jerusalem at war from these accounts. For example, during the battle of Tel Gezer (Mongisard), on 25 November 1175, the Latins, although winning the battle against Salah ad-Din's (Saladin) troops, sustained heavy casualties. Seven hundred and fifty of them were evacuated from the battlefield directly to the hospital in Jerusalem within 24 hours and were treated there.[30]

By the end of the thirteenth century the Crusades period was over. Yet its influence on several aspects of European life, science and culture continued. One of these aspects was medicine, and mainly military medicine.

Napoleon Bonaparte's Military Expedition to the Holy Land (1799)

The French campaign in the Holy Land, 1799, was not only a chapter in the history of military medicine in the Holy Land. Retrospectively it might be appreciated as the first encounter of Europe and the Middle East during modern times. The ties established then have lasted to include many aspects of politics, science and culture. The goal of the French expedition to the Orient was not just the conquest of Egypt and the Holy Land. It was much more prestigious. For the French leaders in Paris, the goal was to deprive the British Empire of some of its most important assets. For young General Napoleon Bonaparte it was another step on his way to prove that he was greater than Alexander the Great.[31]

On 17 May 1798, the French military expedition under the command of General Bonaparte left Toulon harbour on its way to the Near East. It consisted of 35,000 troops, organised in combat and auxiliary units. The medical service assigned to the mission consisted of the combat units' medical officers, mobile surgical units and field hospitals. The chief medical officers of the force were chosen by Bonaparte himself: the chief physician was Rene-Nicolas Desgenettes, a veteran of previous campaigns and a famous medical scholar. The chief surgeon was Dominique-Jean Larrey, an experienced and courageous military surgeon who had distinguished himself in several campaigns and was the man who conceived the idea of the forward mobile surgical unit or the 'Flying Ambulance' ('Ambulance Volante').[32]

The French troops landed in Egypt on 1 July 1798 and during several weeks won the battles against the Mamelukes. In February 1799, after establishing a government in Egypt, Napoleon began the advance through the Sinai desert on his way to the Holy Land. The French expeditionary force included 13,000 soldiers, organised in 4 infantry divisions: cavalry, artillery and engineer units, logistic and medical units.

On 3 March 1799 the French army approached the fortified city of Jaffa. Napoleon did not intend to lay a siege on Jaffa as according to his intelligence, a combined Turkish-British assault was expected in May. If this force had joined the Ottoman force under the command of Djezaar Pasha, the governor of Acre, the enemy might be able to halt the French advance. Thus, the French expeditionary force had to capture the key city of the Holy Land, Acre, before the expected enemy's attack in order to be able to continue the march into Syria. Jaffa was captured by the French troops on 7 March after suffering 242 casualties.[33] About 3,000 defenders found

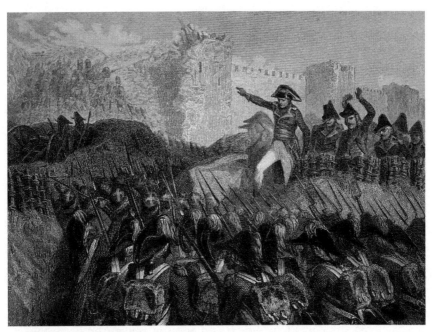

9. Napoleon: Siege of Akko (Acre), 1799.

shelter at Jaffa's citadel. During the following night the civilian population was massacred by French soldiers who were not stopped by their commanders. The next day the defenders at the citadel accepted Napoleon's terms for honourable surrender. Napoleon, who did not wish to free them as it was likely that they would join Djezaar's army in Acre but did not have the ability to hold them as prisoners of war, decided to execute all of them. If Bonaparte had expected that his inhuman act would demoralize the defenders of Acre, he was wrong. Djezaar and his allies understood that they had no choice but to fight the French expeditionary force and to destroy it.[34]

A day after the massacre in Jaffa, the medical officers of several units began to report the appearance of a contagious disease among the troops. The French had encountered this disease already during their advance in Sinai, but then they had suffered only sporadic cases.[35] The disease manifested itself by high fever and enlarged lymph nodes and most cases died of it. For the doctors it was quite easy to diagnose the disease: the giant lymph nodes were defined as buboes and the disease as Bubonic Plague. Napoleon immediately understood the demoralizing effect of the word plague upon his troops and ordered the doctors to deny the existence of this disease. In order to boost the troops' morale, he visited the hospital in a monastery in Jaffa where soldiers were dying from the disease and touched one of the dying patients' buboes with his bare hand. As nothing happened to him, the commanders could spread the rumour that the disease affecting the troops was not the dreaded plague.[36]

On 14 March the French troops began their march in the direction of Acre but the plague followed the troops. In Jaffa Bonaparte left Adjutant General Pierre Joseph Bérardierde Grezieu to run the monastery plague hospital. Twenty-four hours later Grezieu died of the plague. He was replaced by Etienne-Louise Malus who also fell ill but survived the disease.[37] The siege of Acre started on 19 March. The defending force in Acre consisted of about 7,000 soldiers, some Mamelukes who had fled from Egypt, about 2,000 armed citizens and above all a British fleet under the command of Admiral William Smith. When the French Expeditionary Force reached Acre, Chief-Surgeon Larrey ordered the establishment of a field hospital close to the besieged city. Two more hospitals were erected for convalescing patients, one at the castle of Shfar'am (Chefamer) and another one at the hermitage of Mount Carmel. A third hospital was opened at Haifa. Mobile ambulances were attached to the divisions.[38]

On 22 March Larrey wrote a circular concerning the plague epidemic, to all the doctors in the expedition:

> Citizens, I beg you to report, every fifth day, the number of sick in your respective units; The character of the prevalent disease, its progress, and the nature of its termination. This information is necessary to enable the chief officers of the surgical staff to make out such reports as are required by General Bonaparte.[39]

At the same time, the chief physician Desgenettes issued his advice concerning the matter:

> ...it is very advantageous to health to wash at frequent interval feet, hands and face with fresh water and even better to wash them with warm water, into which has been poured a few drops of vinegar or alcoholic spirit.[40]

The siege of Acre lasted about two months. The French tried again and again to use the tactics of undermining the city's walls in order to create a breach and penetrate the city but the defenders managed to anticipate these tactics, to wait for the offenders and to repel them.

During the siege Napoleon dispatched General Jean-Baptiste Kleber's division supported by other small units to establish French control in Galilee and to halt the expected army of the Pasha of Damascus who was marching on Acre.[41] In the battle of Mount Tabor, during 16 April Kleber's division, which was backed by a field ambulance, sustained about 100 casualties who were evacuated to the convent of Terra Sancta in Nazareth, which had been converted into a hospital.[42] After the failure of the assault on the walls of Acre during the night of 9 and 10 May, Napoleon decided to relieve the siege of Acre and to retreat. Later he would write to the Directory in Paris:

> The occasion seemed to favour the capture of Acre, but our spies, deserters, and our prisoners all reported that the plague was ravaging the city and that every day more than sixty persons were dying of it...If the soldiers had entered the city, they would have brought back to camp the germs of that horrible evil, which is more to be feared than all the armies in the world.[43]

The truth, of course, was quite different. The efficient, stubborn and professional defence of Acre, supported by the plague epidemic which affected the French troops, were the real causes of Napoleon' failure at Acre. According to Larrey, during the siege of Acre, the French force sustained 500 killed in action, 2,500 wounded and 700 died of plague. This totalled about a third of the whole force. Larrey reported that during the siege he performed 70 amputations, two of them were disarticulations of the hip joint, which were performed for the first time.[44]

The French troops' retreat from Acre began on 18 May, two months after they had begun to besiege the city. The retreating soldiers were carrying with them hundreds of wounded and sick soldiers. Larrey wrote in his memoirs:

> All the wounded were carried to Egypt; either during the siege or at the departure of the army: eight hundred crossed the deserts, and twelve hundred went by sea, the greater part of whom embarked at Jaffa. On either route we fortunately lost but a small number... General Bonaparte ordered that all the horses belonging to the officers, without excepting his own, should be employed in transporting the wounded, who must otherwise have been left to perish with hunger and thirst, or by the Arabs.[45]

The French troops reached Jaffa on 24 May. Hundreds of wounded soldiers were evacuated by boats to Egypt. There has been no evidence for the famous story concerning Napoleon's order to poison the victims of plague found in Jaffa. Neither Desgenettes nor Larrey, compulsive diary writers themselves and doctors who always acted according to ethical principles, mentioned the event at the time. Three days later the troops began their march to Egypt carrying with them 800 wounded and sick comrades. They reached Cairo on 23 June 1799. In retrospect, it seems that General Bonaparte did not learn much from his failure in the Holy Land. Although in most instances he backed his doctors and supported his wounded and sick troops, he would not regard health as a serious factor in his future campaigns, mainly in Haiti (1801) and Russia (1812).

The Palestine Campaigns 1916 – 1918

The Palestine Campaigns (1916-1918) were a side show in relation to the main front of the Great War in Europe. They were fought by a British Expeditionary Force against the Ottoman army in the Sinai desert, in the Holy Land and in Syria. The structure and function of the British Army medical services in the field during the Great War (1914-1918) were the outcome of two intertwined yet different processes:

a) the first was professional and reflected the advances in the fields of preventative medicine and surgery; they included vaccines given to the troops in order to avoid infectious diseases, better understanding of hypovolemic shock and hemodynamic stabilization, surgical procedures performed under anaesthesia.
b) the second was in the domain of medical organisation, based on the lessons of the Boer War in South Africa (1899-1902).

The cardinal lessons from the Boer War were the need to protect the troops from infectious diseases and the introduction of a new mobile medical unit, the field ambulance, to be used for treatment and evacuation of battle casualties at the front line. The field ambulance was a Royal Army Medical Corps (RAMC) unit which consisted of two sections: an evacuation unit which included stretcher bearers and medical evacuation carts, and a surgical unit that included treatment capabilities including operations.[46] When the Great War in Europe started, the various RAMC units acted according to these principles, which seemed appropriate at the time.

In a few months all activities at the main front drew to a stalemate: the opponent armies became entrenched and the main weaponry used from then on was artillery. Shrapnel wounds caused by artillery were different from those caused by bullets during previous battles. In many cases these injuries were extensive and infected, and demanded urgent surgical treatment. This need created a new type of surgical unit: Casualty Clearing Station [CCS]: a forward surgical unit, located not far from the combat units in which surgery of urgent cases, especially abdominal cases, could be conducted.[47]

From the commencement of war, the task of the British force in Egypt was defensive in order to protect the Suez Canal, the vital route to India and to the oil fields in Mesopotamia. Several forces were dedicated to this mission. A Turkish attempt to raid the Canal Zone in 1915 showed the British Command in Egypt that the best and most efficient way to protect the Suez Canal was by capturing the Sinai Peninsula. During 1916, British cavalry units began to penetrate Sinai. By the end of the year, the whole peninsula was occupied by British cavalry and infantry units.[48] While the troops were staying in the Sinai desert, they were free of diseases except one: Desert Sore. It seemed that any simple scratch turned into an ulcer which healed very slowly. There were two professional approaches to this disease: according to one of them, the Desert Sore was an outcome of malnutrition, probably the lack of vitamin C. According to the second opinion this condition was due to infection with Diphtheroid bacteria. The debate was still at large when the British troops entered the Holy Land and all cases of Desert Sore healed spontaneously.[49]

By January 1917, the strategy of the British was changed from mere defence of Egypt into an initiative to destroy the Ottoman armies in Palestine. The gate to Palestine was Gaza.[50] The First Battle of Gaza began on 26 March 1917. It was fought by infantry and cavalry units supported by artillery. After long hours of fighting, Gaza was almost captured by the British troops when due to misunderstandings, the commander of the British forces in the field decided to retreat. The British losses were quite heavy: 523 soldiers were killed, 2,932 wounded and 512 missing in action. Casualties were treated in the field according to the doctrine and evacuated to hospitals in Egypt.[51] The Second Battle of Gaza was launched on 17 April 1917. Again, the defenders managed to halt the British troops who, eventually withdrew from the town. The British this time sustained 6,444 casualties: 504 killed, 4,359 wounded and 1,576 missing in action.[52] As a result, both the commander of the Egyptian Expeditionary Force (EEF) and the commander of the forces in the field were dismissed.

General Edmund H.H. Allenby, the new commander of the Egyptian Expeditionary Force, came to Middle East from France, where he had been serving as the commander of the 3rd British Army at the Western Front. General Allenby had the reputation of being a tough field commander but also as one who cared for his soldiers and for their health.[53] Allenby had studied the lessons of the two previous failures at Gaza and decided that the future British assault against the Ottoman army would not be directed at the fortified town of Gaza, as expected by the enemy. This time, the target would be Beer Sheba, a remote town beyond the desert, at the Eastern side of the Turkish line. The town should be taken by surprise by the cavalry and Gaza would be the last goal of the offensive and that would begin only after massive artillery shelling, including the use of chemical shells.[54] Allenby was aware of the main limitation of his plan: lack of water for the horses and soldiers along the routes of advance. Thus, water sources were dug in the desert and an adequate water supply was carried by thousands of camels.[55]

The capture of Beer Sheba on 31 October was the start of a well-planned campaign, at the end of which the Turkish defensive line collapsed and Gaza was captured. The principles of the medical plan for this campaign were a central control of medical evacuation at the corps level and the concentration of several field hospitals and mobile surgical units at a central location in order to support all combat units efficiently. From the field hospitals casualties were further evacuated by heavy motor ambulances and by medical trains. During this offensive, known as The Third Battle of Gaza, the British forces suffered 13,099 casualties, of whom 1,346 were killed.[56] The cavalry regiments were not able to pursue the retreating Turkish units due to lack of water for the horses. This allowed the Ottoman army to reorganize quickly after the Beer Sheba-Gaza line had been lost.

From then on, the EEF advanced towards Jerusalem, the Holy City. In spite of strong Ottoman resistance, rough mountainous terrain and extremely cold weather, Jerusalem was captured on 9 December 1917, after being abandoned by the Turkish troops. The British losses from the beginning of the offensive until the fall of Jerusalem, amounted to 21,000.[57] One of the main problems of the British Force on its way to Jerusalem was the treatment and the evacuation of battle casualties. Yet official records indicate that:

> ...the medical services had also performed admirable work under heavy strain, above all the Field Ambulances of the Divisions.[58]

No doubt the mobile surgical units and the CCS's distinguished themselves as well.

Although the occupation of Jerusalem was a source of joy for the British nation, it had not been the strategic goal of the Palestine Campaigns. This had been and still remained the destruction of the Ottoman Army in the Holy Land and this objective had not yet been achieved. However, the EEF could not continue its advance for various reasons, principally because of the situation at the main front in Europe. Allenby was ordered to send all EEF's trained infantry divisions to France and they were replaced by reinforcements from Indian battalions who had no military experience and had to be trained.

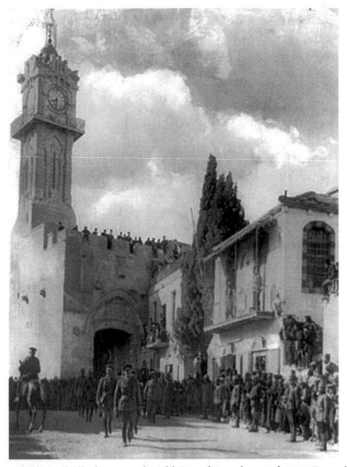

10. General Edmund Allenby enters the Old City of Jerusalem on foot, 11 December 1917.

During the spring and summer of 1918, the EEF units were engaged mainly in three issues: the training of the fresh battalions; the raids to Transjordan and the war against malaria.

The two raids did not achieve their goals; however, it allowed the EEF medical services to support the combat units with the best professional service in the field. During the first raid, the force sustained 988 casualties. Sixty-nine emergency operations were performed at the mobile operating unit near Jericho with low mortality rates.[59] In the second raid, the force suffered 1,076 casualties, 81 of them were operated on at Jericho.[60]

One of the highlights of the medical support for the second raid was the planning of an air drop of medical supplies for units in need. When during the raid a cavalry unit was surrounded by the enemy, sustaining many casualties, airplanes dropped them the needed medical supplies.[61] During the time between the capture of Jerusalem and the last phase of the war, the British forces were concentrated mainly in the Jordan Valley and in the Sharon Valley north of Jaffa. These two areas were heavily infested with anopheles mosquitoes, the transmitters of malaria. General Allenby was aware of the risk of malaria to his troops and saw the fight against the disease as a campaign that should be won. He was one of the very few generals in the history of wars who understood the risks of a disease to the health of the troops and gave full support to the medical services. About a quarter of a million man-days were invested by the EEF soldiers in this campaign which succeeded in diminishing the rates of sickness among the troops.[62]

The last phase of the Palestine Campaigns was the Battle of Megiddo; its goal was the destruction of the VIIth and VIIIth Turkish armies in the Holy Land and the IVth army in Transjordan. Early on 19 September 1918, the XXIst Corps, consisting of five infantry divisions, attacked and destroyed the Turkish line north of the Yarkon River. This allowed the cavalry divisions to break through and to cut Ottoman Army communications as well as destroying the Turkish disorganized retreating units.[63] Ten days after the British attack on the Ottoman fortified line, the cavalry divisions reached the gates of Damascus. On its way, the EEF units destroyed the Ottoman armies on both sides of river Jordan. The actual number of British battle casualties were much less than had been estimated. General Allenby could comment: 'Such a complete victory has seldom been known in all the history of war.'[64]

At Damascus, the British troops found thousands of injured and sick Turkish soldiers who had been abandoned and were in urgent need for medical treatment. It was one of the finest hours of the EEF medical services: its people created medical facilities where they were treating Ottoman soldiers, who became prisoners of war.[65] During the first days of October 1918, Damascus looked like an apocalyptic site as thousands of patients, British and Turkish, were in need of medical treatment due to malaria and typhoid. At the same time another fatal disease reached the area: the Spanish Flu.[66] While Lebanon and Syria were captured by the infantry divisions who marched along the Mediterranean coast, most of the cavalry regiments were stuck in Damascus area due to disease. The only cavalry unit that could continue to advance and to fight the enemy was the 5th Cavalry Division. It pursued the retreating Turkish army, or what had remained of it, up to the Turkish border and the end of the Great War.

At the same time a new epidemic was detected among the Turkish prisoners of war: it was pellagra, a lethal disease whose causes were not identified at that time, but are now known to be a deficiency of the vitamin niacin. It was General Allenby who ordered his Surgeon General, Richard H. Luce, to nominate a Committee of Enquiry in order to reveal the nature of this mysterious disease. Allenby thought that if this epidemic had been contagious, it might hit the British as well. The Committee set to work and found that the cause of pellagra was malnutrition. The committee's work was also highly appreciated by the medical profession:

> The report of the Committee of Enquiry regarding the prevalence of pellagra among Turkish prisoners of war will stand for years to come as a record of one of the best and most scientific inquiries ever accomplished by a nation at war.[67]

In the history of military medicine, the Palestine Campaigns would be always remembered as a rare example of cooperation between commanders and the medical services, guided by a unique commander, General Allenby, who felt responsible for his troops' health.

The Israeli Wars

a) Israel's War of Independence

The Israeli War of Independence started when the Arab States attacked Israel, just after its Declaration of Independence on the 14 May 1948. For the new-born Israel, the imposed war was not a surprise: it was the expected and feared peak of a process tracing back to the many riots, and other events, in which Arabs attacked Jews in various communities around the country. In 1948 these events escalated into an organised war, waged by national armies. The Jewish community, of about 600,000 people, did not yet have a formal military organisation. Its resistance was based on former clandestine organisations, which had acquired some tactical abilities. Most of its military skills were held by Israelis who had volunteered in the British Army during the Second World War.

At the start of the war there was no military medical service and the semi-military organisation, already engaged in fighting, relied on the civilian emergency services, Magen David Adom, MDA, and the civilian services of the Sick Funds. The war affected the Jewish population of Israel significantly as about 6,000 people were killed in the war,1 per cent of the population, around 5,000 of whom were soldiers.[68]

The Israeli combat units were quite small: usually they never exceeded the size of a company or a battalion. Thus, in many units there was no doctor but only medical orderlies. During the war a medical service was established. It recruited physicians who joined the combat units, giving an adequate medical service for most of the soldiers in the field. At the same time the medical service established thirteen military hospitals: several of them, mainly at the Southern and at the Northern fronts, were field hospitals. Others were military base hospitals.

After the War of Independence

During the first years after the war, the military medical service, which had been founded in an *ad hoc* fashion during the war, was replaced by a professional medical corps. The difference between a 'medical service' and a 'medical corps' is fundamental: while a service is engaged in giving appropriate medical treatment to the troops, the medical corps is an integral part of the military organisation. The theoretical roots of the Israeli Defence Forces Medical Corps (IDF MC) were based on the British RAMC experience and tradition. Thus, the MC became responsible for the training of all professionals in service and for the various aspects of organisation, promotion, preventative medicine, etc. Above all, it became responsible for maintaining a proper level of medical readiness and preparedness of the army.

One of the cardinal decisions of that time was the closure of all military hospitals: it was decided that in a state with a small population as Israel was at the time, there was no justification for two systems of hospitalization and that the civilian hospitals would serve also the military population.[69] The impact of that decision was very important: from then on, the Medical Corps' responsibility was only for the troops in the field. During the 1950s, many retaliation actions were taken by Israel against infiltrators who crossed the border and killed and wounded civilians. All units participating in these activities were supported by medical units headed by a doctor. They acquired a lot of combat experience and influenced to a large extent the design of future medical equipment to be used in war. The Medical Corps also became involved in research relevant to the performance of the soldier in the field. The peak of the research at that time was the understanding of water metabolism and performance under harsh climatic conditions. The outcome was the elimination of 'the water restriction regime' which had cost several lives.[70]

During the early 1950s, the 'infiltration' into Israel became more and more organised and caused many casualties and much damage. This hostile activity was backed mainly by Egypt and the retaliation acts of Israel did not affect it. Thus, on 29 October 1956, Israeli forces penetrated the Sinai Peninsula in a military operation to be called the Sinai Campaign, defeated the Egyptian Army and reached the vicinity of the Suez Canal in coordination with British and French forces who attacked the Canal Zone. The destruction of the Egyptian Army was achieved by fast-advancing armoured forces. It was also the first, and the last time, that an airborne battalion was dropped behind the enemy's lines. The elaborate operative scenario challenged the medical corps to a large extent: the detached airborne units were supported by airborne medical teams who treated battle casualties at the front line and managed to evacuate them to rear medical echelons. The armoured units were supported by medical units which could keep pace with the combat units in order to treat casualties at the battlefield.

The Sinai Campaign lasted for eight days. During the operation, 172 soldiers were killed and 817 were wounded. The lessons of the medical corps from this short, yet vigorous, campaign were mainly in the field of organization: from now on, a medical platoon would be an essential component of every battalion and every brigade would include a medical company.

b) The Six-Day War 1967

The *casus belli* for this war was the Egyptian blockade of the Red Sea straits of Israeli vessels. Egypt was joined by Syria and later by Jordan. After three weeks of recruitment of all the reserve units and preparation for war, and the failure of the international community to resolve the issues, Israel attacked. The result was that the Egyptian army was annihilated in four days, the Sinai Peninsula was captured and Israeli forces reached the Suez

Canal. The Kingdom of Jordan lost the areas west of the River Jordan, the West Bank, and Syria lost the Golan Heights. During the War 779 soldiers were killed and 2,593 were injured. Most battle casualties were treated by the medical services in the field. The Israeli Air Force maintained air superiority throughout the war and the civilian population was not threatened. It allowed the various medical echelons supporting combat units, to evacuate battle casualties from the front line directly to rear hospitals by ambulances and helicopters. As a result, field hospitals became redundant.[71]

As an outcome of the Six-Day War, the Israeli Army started to reorganise itself in armoured divisions. Every armoured division was composed of three armoured brigades, an artillery group and a logistic group which included a medical battalion consisting of the medical companies who had been withdrawn from the brigades. As field hospitals were seen to be obsolete they were disbanded, and their surgical teams were incorporated into a surgical company included in the medical battalion.

The War of Attrition

At the end of the Six-Day War, the Israeli Army found itself outstretched from the Suez Canal, through the West Bank to Mount Hermon at the northern edge of the Golan Heights. In Sinai, army units were posted along the eastern bank of the Suez Canal. Egypt could not tolerate the new situation and Egyptian artillery began to shell the Israeli units located on the eastern bank of the Canal. In order to protect the soldiers in these posts and also to hold a line along the canal, 30 strongholds were built along the Suez Canal.

It is difficult to define the exact date when the War of Attrition began, as sporadic Egyptian artillery shelling started soon after the Six-Day War. However, it was declared over on 7 August 1970, due to an agreement between Egypt and Israel. The constant Egyptian artillery shelling of the strongholds inflicted many casualties on the Israeli troops. These injured soldiers received proper medical treatment at the strongholds, as at every such post a doctor was always present. However, many casualties required more definitive professional treatment, including major surgery and had to be urgently evacuated to a hospital.

Two problems were soon identified. First, evacuation of casualties from the front line was at most times under fire, so casualties were evacuated from the stronghold either in an armoured carrier and later in special tanks designed for medical evacuation. Such carriers would evacuate casualties to a close and relatively safe spot where a helicopter could land and further evacuate them to the rear. According to the Israeli medical doctrine, air evacuation of a casualty is a medical process and not just transportation. This required the presence of a doctor on the helicopter assigned for medical evacuation. Secondly, the distance from the Sinai front line was very far from civilian hospitals in Israel and time was often a crucial factor in the prognosis of casualties. The solution was the establishment of a Field Hospital in the middle of the Sinai desert, sited near an airstrip and beyond enemy artillery range. The hospital consisted of an operating theatre, a small laboratory and a blood bank service. Its personnel consisted of reserve surgeons, anaesthesiologists and nurses who were summoned regularly for active reserve duty. Such teams always maintained the hospital preparedness. The toll of the War of Attrition in Sinai was 367 killed and 999 injured. Most of the casualties got initial treatment at a stronghold, or in the field, and were evacuated to the field hospital in the Sinai desert. Later they were evacuated by regular airplanes to hospitals in Israel.[72]

The 1973 October (Yom Kippur) War

On 6 October 1973, the Jewish Day of Atonement, Egypt and Syria began a coordinated war against Israel. Although Israel had been surprised initially, eighteen days later the war was over after an Israeli victory. The strategic surprise cost Israel a high price. During the war 6,409 battle casualties were treated by the Israeli military medical services and 2,653 were injured in action and died of their wounds. However, for the Israeli Medical Corps it was one of the peaks of their performance.

During the first phase of the war, at the Southern front, all the strongholds along the Suez Canal, but one, were captured by Egyptian troops who had crossed the canal. The soldiers in these posts were either killed or taken as prisoners of war. Many of them were wounded. Most of the casualties, who during these days were treated by the various medical echelons at the front, belonged mainly to units which attempted to rescue their comrades from the strongholds. During the second phase of the war, most of the casualties were inflicted either by Egyptian artillery or during battle engagements in the field. Most of these engagements were between armoured units and, typical to armoured warfare, about 10 per cent of the casualties sustained burns.

Battle casualties were treated first at the front line, either by themselves or by a comrade and then treated by the medical echelon at the unit level. From there, injured soldiers were evacuated, either by ambulances, armoured personnel carriers or helicopters to the main Field Hospital at the centre of Sinai, which had been established during the War of Attrition. The Sinai Field Hospital operated as an Evacuation Hospital with its main task being to assess casualties, redress their wounds, to stabilise their hemodynamic status and to perform resuscitation when it was necessary. Most of the casualties admitted to the hospital were then evacuated by air to hospitals in Israel. Out of about 4,000 cases passing through the hospital during 18 days of active fighting, only 51 needed urgent life-saving major surgery.[73]

The professional innovation in the work of the Sinai evacuation hospital located behind the southern front, was in post-operative care. Since the First World War it had been the rule that soldiers who had undergone surgery, especially the post-laparotomy cases, should be held at the hospital for at least a week. In Sinai in 1973, the post-operative cases were evacuated by air to hospitals in less than 24 hours after surgery and no complications were noted. Early post-operative evacuation allowed the Field Hospital to always be ready for new casualties and not be overwhelmed by them.[74]

The First Lebanon War, 1982

This war was initiated by Israel against terrorist organisations based in Southern Lebanon. The active phase of the war took place from 5 June to 28 July 1982, but the involvement of Israel in Southern Lebanon lasted for a much longer period of time. During the active fighting about 1,500 soldiers were injured and 670 more were killed. This war was different from previous Israeli military conflicts. While most of the former battles had been fought by armoured units in the open, the Lebanese arena was characterised by mountainous terrain and built-up areas. Both battlegrounds were not the usual arenas for armoured troops, and it was the infantry who fought the enemy in most encounters. This manifested itself by the types of injuries which were inflicted upon the combat units: only 3.9 per cent of the casualties suffered from burns as compared to almost 10% during the 1973 war; 11.6% of the casualties were hit by bullets and 2.3% suffered from blast injuries.[75]

Military medicine during the Lebanon War, 1982 manifested itself mainly in three areas:

1) Finding solutions for the treatment and evacuation of injured soldiers during the most complicated and demanding form of fighting: military operations in urbanised terrain. One of the innovations was the evacuation of casualties from the combat zone in tanks, dedicated to

this mission where 85% of injured soldiers were evacuated by air from the front line, most of them in less than an hour.

2) The Israeli troops fighting against terrorists inside towns and villages were exposed to demolition charges and to the blowing up of buildings. Under these circumstances the medical services had to take care of casualties who suffered from multiple injuries and cases of the Crush Syndrome, traumatic rhabdomyolysis. This syndrome is the outcome of skeletal muscle injury, and the resultant release of muscle cell contents into the blood stream. The collapse of a building due to an explosion causes immediate death among the majority of the victims due to the blast effect causing severe damage to vital organs. The survivors whose extremities are pinned under heavy rubble are the ones at risk of developing the syndrome and are candidates to develop acute renal failure after being extricated from under debris. A simple method of treatment, involving early and massive volume replacement on site, followed by forced alkaline solute diuresis, was developed in Israel and was given to those who had been trapped under rubble and was found to be very effective.[76]

3) It was estimated that the civilian hospital of Upper Galilee, the main hospital close to the Lebanese front, might be overwhelmed by battle casualties. In the worst scenario, when it may also admit civilian casualties, it might be unable to cope with the situation. It was planned, for the first time, to augment the hospital with a reserve military surgical unit. This was a unique unit which consisted of veterans of the evacuation hospital of Sinai, who had acquired a lot of military medical experience during the 1973 War. As the war started, the unit augmented the hospital. The integration between these two different bodies was successful.[77]

Conclusion

It seems that the Holy Land has seen too much war and suffering. Although it has contributed much to the development of military medicine, we should hope that the future of this country will be different; or in the prophet's words, 'Nation shall not lift up sword against nation, neither shall they learn war any more.'[78]

Notes

1. Garrison, F.H., *Notes on the History of Military Medicine* (Washington D.C.: Association of Military Surgeons, 1922), pp.1-3.

2. Dolev, E. and Llewellyn, C.H., 'The Chain of Medical Responsibility in Battlefield Medicine', *Military Medicine*, 1985, 150, pp.471-75.

3. Ibid.

4. Michaeli, D., 'Medicine on the Battlefield', *Journal of the Royal Society of Medicine*, 1979, 72, pp.370-72.

5. *Book of Chronicles II*, Chapter16, verse 12.

6. Dolev, E. and Nerubay, J., 'Battle Wounds in the Bible', *Korot: Israel Journal of the History of Medicine and Science*, 1982, 8, pp.35-37; *Book of Samuel II*, Chapter 2, verse 23; *Book of Kings I*, Chapter 22, verses 34-35; *Book of Kings II,* Chapter 9, verse 24.

7. Majno, G., *The Healing Hand* (Cambridge MA: Harvard University Press, 1975), pp. 90-111.

8. *Book of Isaiah*, Chapter 1, verse 6.

9. Kottek, S.S., 'Hygiene and Health Care in the Bible', in Wasermann, M. and Kottek, S.S. (Eds), *Health and Disease in, the Holy Land* (Lewiston NY: The Edwin Mellen Press, 1996), pp.37-68.

10. Garrison, *Notes on the History of Military Medicine*, pp.42-46.

11. Hippocrates as cited by Connell, C., 'War's Medical Legacy', *Stanford Medicine Magazine*, summer 2007 (Loeb Classical Library, no. 482).

12. Garrison, *Notes on the History of Military Medicine*, pp.62-67.

13. Majno, *The Healing Hand,* pp. 381-92.

14. Rimon, O., 'Surgical Instruments from the Roman Period' in Rimon, O. (Ed.), *Illness and Healing in Ancient Times* (University of Haifa, 1996), pp.17-21.

15. Garrison, *Notes on the History of Military Medicine,* pp.79-81.

16. Leo, *Tactica* (Leiden: Epilogue, 1612), p. 381, cited by Garrison, *Notes on the History of Military Medicine*, p.80.

17. Miller, T.S., 'Byzantine Hospitals' in Scarborough, J. (Ed.), *Symposium on Byzantine Medicine* (Dumbarton Oaks Papers no. 38, DO Publication Office, Washington DC, 1984). pp.53-63.

18. Dols, M.W., *The Black Death in the Middle East* (Princeton University Press, 1977), pp.21-23.

19. Dolev, E., 'Medicine in the Crusaders' Kingdom of Jerusalem' in Wasermann and Kottek, *Health and Disease in the Holy Land*, pp.157-172.

20. Ibid., pp.157-172.

21. Ibid.; Dolev, E. and Knoller, N., 'Military Medicine in the Crusaders' Kingdom of Jerusalem', *Israel Medical Association Journal*, 2001, 3, pp.389-92.

22. Ibid.

23. Dolev, 'Medicine in the Crusaders' Kingdom of Jerusalem', pp.157-172; Hume, E.E., *Medical Work of the Knights Hospitallers of Saint John of Jerusalem* (Baltimore: Johns Hopkins University Press, 1940), pp.4-8.

24. Miller, T.S., 'The Knights of St John and the hospitals of the Latin West', *Speculum*, 1978, 53, pp.709-33.

25. Delaville Le Roulx, J., *Cartulaire Generala de l'ordredes Hospitallers de S W, Jean De Jerusalem*, 1100-1310 (4 vols, Paris, 1894-1906).

26. Dolev, 'Medicine in the Crusaders' Kingdom of Jerusalem', pp.157-172.

27. Ibid.

28. Mitchell, P.D., *Medicine in the Crusades* (Cambridge: Cambridge University Press, 2004), pp.178-180.

29. William of Tyre, *A History of Deeds Done Beyond the Sea*, Ed. and trans. by Babcock, E.A. and Krey, A.C. (New York: Columbia University Press, 1943): Book III, 16, 17. Book IV, 17. Book VI, 2, 10. Book X, 8, 26, 28, Book XI, 31. Book XII, 31. Book XIV, 3. Book XV, 27. Book XVIII, 17, 25.

30. Dolev and Knoller, 'Military medicine in the Crusaders' Kingdom of Jerusalem', pp.389-92; Hume, *Medical Work of the Knights Hospitallers of Saint John of Jerusalem*, pp.4-8.

31. Strathern, P., *Napoleon in Egypt* (London: Vintage Books, 2008), pp.314-15.

32. Richardson, R.G., *Larrey:* Surgeon *to Napoleon's Imperial Guard* (London: John Murray, 1974), pp.32-38.

33. Larrey, D.J., *Memoirs of Military Surgery and Campaigns of the French Armies*, vol. I: 'Campaigns in Egypt and Syria', Trans. by Hall, R.W. (Baltimore: Joseph Cushing, 1814); The Classics of Surgery Library, Birmingham, Alabama, 1985, p.163.

34. Herold, J.C., *Bonaparte in Egypt* (London: Readers Union/ Hamish Hamilton, 1964), pp.273-80.

35. Ibid.

36. Ibid.

37. Strathern, *Napoleon in Egypt*, p.331.

38. Larrey, *Memoirs of Military Surgery and Campaigns of the French Armies*, p.167.

39. Richardson, *Larrey:, Surgeon to Napoleon's Imperial Guard*, p.64.

40. Strathern, *Napoleon in Egypt*, p.345.

41. Herold, *Bonaparte in Egypt*, p.292.

42. Larrey, *Memoirs of Military Surgery and Campaigns of the French Armies*, p.172.

43. *Napoleon's Correspondence*, vol. V, p. 440 (cited by Herold, *Bonaparte in Egypt*, p.307).

44. Larrey, *Memoirs of Military Surgery and Campaigns of the French Armies*, pp.174-5.

45. Ibid., p.178.

46. Dolev, E., *Allenby's Military Medicine* (London: I.B. Tauris, 2007), pp.5-11.

47. Ibid., pp. 12-13.

48. Wavell, A.P., *The Palestine Campaigns* (London: Constable, 3rd edn., 1933), pp.38-51.

49. Dolev, *Allenby's Military Medicine*, p. 33.

50. Wavell, *The Palestine Campaigns*, p.67.

51. Dolev, *Allenby's Military Medicine*, p.34.

52. Ibid., p. 38.

53. Ibid., pp.52-54.

54. Ibid.

55. Wavell, *The Palestine Campaigns*, pp.101-108.

56. Dolev, *Allenby's Military Medicine*, pp.63-69.

57. Ibid., p.105.

58. Falls, C., 'Military Operations, Egypt and Palestine: from June 1917 to the End of the War' in *History of the Great War Based on Official Documents* vol.I (London: HMSO, 1930), p.264.

59. Dolev, *Allenby's Military Medicine*, p.117.

60. Ibid., p.127.

61. Ibid., pp.126-127.

62. Dolev, E., 'I am Campaigning against Malaria', *Korot: Israel Journal of the History of Medicine and Science*, 2011-12, 21, pp.75-88; Pirie-Gordon, H., *A brief record of the*

advance of the EEF under the command of General Sir Edmund H H Allenby, July 1917 to October 1918 (London: HMSO, 1919), pp.104-105.

63. Wavell, *The Palestine Campaigns*, pp.203-208.

64. Allenby's letter to the troops 26 September 1918, cited by Dolev, *Allenby's Military Medicine*, p. 159.

65. Dolev, *Allenby's Military Medicine*, pp.161-64.

66. Ibid., p.167.

67. Ibid., pp.173-175.

68. Hurwich, B., *'The Fifth Front': the Israeli Soldier: Military Medicine in Israel. Volume II: The War of Independence 1947-1949* (Ministry of Defence, 2000), pp.398-400 (Hebrew).

69. Nadav, D., *White and Khaki: The History of the Israel Medical Corps 1949-1967* (Ministry of Defence, 2000), pp. 36-39 (Hebrew).

70. Sohar, E., Michaeli, D., Waks, U. and Shibolet, S., 'Heatstroke caused by Dehydration and Physical Effort', *Archives of Internal Medicine*, 1968, 122, pp.159-61.

71. Dagan, D., 'Six Days of War', *Journal of Israeli Military Medicine*, 2017, 14, pp.5-6 (Hebrew).

72. Gimmon, Z. and Adler, J., 'Medical Support during the Sinai War of Attrition (1968-1970) from a 30-year Perspective', *Harefuah*, 2000, 138, pp.74-75 (Hebrew).

73. Pfeffermann, R., Rozin, R.R., Durst, A.L. and Marin, G., 'Modern War Surgery: Operations in an Evacuation Hospital during the October 1973 Arab-Israeli War', *Journal of Trauma*, 1976, 16, pp.694-703.

74. Rozin, R., Klausner, J.M and Dolev, E., 'New concepts of forward combat surgery', *Injury*, 1988, 19, pp.193-97; Dolev, E., 'Early Evacuation of Patients from the Battlefield after Laparotomy: Experiences in Vietnam, Israel and the Falklands', *Military Medicine*, 1987, 152, pp.57-59.

75. Dolev, E., 'Medical Services in the Lebanon War, 1982: an Overview', *Israel Journal of Medical Science*, 1984, 20, pp.297-99; Dannon, Y.L., Nili, E. and Dolev, E., 'Primary Treatment of Battle Casualties in the Lebanon War, 1982', *Israel Journal of Medical Science*, 1984, 20, pp.300-302; Gasko, O.D., 'Surgery in the field during the Lebanon War, 1982: Doctrine, Experience and Prospects for Future Changes', *Israel Journal of Medical Science* 1984; 20, pp.350-354.

76. Better, O.S., 'Rescue and Salvage of Casualties Suffering from the Crush Syndrome after Mass Disasters', *Military Medicine*, 1999, 164, pp.366-69; Michaelson, M., Taitelman, U., Bshouty, Z., Bar-Joseph. J. and Bursztein, S., 'Crush Syndrome: experience from the Lebanon War, 1982', *Israel Journal of Medical Science*, 1984, 20, pp.305-307.

77. Rozin , R., 'Integration of Military Unit and Civilian Hospital during Mass Casualty Situation: Experience during the 1982 Lebanon War', *Military Medicine*, 1986, 151, pp.580-82.

78. The *Book of Isaiah*, Chapter 2, verse 4.

6

Health and Medical Services in Ottoman Eretz Israel

Miri Shefer-Mossensohn

[Author's note: To make the article accessible for English readers who are not familiar with Ottoman Turkish and Arabic, historical terms and names have been transliterated into a modified Latin alphabet and under-dots on consonants and macrons on vowels have been eliminated. This article is a revision and an update of my 'Communicable Disease in Ottoman Palestine: Local Thoughts and Actions', Korot, 21 (2011-2012), pp.19-49.]

Health and medical services in Ottoman Eretz Israel (1517-1917) were varied and very complex. Scholars who have investigated this topic based on Jewish and European sources commonly claim that prior to the nineteenth century and the advent of western medicine into the Middle East, no real understanding of diseases existed; hence no treatment schemes were enacted, nor was the will to prevent or treat even present. Instead, fatalism was the norm. Many European observers – and in the nineteenth century Americans as well – viewed Ottoman Eretz Israel as backward, dirty and unhealthy.[1]

Local Arabic and Ottoman sources, however, provide an impression of the inhabitants of this Ottoman province as active players in the realm of health and medicine. These sources are chronicles, accounts of Ottomans passing in the region, the Sultan's decrees, and biographical dictionaries that preserve the memory of noted dignitaries of the time.

An especially invaluable material is the *sijills* (records or protocols from the Muslim court) given this unique function of the Ottoman qadi (Muslim judge) as an Ottoman official. He acted as the mayor in charge of municipal planning, maintenance, social welfare and hygiene; a notary; the police commissioner; and a part-time purser for the Ottoman government. Until the nineteenth century the qadi court was the main urban-civil institution in Jerusalem. The outcome, in Jerusalem for example, is nearly 600 leather-bound volumes that cover the court registers of the sixteenth through to the nineteenth centuries. The entries were written in Arabic, with Ottoman-Turkish reserved for copies of the Sultan's writs, and cover all sections in the Jerusalem population, including many non-Muslims and villages around Jerusalem who were routinely recorded as settling their affairs before the Muslim judge in town.[2]

The paper trail from the imperial bureaucracy is another most valuable source used here, as the local courts were in constant dialogue with the central administration. The Ottoman Empire produced a massive paper archive recording its administrative activities, now at the Ottoman Prime Ministry Archives (Başbakanlık Osmanlı Arşivi [BOA]) in Istanbul. During the early modern period a major source was the imperial orders from the mühimme defterlei (literally: Registers of Important Affairs), which is copies of orders issued to Ottoman officers throughout the provinces. These orders were presented as personal responses of the Sultan to petitions or reports from a certain locale and outline a policy to be followed.[3] During the nineteenth century the organization of the central bureaucracy changed. Now the administrative, diplomatic and military concerns of the imperial centre regarding Palestine were dealt with by various specializing ministries.

This is not to say Ottoman and Arabic sources did not see the piles of dirt, ruined buildings and carcasses of dead animals, smell sewage flowing in the streets, or experience scarcity of water in summer that outsiders observed. However, Arabic and Ottoman sources reveal locals devoted time and thinking to understanding disease and took actions to ward off illness. From their standpoint, they certainly did not neglect their health. The medical successes may have been mediocre, but not different or worse than the medical standard that existed elsewhere. Language barriers prevented many scholars from accessing these local sources.

A number of factors have led to a difference between the images that appear from the various sources. Arabic and Ottoman sources relate a medical course of action, which was a health regime that carried its logic to locals, even when outsiders could not follow its rationality. European observers' accounts were interpretations of reality and not necessarily a documentation thereof. On top of literary forms and norms that the writers had to comply with, they were torn between conflicting emotions. The authors, both Jews and Christians, were conditioned by religious sentiment and longing for the biblical past. They had misconceptions about the 'Orient' generated by Biblical lore, Crusader myths and the reality of early modern Ottoman-European encounters. The outcome is conflicting images of either a romanticized Holy Land or a disappointed look at a backward and barbarous terrain.[4]

The Early Modern Period

What did the inhabitants of Ottoman Palestine think and do about disease? Local inhabitants did not write about their diseases (or at least no such writings survived, as far as we know), but contemporary sources pertaining to the early modern period reveal the contemporaneous intellectual climate in Palestine. We encounter a great diversity of opinions and practices.

Medicine and health in the Ottoman period were 'systems' of a variety of health-promoting beliefs and actions, scientific knowledge and skills of various types of healers. Lawrence I. Conrad has identified three sub-systems within the larger medieval Muslim medical system: folkloristic popular medicine, religious medicine ('Prophetic medicine') and mechanistic medicine based on Galenic humoralism. These three were the building blocks of the Ottoman medical system as well. Each of them had its own body of medical knowledge, unique disease theory and characteristic therapeutic techniques. Each medical tradition boasted a different source of legitimacy for its truth and efficacy: humoralism was inherited from Greek Antiquity and rested on its scientific authority; folk medicine was sanctioned by custom and consensus from below; and Islamic religious medicine originated from (and was therefore sanctioned by) the sayings of the Prophet Muhammad.[5]

The medical reality, both on the theoretical and clinical levels, was of considerable overlap, even ambiguity, in knowledge and technology. Both healers and patients did not consider the various traditions as mutually exclusive. We may even suspect that many healers and patients did not concern themselves with such categorization in day-to-day medical routine. The main criterion, maybe the only one at times, was the presumed efficacy of a treatment. Yes, to some other healers and patients, the etiological theorization was meaningful. Furthermore, the multitude of medical explanations and practices framed the medical market as competitive, which made patients and healers sensitive to alternatives.

Knowledge and clinical practice did not cross only medical traditions but also religious and ethnic communities. Following Justin Stearns, an historian of the pre-modern Islamic world, we should assume similarities between the religious communities that made up the varied religious and ethnic population in this province. The previous commonplace wisdom maintained that religious communities cultivated different perceptions and practices. For instance, scholars argued that Christians and Jews were more likely to accept contagion theory and flight from the plague. Muslims in general, for scriptural or theological reasons, were assumed to be less open to fleeing from the plague or to the (presumed) overwhelming empirical evidence for the plague's contagious nature. Rather, Muslims believed, or so it was presumed, that the epidemic had been decreed by God and that it was not contagious. It was further commonly asserted that any Muslim opposing these tenets must have been considered a heretic, and would have been punished by the community.[6] However, Stearns showed these also included a considerable number of shared attitudes across the Abrahamic religious communities. Furthermore, Stearns argued convincingly that within the Muslim community a vocal minority openly expressed a belief in the transmission of disease.[7] Stearns analysed mainly views and practices in the western Mediterranean, particularly in the Muslim and Christian communities, but his findings are applicable to the eastern shores of the Mediterranean.

Illnesses

Many medical maladies existed in Ottoman Palestine. The evidence is descriptive and based on impressions. Contemporary historians cannot extract from them proper statistics of the ailments of that era, but they relate to the health regime and point to some of the main medical concerns of the time.

The reality was of high mortality and early death. This is not to say that people did not reach old age, but there were many medical circumstances and natural disasters that caused young, even very young, children to pass away. Children died in infancy; mothers died in childbirth; many pregnancies did not reach term. The presence of death intensified in the time of plague, but plague was endemic to the region and claimed victims not just in times of severe outbreaks.

Some Ottomans, regardless of their specific religious affiliation, placed the origin of disease with God. Muslims framed their thinking in quotations from the *Qur'an* and Hadiths (sayings attributed to Muhammad). Drawing on the Muslim scriptures and the mythological legacy, especially Biblical lore, disease was understood as bearing an ethical-moral lesson: a punishment from God, a reward (in the form of martyrdom) for the pious, or a sign of the Day of Judgment. Such responses highlighted the religious significance of disease. Other writers of the time described the plague as contagious. Their concept of contagion referred to transmission through contact or proximity as well as the corrosion of inanimate objects and even the transmission of malignancy by gaze (the Evil Eye). This line of explanation does not contradict the first type of response that highlighted the role of God. However, some prophetic sayings suggest opposing course of actions: in some, Muhammad advised not to enter a territory affected by the plague, but another saying attributed to Muhammad forbade fleeing.[8]

Disease was deemed normal. The normalcy of the plague appears in a court case in Jerusalem in mid-February 1764, regarding the alleged disappearance of a deposit of silk and soap from the Jaffa port. The litigants are Musa al-Kazimi, a Jew, who complained against another Musa, an Orthodox Christian, who rents draft animals. The Jew contracted Musa a few years prior to deliver a crate full of silk, hats and soap to a third person, one Anton from Izmir, at the port of Jaffa. He claimed the cargo never arrived and demanded that Musa return it. Musa the defendant, on his part, confirmed he was hired for such a task but argued that the delivery was handed over to Anton, as requested. In his defence, Musa raised three claims, one of them medical: he was sick with the plague and could not deliver the crate himself, so he passed the crate to his assistant to carry out the delivery from Jerusalem to Jaffa. Musa also supplied eyewitnesses who testified they saw the transaction on the Jaffa wharf. The judge then rejected the claim and forbade Musa al-Kazimi to pursue the matter further.[9]

It is anyone's guess whether Musa, the animals' drafter, was indeed ill with this specific malady or whether he was ill at all. He was not requested to bring evidence or supply an eyewitness to verify his medical condition. Yet it was important for Musa to insist he contracted that specific illness, as he repeats it twice. Musa wanted to explain the reason he could not perform the task he was paid for. Being sick with the plague (rather than a lighter malady) was apparently an accepted excuse for deferring the delivery to someone else.

Several aspects of this case attest to the perception of the plague as routine. Firstly, although the plague was considered a grave medical condition, it was normal to fully recuperate from it: several years later we find Musa completely healthy (at least he does not claim otherwise). Secondly, the judge, who is in charge of communal well-being (in the medical-physical sense as well) does not seem concerned to hear about a past victim of the plague or to be in his company. And thirdly, for everyone concerned, a plague is a normal event that does not necessarily require a radical response: despite an active case of a plague, the transaction was carried out.

In many cases of the plague civil and commercial life did not stop. Evidence exists from eighteenth-century Aleppo for a pattern of self-imposed confinement, at least by some social sectors. It appears that such initiatives were taken in severe and violent outbreaks of the plague but not necessarily routinely, and certainly not in Jerusalem.[10] Here, for instance, inter-city movement between Jerusalem and Jaffa continued.

Likewise, inter-faith contacts too were more or less intact, although times of crisis, such as plagues, could set off a wave of inter-communal strife.[11] The on-going proximity and the similar responses to the plague (none had a specific protective and effective measure) explains why all communities suffered the same morbidity rate in times of disease.[12] There were different patterns of disaster behaviour, but in many cases they had to do with individual perceptions and motivations rather than communal preferences. Religious faith was one (but only one) factor that mattered. Yet Yaron Ayalon shows that although inter-confessional boundaries could be loose, in times of crisis Ottomans turned to their religious community for aid. They relied on the norm to give and donate, and communal charitable institutions functioned as relief agencies. Non-Muslim Ottomans had fewer opportunities or possibilities than Muslims, even though most daily affairs were quite similar.[13]

Physicians and Healers

Despite what seems a gloomy situation, disease was not just normal but was also perceived to be curable. The local population availed itself to a host of healers. One group of healers were physicians associated with the humoral medical system. Conversely, the humoral terminology is used, and these healers are referred to as either physicians (*ṭabībs*, *ḥakīms*), ophthalmologists (*kaḥḥāls*) and surgeons (*jarrāḥs*). There was also a host of other providers of medical services: herbalists, pharmacists, circumcisers, bonesetters, cuppers and faith healers who prepared amulets, exorcists and more.

There were also female healers. Women were not only involved in the traditional female healing occupations of midwives (*dayas*) and wet nurses (*qabilas*). Indeed, evidence reveals that women healers enjoyed diverse professional training, qualifications, and expertise and dealt with male and female patients and colleagues alike. This medical reality is attested by many cases of medical malpractice where male healers treated women or female healers treated men. The plaintiffs and the judges did not bring up the claim that a woman treating a man (or vice versa) is something inherently wrong, even in cases which involved intimate body parts or pregnancies and deliveries.[14] The social convention seems to have allowed for a broad range of medical possibilities.

Treatments

Several possible channels existed in the quest for health. One course of action involved the herbal remedies of traditional medicine, whether based on humoral principles or local customs. The Cabbalist and healer Rabbi Hayyim Vital (1543-1620) wrote a treatise on practical healing. It included many recipes, including those believed to be anti-plague. Some were assumed to be preventive; others curative. His recipes included plants, such as onions or prunes, specific dietary items such as veal and almond milk, and numerous others. Some of the advice seems more bizarre, like dry human faeces.[15]

Rabbi David de Silva's eighteenth-century treatise *P'ri Megaddim* provides a more learned-medicine type of advice. This Jewish physician was also educated in Europe (he might have received a diploma in Leiden, Holland, as well as studying with several European Jewish physicians); his text reveals European medical phrases of that period, attesting to his European medical background. However, the *materia medica* covered situates these phrases well within the framework of Arabic-Greek medicine. Furthermore, humoral medical principles guided his approach.[16] Rabbi de Silva specified two plants he himself applied in remedies for the plague. One was Aloe, whose properties are hotness and dryness. A small quantity helps to balance the humours; a slightly larger quantity kills worms and strengthens post-partum ailments in women. De Silva recommended using the larger quantity during the plague.[17] A second useful herb di Silva noted came from the Callitris tree (a member of the cypress family), which, he claimed, is hot and dry as well, and thus highly beneficial to ailments associated with coldness. He considered it to help the stomach, crush kidney stones, reduce haemorrhaging and to freshen breath odour, among other properties, positing that leaves and fruit are also antibodies for all poisons, including a snake bite and the plague.[18]

Another contemporaneous course of action depended on belief in local saints and holy sites (trees, springs and rocks) to provide cures. Evliya Çelebi (c. 1611-85), an Ottoman literati and courtier and arguably the most renowned Ottoman traveller, visited Palestine in 1648-50. The importance of Evliya's account is that it supplies us with patterns of conceptions and attitudes prevailing in Ottoman society, providing a view of the Ottoman mind from within.[19] Among other things that attracted his attention were health and patterns of daily life and hygiene practices.

On his excursions in Ottoman Palestine, Evliya enumerated the various hammams (baths) and cold and hot springs throughout the countryside as told by local informants. He commented on the purity of the water and its sweet taste, noting its therapeutic virtues. Some of the springs were identified with a specific prophet or holy figures (for instance, Jacob, Jesus, etc.), and others were associated generally with their location. Certain sites offered general cure: people who immerse themselves in these waters for seven or forty consecutive days (symbolic numbers, of course) heal from whatever ailment bothers them, regain their strength and even put on some weight and immunize themselves from future predicaments. Other sites offered more specific help, like alleviating stomach aches, rheumatism, leprosy, skin rashes, fertility problems and heart disease.[20]

Evliya reports that thousands of local pilgrims of all religious faiths in Palestine frequented such sites annually. His numbers may seem suspiciously generous (Evliya is known for his tendency to exaggerate and embellish), but they are corroborated by the Ottoman bureaucracy. A decree of the Sultan issued to the governor of Damascus (Ottoman Palestine was the southern part of that province), in the summer of 1560 discussed the curative waters in Tiberias. The context was a proposal by Doña Gracia Nasi, a wealthy Spanish-Jewish merchant in Istanbul, to Sultan Süleyman to revive Tiberias and resettle it with Jews, as the hot baths attract 1,000-3,000 pilgrims per year visiting there. Once the buildings were renovated, the number of pilgrims was expected to increase greatly and should bring great revenues to the imperial treasury.[21]

The common perception behind the various approaches to health and medicine regarding medication and hygienic routine arose from the assumption that the plague is curable. There was another, alas less optimistic, perception. Indeed, one was to confront disease by fleeing in times of epidemic. In June 1579 a detailed complaint was entered into the Muslim court registers of Jerusalem. The local Muslim community filed against a new group of Egyptian Jews residing in town. The list refers to numerous incidents the Muslims considered to be transgressions of law and custom. These complaints address inter-faith communal relations, the financial situation in Jerusalem and the possible over-taxing of town food and water resources by Jews. According to the complaint, these Egyptian Jews used the spring pilgrimage to Jewish holy sites (the Passover pilgrimage) as a pretext to enter Jerusalem when in fact they sought to escape the plague (*al-wabaawal-ta'un*) that infested Cairo at the time.[22] This complaint reveals the common practice of escaping the plague by relocation temporarily to another region. The Muslim plaintiffs regard the Egyptian Jews' arrival in Jerusalem to escape the plague to be obvious. Likewise, Jews in Salonica referred to leaving the city limits during the plague as a well-established tradition 'from ancient times' (*kadimden*).[23]

Transmission of Disease

Regarding routes of transmission and distribution of diseases in Ottoman Eretz Israel, plagues travelled up and down the Syrian coast from Damietta in Egypt to Beirut in Lebanon, transmitted from one port to another, then southward by land and sea to Sidon, Acre, Nazareth, Nablus and Jerusalem. Alternatively, a plague could begin in Aleppo – a Middle Eastern gateway to and from the Silk Road – travel to Damascus (the northern starting point of the annual pilgrimage to Mecca and Medina), and west to the coast or south toward Safed and Jerusalem.[24]

The Ottoman imperial bureaucracy monitored outbreaks of plagues, restricted movement in order to keep governance, agriculture and trade intact, and also implemented some anti-plague measures as a means of controlling and scrutinizing its spread. Taken together, these pieces of evidence show Ottoman awareness of the possibility of communicable disease – although they adopted quarantine policies only in the eighteenth century and fully implemented them in the nineteenth.[25]

Medicine and Health in Ottoman Eretz Israel in the Long Nineteenth Century

Medicine as a theory and clinical reality radically changed in the Middle East during the long nineteenth century. One obvious change involved advancements in technology and scientific knowledge, and these filtered into the Ottoman Empire as well. The Ottoman elite which traditionally patronized mainly humoral medicine, started to disseminate Western medical knowledge, education and institutions.[26] New transportation devices brought about global dangers and increased the urgency of monitoring and controlling epidemics. It was especially cholera and typhus which were particularly threatening.

The Ottoman Empire at the time was busy with the emergence of a new state and its re-ordering. This was the aim of the *Tanzimat* project, literally meaning re-organization. The reforms introduced institutional changes that affected state and social organs. Medicine and medical institutions were included, although the ultimate aim was not necessarily to improve the well-being of citizens, but rather to improve state management. With health intentionally and successfully transforming into a mechanism of state control, medicine in general and disease in particular attracted much attention on the local and imperial levels during this period.

Alongside the significant internal change, there were also no less dramatic changes in the international context. Western presence was gaining significance in the Ottoman Empire in general and Eretz Israel in particular. In the medical realm, Western influence materialized through several avenues. One avenue was in the form of Western physicians who practised modern medicine. European physicians were known in this region throughout the Ottoman period: they were members of foreign consulates, trade companies or adventurers. Jews who studied in European universities and then migrated to Eretz Israel were another group of European-educated physicians practised here. But the new circumstances of the nineteenth century raised the volume and visibility of these Western and Western-educated physicians considerably.

Another avenue for modern medicine to impact the region was the education of students from the region in modern medical schools. They either went to study medicine at universities abroad or in modern institutions in the Middle East. For young men in late Ottoman Palestine/Eretz Israel, the Beirut colleges, which also included medical schools, were the magnet such as Saint-Joseph University and especially the Syrian Protestant College (which in 1920 became the American University of Beirut).[27]

Yet another avenue for Western medical presence in the region in the late Ottoman period was the establishment of numerous hospitals. Some institutions were identified with specific countries who patronized them (British, Scottish, German, French, American, Prussian, Russian, Habsburg and Italian) or with religious communities (Jewish, Catholic, Protestant and Evangelical missionary establishments). In Palestine, as elsewhere, medical facilities and scientific progress were used as one of the means to further Western material gains and not just health and wellbeing to the local population.[28]

In Eretz Israel, as in other Ottoman provinces, the local administrative councils (*majlis al-idara* in Arabic or *meclis-iidare* in Turkish) were responsible for taking active measures against public health hazards and agricultural diseases. Starting in the 1860s and 1870s the imperial government fostered these various municipal councils, organized hierarchically by a mixture of appointments and elections and granted with certain responsibilities. The role of the councils was to clean and illuminate the streets, to provide medical attention and medicine to the needy free of charge, to supervise prices of foods and to install and maintain public toilets. However, these bodies had limited authority (they functioned more in an advisory capacity) and were prohibited from spending beyond their annual income raised from taxes, dues and a governmental subsidy. Thus, their services were quite restricted. This was the case in Haifa, for instance.[29]

The Jerusalem municipality also had quite extensive responsibilities. Of all of these the municipality was most concerned with health and sanitation. Public cleanliness was imperative for maintaining public health and preventing the spread of disease. This was particularly true in the Old City, because of its cramped quarters and tightly-packed commercial alleys, but was relevant to all neighbourhoods including the extramural ones. Hence, the council doubled its cleaning budget at the beginning of the twentieth century and opened a municipal medical clinic. In 1912 a municipal hospital was founded as well, competing with the numerous private hospitals many of which belonged to the European Christian and Jewish communities. The municipality also extensively utilized the new press to report on its accomplishments and engage residents in various health measures. Newspapers reminded residents not to throw rubbish on the street. They announced the outbreak of epidemics such as cholera and spinal meningitis and urged the inhabitants to purify their wells and avoid eating spoiled meat and fish.[30]

The local Ottoman governor (*mutassarıf*) of the Jerusalem district was above the municipality in the provincial administrative hierarchy. The collection of letters and telegrams of Ali Ekrem Bey (1867-1937), the governor between 1906 and 1908,[31] demonstrate his concern with health and natural resources, from the position of these issues and their impact on the interests of the empire in the region. A few months later, in the autumn of 1907, Ali Ekrem Bey reported to the Ottoman imperial palace that he had taken steps towards the surveying and eventual exploitation of Dead Sea resources, the revenues of which were to accrue to the Sultan's privy list. Apparently, at this point he was more concerned with locating exotic plants and animals for the Sultan's private collection rather than unearthing natural resources such as minerals, although the existence and economic potential of the latter was already known.[32]

Ali Ekrem Bey was right to assume that health, epidemics and natural resources in Palestine were of interest to the central bureaucracy. The central administration, like the local inhabitants and governmental bodies, associated infrastructure with modernity. This was especially true in

Palestine, which drew considerable international attention. Running water, sewer systems and clean roads were considered an aspect of civic and commercial development. Water, fresh food, medications, hospitals and the whole parcel of public health services were crucial for the state and population's well-being, but also for the state's image.[33]

Indeed, the connection between public health services in Ottoman Palestine and self-image and pride is present in the documents prepared by the Ottoman central administration in Istanbul. The bureaucracy evolved during the nineteenth century and became more professional. One by-product was that the later nineteenth-century edicts come from specialized ministries, such as the Ministry of Interior (*Dahiliye Nezaret*), which issued orders regarding quarantines to prevent epidemics from spreading between provinces. This was the concern of a 1908 order to place ships arriving at the Jaffa port in isolation if their port of origin is known to suffer from contagious disease. The Health Inspector clarified that passengers and boatmen are not to go ashore, nor could local people embark before health measures were implemented in these ships.[34]

Indeed, one new health characteristic of the late Ottoman period in the region was the introduction of quarantine measures. This was the outcome of the Tanzimat-period centralization and the implementation of new medical knowledge and practice in the region. Before the middle of the nineteenth century the Ottoman Empire did not use quarantines in its formal health policies. Ottomans were familiar with such preventive practices in the Mediterranean Sea and the Italian cities since the early modern period but refrained from carrying it out in their own domains. Partly, the reason to the delay in quarantine measures in the Ottoman empire was that until the nineteenth century there was no scientific proof of the efficacy of quarantines. Ottoman medical theory did not unequivocally support the possibility of contagion. There was, however, also social motivation to reject quarantines. Quarantine measures increased fears of plague and its consequences, causing widespread discontent, rebellion and escape from the regime. Fear of social separation from families and being cut off from institutions of death counted as more troublesome for the locals and for the bureaucracy than the fear of biological-physical death.[35]

During the nineteenth century the Ottoman Empire started to implement quarantines as part of its official health policies, within the empire and on the borders. Such policies were instigated already during the eighteenth century but were sporadic.[36] The application of quarantines during the nineteenth century, however, was the product of the intellectual and political climate that allowed for the introduction of proactive anti-disease measures on a large scale.[37]

With regard to Ottoman Palestine, in 1864, the governor of Jerusalem was notified of cattle disease in Egypt. He ordered quarantine measure in the environs of Gaza, Jaffa, Ramla and Lydda. Units of two or three soldiers were dispatched to each place to inspect that no animals ran away and assess whether any animal displayed epidemic symptoms. They were ordered to kill and properly bury afflicted animals.[38] In 1865, local measures taken in Jaffa and Gaza to prevent the spread of cholera were reported to Istanbul and their initiators were awarded a medal.[39] In 1901, a letter was sent to the Ministry of Military Schools, which included also a medical school. The letter regarded the precautions required to prevent the spread of epidemics in Jerusalem from reaching Beirut. Jerusalem was instructed to subordinate to the inspection officers in Beirut, who would be adopting responsibility for the region.[40]

Alongside the major inroads Western medicine had made in the region, there was also noticeable continuity of existing pre-nineteenth century medical beliefs and practices. For example, pilgrimage to natural sites and graves of holy figures when looking for a cure continued well into the modern period alongside the growing spread of Western medicine.

The evidence of the resilience of traditional medical practices comes, for instance, from Tawfiq Canaan (1882-1964), a Christian Palestinian from Beit Jala and a medical doctor who was educated in Beirut at the Syrian Protestant College. He practised medicine in hospitals in Jerusalem, including Shaarei Zedek. He specialized in Germany in tropical medicine in general and medicine in particular and continued his contacts with the German health establishment after his return to Jerusalem. Under the Ottomans, and later the British mandate, he managed the local Health Bureau.[41] Canaan, however, was also an ethnographer. His unique position as a practising local physician with Western education, but also equipped with avid interest in and respect for indigenous customs, allowed him to document traditional health practices, such as the continued existence of many shrines throughout the region.[42] Some of the specific health-related rituals, ceremonies and customs around sacred trees, stones and waters thrive through to the present day.

Conclusion

The cyclical condition of health and illness was a routine part of everyone's life in Eretz Israel during the Ottoman period. It was dealt with as a normal and natural phenomenon. Furthermore, not just the health risks were similar but also the specific health beliefs and practices were a shared experience, regardless of social standing, religious affiliation and ethnic origin. The various historical records discussed above point to a society that framed maladies into routine life. Ottoman Palestine experienced repeated natural disasters that remained fresh in the individual and collective memory: disease, earthquakes, famine, draught, heat waves or cold and damp winters. The late eighteenth century also introduced political turbulence that lasted well into the nineteenth century and exacerbated natural problems. The advantage of this unhappy occurrence was that locals were not surprised by the presence of disease. Many had a point of reference from their own experience. This state of mind could lead to fatalism, but it did not for the local population of Eretz Israel took its health seriously.

In the wake of the Covid-19 pandemic the plague precautions of an earlier era strike a familiar chord: 'The fear of social separation from families…counted as more troublesome for the locals and for the bureaucracy than the fear of biological-physical death.'

Notes

1. Some representative examples of this scholarship are Kass, A. M., 'Western Medicine in Nineteenth-Century Jerusalem', *Journal of the History of Medicine and Allied Sciences*, 44 (1989), pp. 447-461; Levy, N., *The History of Medicine in the Holy Land: 1799-1948* (B'nei Braq: Hakibbutz Hameuchad, 1998); Perry, Y. and Lev, E., *Modern Medicine in the Holy Land: Pioneering British Medical Services in Late Ottoman Palestine* (London and New York: I.B. Tauris, 2007). A noted exception to include Ottoman sources is Singer, A., 'Ottoman Palestine (1516-1800): Health, Disease, and Historical Sources' in Waserman, M. and Kottek, S.S. (Eds), *Health and Disease in the Holy Land: Studies in the History and Sociology of Medicine from Ancient Times to the Present* (Lewiston: Edward Mellen Press, 1996), pp.189-206.
2. The foremost scholar of the Ottoman Jerusalem court records is Amnon Cohen. He presented the Jerusalem court registers in Cohen, A., *Ottoman Documents on the Jewish Communities of Jerusalem in the Sixteenth Century* (Jerusalem: Yad Izhak Ben-Zvi, 1976), pp.9-13; for the English summary see vii-x.
3. Faroqhi, S., 'Mühimme Defterleri', *Encyclopaedia of Islam, Second edn.*; Heyd, U., *Ottoman Documents on Palestine, 1552-1615* (London: Oxford University Press, 1960), The Firman According to the Mühimme Defteri, pp.3-31.
4. Ze'evi, D., 'Women in 17th-Century Jerusalem: Western and Indigenous Perspectives', *International Journal of Middle East Studies*, 27 (1995), pp.157-73.
5. Conrad, L.I., 'Medicine: Traditional Practice', *The Oxford Encyclopedia of the Modern Islamic World* (New York: Oxford University Press, 1995), pp.85-8.

6. An example is Barel, D., *An Ill Wind: Cholera Epidemics and Medical Development in Palestine in the Late Ottoman Period* (Jerusalem: Mosad Bialik, 2010), pp.28-29 (Hebrew).
7. Stearns, J.K., *Infectious Ideas: Contagion in Pre-Modern Islamic and Christian Thought in the Western Mediterranean* (Baltimore: Johns Hopkins University Press, 2011); idem. 'Contagion in Theology and Law: Ethical Considerations in the Writings of Two 14th Century Scholars of Naṣrid Granada', *Islamic Law and Society*, 14 (2007), pp.109-29; idem. 'New Directions in the Study of Religious Responses to the Black Death', *History Compass*, 7 (2009), pp.1,363-75; idem. 'Public Health, the State, and Religious Scholarship Sovereignty in Idrīs al-Bidlīsī's Argument for Fleeing the Plague', in Benite, Z., Geroulanos, S. and Jerr, N. (Eds), *The Scaffolding of Sovereignty: Global and Aesthetic Perspectives on the History of a Concept* (New York: Columbia University Press, 2017), pp.163-85.
8. Akasoy, A., 'Islamic Attitudes to Disasters in the Middle Ages: A Comparison of Earthquakes and Plagues', *The Medieval History Journal*, 10 (2007), pp.387-410.
9. Cohen, A., Simon-Pikali, E. and Salama, O., *Jews in the Moslem Religious Court: Society, Economy and Communal Organization in the XVIII Century; Documents from Ottoman Jerusalem* (Jerusalem: Yad Izhak Ben-Zvi, 1996), pp.302-304.
10. Marcus, A., *The Middle East of the Eve of Modernity: Aleppo in the Eighteenth Century* (New York: Columbia University Press, 1989), pp.258-260; Buchman, Y., 'Life in the Shadow of the Plague', *Jerusalem and Eretz-Israel*, 2 (2004), pp.51-75.
11. Campos, M.U., *Ottoman Brothers: Muslims, Christians, and Jews in Early Twentieth-Century Palestine* (Stanford: Stanford University Press, 2011), p.11.
12. Masters, B., *Christians and Jews in the Ottoman Arab World: The Shifting Boundaries of Political Communities 1516-1918* (Cambridge: Cambridge University Press, 2001), p. 54: Marcus, *The Middle East of the Eve of Modernity*, p.259.
13. Ayalon, Y., *Natural Disasters in the Ottoman Empire: Plague, Famine, and Other Misfortunes* (New York: Cambridge University Press, 2015).
14. See some of the cases in published Jerusalem records, such as Cohen, A. et al., *Jews in the Moslem Religious Court*, pp.324–25 (case 279), 328 (case 286) (Hebrew).
15. Buchman, Y. and Amar, Z. (Eds), and comment, *Practical Medicine of Rabbi Hayyim Vital (1543-1620): Healer in the Land of Israel and Vicinity* (Ramat Gan: Bar Ilan University, 2006), pp.70-96.
16. Amar, Z. (introd. and annot.), *P'ri Megaddim by R. David Silva, Physician in Jerusalem* (Jerusalem: Yad Ben-Zvi Press, 2003), 16, pp. 33-35.
17. Ibid., p.131.
18. Ibid., p.169.
19. Dankoff, R., *An Ottoman Mentality: The World of Evliya Çelebi* (Leiden: Brill, 2004).
20. Çelebi, E., *Seyahatname*, vol. 2 (İstanbul: Yapı Kredi Yayınları, 2011), 9 (Eds. Yücel Dağlı, Seyit Ali Kahraman, and Robert Dankoff), pp.217-19, 223, 225, 229; For the English translation see, *Evliya Tshelebi's Travels in Palestine (1648-1650)*, St. H. Stephan, trans. (Jerusalem: Ariel Publishing House, 1980), pp.12-13, 43-44, 51-52.
21. Heyd, U., 'Turkish Documents on the Rebuilding of Tiberias in the Sixteenth Century', *Sefunut*, 10 (1966), 202 (Hebrew); ibid., *Ottoman Documents on Palestine*, document 89, pp.140-42; Singer, 'Ottoman Palestine (1516-1800): Health, Disease, and Historical Sources', p.202.
22. 25 Rabi' al-Thani, 978 [21 June1579]; Jerusalem *Sijill*, volume 58, document # 444. The document was first published in 'Ovadia Salama, Slaves Owned by Jews and

Christians in Ottoman Jerusalem', *Cathedra*, 49 (1988), p.62 (for a facsimile production) and p.68 (for discussion) (Hebrew). A more elaborate discussion appears in Amnon Cohen, A., 'The Importance of Arabic for Jewish History: Anecdotes from Ottoman Jerusalem', *Cathedra*, 50 (1988), pp.70-72 (Hebrew). An English summary and a facsimile reproduction can be found in Cohen, A., *A World Within: Jewish Life as Reflected in Muslim Court Documents from the Sijill of Jerusalem (XVIth Century)* (Philadelphia, PA: Centre for Judaic Studies, University of Pennsylvania, 1994), p.167, F/302.

23. BOA, Mühimme Defteri [MD], 19/20/417. Published by Yılmaz, C. and Yılmaz, N. (Eds), *Osmanlılarda Sağlık/Health in the Ottomans* (İstanbul: Biofarma, 2006), 2, p.60-61 (document 133); Varlik, N., 'Plague, Conflict, and Negotiation: The Jewish Broadcloth Weavers of Salonica and the Ottoman Central Administration in the Late Sixteenth Century', *Jewish History*, 28 (2014), pp.261-88.

24. Singer, 'Ottoman Palestine (1516-1800): Health, Disease, and Historical Sources', p.198.

25. Varlik, N., *Plague and Empire in the Early Modern Mediterranean World: The Ottoman Experience, 1347-1600* (Cambridge: Cambridge University Press, 2015); Ayalon, *Natural Disasters in the Ottoman Empire*; Bulmuş, B., *Plague, Quarantines and Geopolitics in the Ottoman Empire* (Edinburgh: Edinburgh University Press, 2012).

26. Some examples from older and current scholarship: Gallagher, N.E., *Medicine and Power in Tunisia, 1780-1900* (Cambridge: Cambridge University Press, 1983); Fahmy, K.,'Women, Medicine and Power in Nineteenth-Century Egypt' in Abu-Lughod, L. (Ed.), *Remaking Women: Feminism and Modernity in the Middle East* (Princeton: Princeton University Press, 1998), pp.35-72.

27. On Saint-Joseph University: Herzstein, R., 'The Foundation of the Saint-Joseph University of Beirut: The Teaching of the Maronites by the Second Jesuit Mission in the Levant', *Middle Eastern Studies*, 43 (2007), pp.749-59; idem. 'Saint-Joseph University of Beirut: An Enclave of the French-Speaking Communities in the Levant', 1875 – 1914, *Itinerario*, 32 (2008): pp.67-82. On the American University of Beirut, see for instance Zachs, F., 'From the Mission to the Missionary: The Bliss Family and the Syrian Protestant College (1866-1920)', *Welt des Islams*, 45 (2005), pp.255-91.

28. Schwake, N., 'Hospitals and European Colonial Policies in the 19th and Early 20th Centuries' in Waserman and Kottek (Eds), *Health and Disease in the Holy Land*, pp.231-62; Perry and Lev, *Modern Medicine in the Holy Land*; Lev and Amar, Z., 'The Turning Point from an Archaic Arab Medical System to an Early Modern European System in Jerusalem according to the Swiss Physician Titus Tobler (1806-1977)', *Canadian Bulletin of Medical History*, 21 (2004), pp.159-80.

29. Yazbak, M., *Haifa in the Late Ottoman Period, 1864-1914: A Muslim Town in Transition* (Leiden: Brill, 1998), pp.35, 38, 77, 79-81, 110.

30. Campos, M.U., *Ottoman Brothers, Muslims, Christians and Jews in Early Twentieth-Century Palestine*, pp.169-70.

31. On Ali Ekrem Bey and his collection of papers in the Israeli State Archives, see Kushner, D., 'Ali Ekrem Bey, Governor of Jerusalem, 1906-1908', *International Journal of Middle East Studies*, 28 (1996), pp.349-62.

32. Kushner, D., *A Governor in Jerusalem: The City and Province in the Eyes of Ali Ekrem Bey, 1906-1908* (Jerusalem: Yad Izhak Ben-Zvi, 1995), pp.122-23, 126-29.

33. Following Campos, p.174.

34. BOA, DH.MKT, 2657/98; published by Osmanlı Belgelerinde Filistin, 115-16 (document 18).

35. Mikhail, A., *Nature and Empire in Ottoman Egypt: An Environmental History* (Cambridge: Cambridge University Press, 2011), p.233.

36. Panzac, D., 'Politique sanitaire et fixation des frontières: L'exemple Ottoman (XVIIIe–XIXe siècles)', *Turcica*, 31 (1999), pp.87–108.

37. For quarantine measures in the Ottoman Middle East within international anti-pandemic endeavours, see Robarts, A., *Migration and Disease in the Black Sea Region: Ottoman-Russian Relations in the Late Eighteenth and Early Nineteenth Centuries* (London: Bloomsbury, 2017); Huber, V., *Chanelling Mobilities: Migration and Globalisation in the Suez Canal Region and Beyond, 1869-1914* (Cambridge: Cambridge University Press, 2013); Bulmuş, B., *Plague, Quarantines and Geopolitics in the Ottoman Empire* (Edinburgh: Edinburgh University Press, 2012); Ayalon, *Natural Disasters in the Ottoman Empire*.

38. Başbakanlık Osmanlı Arşıvı [BOA], A.MKT.MHM, 309/19; published in *Osmanlı Belgelerinde Filistin / Palestine in Ottoman Documents* (İstanbul: T.C. Republic of Turkey, General Directorate of State Archives, 2009), pp.87-90 (document 10).

39. BOA, A.MKT.MHM, 341/19; published in *Osmanlı Belgelerinde Filistin*, 91-94 (document 11).

40. BOA, DH.MKT, 2459/119; published in *Osmanlı Belgelerinde Filistin*, 113-14 (document 17).

41. Lapp, P.W. and Albright, W.F., 'Tawfiq Canaan in Memoriam', *Bulletin of the American Schools of Oriental Research*, 174 (April 1964), pp.1-3; al-Nashef, K., 'Tawfiq Canaan: His Life and Works', *Jerusalem Quarterly File*, 16 (2002), pp.12-26; Tamari, S., 'Lepers, Lunatics, and Saints: The Nativist Ethnography of Tawfiq Canaan and His Jerusalem Circle', *Jerusalem Quarterly File*, 20, (2004), pp.24-43; al-Ju'beh, B., 'Magic and Talismans: The Tawfiq Canaan Collection of Palestinian Amulets', *Jerusalem Quarterly*, 22-23 (Fall-Winter 2005), pp.103-108.

42. Kan'an, Tawfiq, *Haunted Springs and Water Demons in Palestine* (Jerusalem: Palestine Oriental Society, 1922); idem., *Mohammedan Saints and Sanctuaries in Palestine* (London: Luzac, 1927).

7

Medicine in British Palestine, 1919-1948

Kenneth Collins

Introduction

At the beginning of the British Mandate health care was often undeveloped with health clinics and hospital facilities, sometimes provided by European religious societies, only available in the larger towns, especially in Jerusalem. Consequently, life expectancy was low, infant mortality was high and there was a high susceptibility to diseases such as malaria. trachoma and leprosy. In this chapter, we will examine health policy, developments in the delivery of care and changes in medical outcomes during the roughly 30 years of the British Mandate for Palestine. The Mandate Government health records, although assembled for shipment to Britain in 1948, have in the main not survived although many annual reports, such as those published by the Palestine Government Department of Health and the Jewish health bodies, are available and have been widely consulted.

Many of the issues which coloured the practice of medicine and the delivery of health care in the Jewish community during the British Mandate are seen through many different perspectives. One such example is the management of trachoma, a troublesome eye disease and common during the Mandate era, associated with the poverty, poor hygiene and blindness. This chapter reviews how trachoma was handled in the Yishuv (Jewish community in Eretz Israel) during the Mandate era, based on extensive archival material, principally from Jewish and Zionist sources.

Medicine and Hospitals in Ottoman Palestine

As many of the medical organisations functioning in the early years of the Mandate were founded in the Ottoman era, a short account of this period is necessary. Such facilities as existed for the Jewish community at the

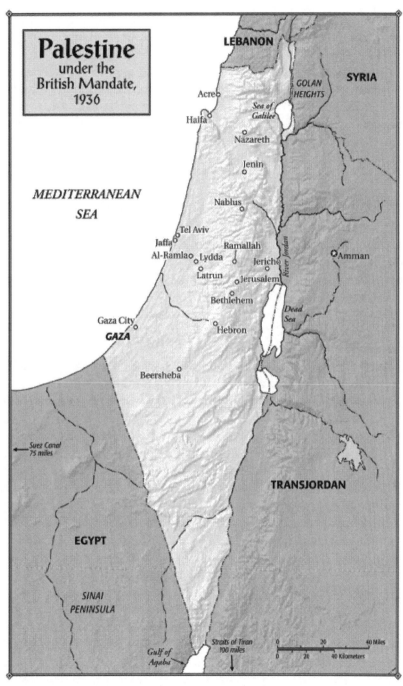

11. Palestine Mandate Map.

beginning of the Mandate had been created not just to provide care for the Jewish sick but also to keep them out of the clinics and hospitals of the Christian missionaries.

Concern about the medical missions led to the initiative of Sir Moses Montefiore in 1843, sending Dr. Simon Frankel, of Breslau, who had studied medicine in Munich, to set up a dispensary. A hospital was also established but soon closed and Montefiore planned, with substantial help from Judah Touro, to build a hospital outside the Old City. These plans did not come to fruition but, in the meantime, the Rothschild Hospital was established within the Old City, in a building owned by the Sephardi community, although a new building was erected outside its walls in 1888.

The Bikkur Holim Society was established in 1837 to provide nursing care in peoples' homes. In 1865 a house was purchased for use as a hospital and dispensary, receiving some support, firstly from Sir Moses Montefiore and then from Jewish communities in Germany. The facilities gradually developed during the last half of the nineteenth century and with good management plans were prepared for a more substantial hospital in 1910 when the corner-stone was laid. However, with the outbreak of war building plans were delayed and the new building opened only in 1925, in its present site on Rehov Strauss.

Another Jewish hospital in Jerusalem, Shaarei Tzedek, was opened on Rehov Yafo in 1902 on the initiative of Dr. Moshe Wallach, who had arrived in Jerusalem as a young medical graduate who had studied at the Universities of Berlin and Wurzburg. In 1890, just a year after his graduation, he was selected by a Jewish charity in Frankfurt to open a modern hospital in Jerusalem. After setting up a clinic in the Old City and some work at Bikkur Cholim he returned to Europe to raise funds in Germany and Holland. With this, he purchased land on what became Jaffa Road, and arranged for the building of a spacious hospital, which opened in 1902 with 20 beds and space for clinics, offices and a pharmacy. With his deeply religious leadership, the hospital was run on strictly Orthodox lines.

When the Rothschild Hospital relocated outside the Old City in 1888, its former premises were returned to the Sephardi community, in the form of the Misgav Ladach Society, which had been formed a decade earlier by wealthy Jews from Salonica. Beginning as a *kupat cholim*, an insurance style sick fund, it first opened a dispensary and in 1889 hospital facilities were established within the building. Though funded by the Sephardi community, it treated Ashkenazi Jews and some Arabs too. Despite financial difficulties during and after the First World War, it remained active

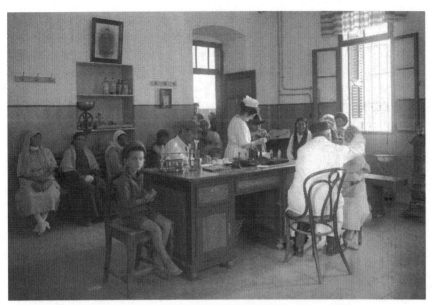

12. Outpatient Clinic at Shaarei Tzedek Hospital, Jerusalem, around 1910.

as the only Jewish hospital in the Old City until it was destroyed in 1948 during the War of Independence, when the Jewish community was evacuated. The hospital then reopened in Katamon in western Jerusalem, where it operated for 40 years as a maternity hospital, eventually becoming a Kupat Cholim hospital after substantial renovation, in 2005.

Other Jewish hospitals were established in towns with a significant Jewish population. These included Jaffa in 1891, Tiberias in 1897 and Tzefat (Safed) in 1912. The hospital in Jaffa, Shaar Zion, was the first in the country to employ women doctors and the first moves to set up an association of Jewish doctors were also based there in 1912.

One of the leading hospitals provided by missionary groups was the Scottish Mission Hospital in Tiberias, founded in 1885 by Dr. David Torrance. He, and subsequently his son, Dr. Herbert Torrance, both Glasgow graduates, were to run this facility until 1953.[1] In 1885, Tiberias would have seemed to be unbearably hot in the summer, with the town poverty-stricken, dirty and disease-ridden. While there was an initial hope that treatment might lead to conversion, it became quickly clear this was not going to happen. The Jewish community in Tiberias, as well as the smaller Arab Muslim population, came to rely on the Torrances and the Scottish Hospital, attracted by the standards of care and the level of compassion it provided. In its early years, Arab patients often walked dozens of miles to the hospital from remote areas, many times suffering from a variety of serious complaints. The Scottish Mission Hospital provided maternity services to the population of the Galilee, well into the State era.

Other Christian medical centres were to be found in Tzefat, Hebron, Jaffa and Nazareth as well as in Jerusalem, provided by both the Catholic Church and the various Protestant denominations. The high prevalence of eye diseases, the scourge of the local population, encouraged the English branch of the Order of St. John of Jerusalem to build a hospital. Following agreement of the Sultan in 1882, an Ophthalmic Hospital and Dispensary was established with the support of the Prince of Wales, later Edward VII.

The Catholic Order of John supported a mobile clinic at Tantur, near Jerusalem, to care for the local Bedouin population and a permanent hospital was established in 1876, although its activities declined during the Mandate years and it was used as a detention centre for Italian missionaries during the Second World War. A leprosy hospital, Jesus-Hilfe, was founded in 1867, and supported by German Protestants on the initiative of Baroness Augusta Keffenbrinck-Ascheraden and, designed by Conrad Schick, it moved to its present site in Talbiye, Jerusalem, in 1887. Other Jerusalem hospitals, supported by the Christian churches included the Marienstift Kinderhospital, a childrens' hospital, associated with Dr. Max Sandreczki and his wife Johanna. The Archduke of Mecklenburg Schwerin and his newly-wedded wife, Princess Marie, agreed to support the hospital, which opened the year after their pilgrimage to Jerusalem in 1871. It was agreed that there would be no attempt at proselytism and that the hospital would serve all the children of the Holy Land regardless of ethnic or religious affiliation. Sandreczki recorded the high mortality rates and described local conditions as possessing 'a filthy environment, (with) ignorance and apathy of parents'. The hospital operated from 1872 until1899 when it closed with Sandreczki's suicide, having run out of funds and being regarded as an alien institution in a traditional society.

The Templers, members of a German Protestant sect, settled in seventeen locations in Palestine, notably in Haifa, Sarona, near Jaffa but now in central Tel Aviv, and Emek Refaim in Jerusalem. They brought doctors into the country and established pharmacies, clinics and even a small hospital in Jaffa. Their activities ceased when their Nazi affiliations became clear during the 1930s and the community was deported to Australia.

These hospitals carried a significance beyond their importance to the local population. Religious groups, both Christian and Jewish, as well as European nations, British, French, German and Italian, saw their presence in the Holy Land as making a political and national statement built often for politics and nationalist pride and containing elements of patriotic rivalry. Even within the Jewish community, the leading Sephardi philanthropist in the nineteenth century was the British Sir Moses Montefiore while funding from the Rothschilds came from members of the French family.

The early Zionist movement was deeply concerned about health issues and many of their leading figures were physicians. One of the aims of the Zionist movement, incorporated by all its divisions, was the desire to change the poor physical image of the 'ghetto' Jew, a notion reflected in the expression 'muscular Judaism' coined by Dr. Max Nordau (1849-1923) at the Second Zionist Congress held in Basel in 1898. Nordau aimed to improve the mental and physical health amongst the masses of East European Jews as part of the national revival implicit in the Zionist movement. This led to the encouragement of gymnastics and other sporting activities and the establishment of Jewish sports clubs like Bar Kochba and Maccabi.

Dr. Leon Pinsker (1821–1891) was the founder and leader of the Hovevei Zion movement. Russian antisemitism had convinced him that only a Jewish national consciousness leading to political independence, as he described in his famous pamphlet *Auto-Emancipation*, could solve the crises facing the Jewish people. Dr. Franz Oppenheimer (1864 – 1943) was a political theorist as well as a physician and provided some of the early support for the early Jewish communal villages in Palestine. As early as the 6th Zionist Congress in 1903, he had delineated his objectives for the Zionist movement to be based on communal agricultural settlements, with the land held by the settlers and to be populated by Jewish migrants especially from Galicia, Rumania and Russia.

Dr. Shaul Tchernichovsky (1874-1943) studied medicine in Heidelberg and Lausanne. From then, he combined his activities as a doctor with writing poetry. He was active in writers' organisations, was a member of the Committee of the Hebrew Language and edited the Hebrew terminology manual for medicine and the natural sciences. Dr. Hillel Yaffe (1864–1936) immigrated to Palestine in 1891. His medical legacy was his work in treating malaria which involved treating the environment as much as his patients, inevitably involving him in research and political activism. Dr. Helena Kagan (1889-1978) broke new ground in a lengthy and devoted medical career in the fight against rheumatic fever, malnutrition and asthma in children. She was involved in the founding of Tipat Chalav clinics and the WIZO daycare centres and was head of paediatrics at the Rothschild-Hadassah hospital until 1925, later operating a private clinic in her home. She received numerous awards in recognition of her unique contribution to society and the community including an honorary doctorate from the Hebrew University and the Israel Prize.

Health Policy During the British Mandate

Health services improved during the three decades of British rule although Government funding for health was not seen as a priority. Developments in the Jewish community were often funded by the Jews themselves or were supported by Jewish communities abroad, especially in the United States. Rural Arabs tended to rely on traditional folk healers, while in larger towns they had to accept the lower level of health care provision which was provided by the Mandate Government.

The Palestine Government Department of Health (GDH) did not aim to provide comprehensive health facilities. The Government's emphasis on security and public works meant that spending on health was often constrained. Government policy focused on control of infectious diseases with some degree of success. However, funding needs of public works and health overlapped such as in the continued difficulties in providing an adequate sewage and sanitation system.[2] The GDH sought to involve local communities in health care, with clinics mainly in Arab centres or cities with a mixed population hoping that they would be able to take over the work. Immunisations against such diseases as typhoid, cholera and smallpox began in the 1920s

Training nurses and doctors to care, e.g. for trachoma in the schools and rural areas, was a priority for the Government but its delivery was difficult and the contrast between the services offered by GDH and the Jewish services of the Hadassah Medical Organization and Kupat Cholim, the Jewish workers' sick fund, inevitably led to ethnic health disparities. In 1935, when the Jewish population of Palestine was less than a third of the total, the expenditure by the Jewish health bodies was double that of the Government Department of Health.

The differences were perhaps inevitable as Jews were predominantly urban, where most hospitals and clinics were located, while Muslims were found mainly in smaller towns and villages. While Jewish and Christian patients could rely on a variety of medical options, provision for Muslim patients did not really develop until around the Second World War. The Mandate authorities created an expectation of better health, mainly through trying to eliminate such infectious disease as malaria, typhoid, typhus and dysentery. Again, Jewish patients benefitted more from such policies. Malaria, for example, had virtually disappeared in the Yishuv by the end of the Mandate while there were still thousands of Arab patients with the disease. Thus, expectations often did not match reality as the facilities to meet the fall in infant mortality and rise in life expectancy were slow in coming.

Within the Jewish sector there was, from the start, an emphasis on health improvement as an early priority of the Zionist movement was in creating a healthier and fitter Jew. In June 1918, even before the end of the First World War, the first Jewish post-war health care facilities began with the arrival of the American Zionist Medical Unit (AZMU) with 20 doctors and 20 nurses. This Unit developed into Hadassah, supported by American women Zionists, and as we shall see became a vital component in the creation of a modern health system. Thus, health and hygiene helped the development of Zionism and brought benefit to the Jewish national project. Jewish historians often described idealistic Zionist pioneers working under austere conditions on the land and creating a new society in heroic terms. With this came the development of institutions to provide the Yishuv, the Jewish community in pre-state Israel, with the key health components of a welfare state.

We have noted the Government reluctance to provide funding for the level of health care demanded by both Arabs and Jews. It considered that the level of taxes raised in Palestine did not justify a greater Government investment while the expectations of the two communities diverged so much that a single system would be impractical.[3] By the end of the Mandate Government hospital beds made up just around a third of the total with a slightly higher proportion in the Jewish hospitals and the remainder mainly consisting of mission hospitals. Government hospital provision gave priority to its own officials and members of the military further limiting access by the general population. While municipal health provision was provided the Government always suspected that Arab communities in more prosperous areas could contribute more.[4]

During the 1930s the Jewish population received a greater share of the health budget than their share of the working population would justify, although the sum was less than their tax payments would justify. As the Jewish population proved to be more resourceful in funding health care, the disparity between the two communities continued to increase. Health disparity showed quickly in such measures as crude deaths rates.[5] There was little change in Muslim crude death rates during the Mandate with levels falling marginally, from 23.1 to 22 per 1,000 of population, between 1923 and 1942. By way of comparison, the lower figures for Jews, 13.7, and Christians in 1923, 16.2, had fallen further to 7.9 (for Jews) and 11.2 (for Christians) by 1942.

As the Jewish population came to be concentrated in the largest cities and in compact rural areas, delivery of care was much easier than in small and relatively inaccessible Arab villages. However, the increasing activity of Jewish health bodies did have a beneficial effect on the wider population. Thus, the facilities of the American funded Hadassah Medical Association ran hospitals and clinics open to both Jews and Arabs and the Joint Distribution Committee, the 'Joint', also American funded, provided the Government with funds to be used in the fight against malaria. Political instability also contributed to the unevenness of health care delivery. The massacre of Jews by Muslims in Hebron in 1929 and its aftermath, and conditions during the Arab Revolt of 1936-1939, made conditions for doctors and nurses fraught with danger as they tried to run clinics in different centres.

From 1933 to 1938 more than 1,200 Jewish doctors immigrated as the Nazi threat in Europe increased. They brought new approaches to health care, based on their clinical training and experiences in Germany and they soon entered the Kupat Cholim system, sometimes after a period in private practice. Given the numbers, one doctor to 300 Jews, employment was often precarious and there were regular complaints that Jewish physicians were not well represented in Government employ. However, as the population increased hospital care expanded: the beginnings of the Beilinson and Assuta Hospitals can be identified during this period and, eventually, the greater availability of Jewish physicians led to their employment in Government hospitals. Jewish doctors were under-represented in Government health employ as barriers, both financial and linguistic, affected their recruitment although Jewish and Arab nurses functioned together through the Mandate.

Medical Care in the Arab Population

In her review of Arab Health care during the British Mandate, Sandy Sufian noted that this large topic has not received much scholarly attention, for a variety of reasons often related to concentration on other topics in the Palestinian narrative rather than health-care.[6] Nevertheless her brief account of Arab health care during the Mandate indicates that the Government did not see Arab health as a funding priority. Indeed, Government health funding dropped during the Mandate as a proportion of its annual budget and its emphasis on clinical care came at the expense of dealing with prevalent infectious diseases.[7]

Hospital care was mainly provided by Government hospitals or by the variety of Christian missionary institutions, often created in Ottoman times. As these hospitals were concentrated in the urban centres, rural Arabs had limited access to facilities that were available. As we have seen, some of the health bodies of the Jewish community, the Hadassah Medical Organisation and Kupat Cholim, provided care to the Arab population. While useful in many parts of the country, this did not reach the level of widespread provision. A certain level of health care contact between the Arab and Jewish population did exist but could be affected during periods of tension such as during the Arab Revolt of 1936-1939. However, no separate Arab health care system was established during the Mandate. This can be partially attributed to financial considerations and a lack of support from the Government.[8]

Western medicine also had to compete with the traditional practices of unqualified healers who prescribed herbal remedies and practices to ward off the 'evil eye' to which children were especially prone. Gradually, the number of Arab physicians in the country increased although, due to Jewish immigration, the Jewish doctors numbered around 90 per cent of all medical practitioners at the end of the Mandate. By this time a Palestine Arab Medical Association had been established and many of the Arab doctors were training in the various medical specialities in medical schools abroad. Sufian also points to the role that Palestinian physicians played in nationalist causes. Tawfiq Canaan, in his evidence to the Anglo-American Commission of Inquiry in 1946, disputed the claim that Zionism had improved the health and welfare of the Arab population or that it had extended medical facilities to the Arabs 'on a large scale'.[9] While Jews were building the medical institutions necessary for independence, the Arab population was focused on opposition to Jewish independence.

The Beginnings of Health Organisations: Kupat Cholim and Hadassah

Kupat Cholim

No understanding of the provision of health care during the Mandate is complete without examining the role played by both Kupat Cholim and Hadassah. Kupat Cholim, the Workers' Health fund in Eretz Israel, is now known as Kupat Cholim Clalit following the entry of other health providers in Israel in recent years., The vision was to create a health organisation that embodied the ideals of social values of justice and equality as perceived by the members of the Second Aliyah. [The Second Aliyah took place between 1904 and 1914, and brought around 35,000 Jews to Ottoman-Palestine, mostly from the Russian Empire, though some also from Yemen.]

The organisation had its beginnings in 1911 as the Judea Workers' Health Fund, meeting the need of Jewish workers for an affordable health system. By 1920, with the beginnings of the Mandate, Kupat Cholim had been formally established. The first health funds aimed to meet the requirements of the Jewish agricultural workers, and indeed the agricultural labourer, played a core role in shaping Kupat Cholim's development. The first impulses in setting up the organisation were based on the simple mutual-aid welfare societies which existed in most Jewish communities in Eastern Europe, and were taken by the masses of Jewish immigrant to Britain and North America. This was buttressed by the adoption of European models of health care insurance for the working population.

Given the absence of government initiatives in creating a health care framework, Kupat Cholim was forced to operate initially as an independent provider although, increasingly, its structural base was to lie within the Histadrut, the trade union organisation representing Jewish labour. Thus, from the start Kupat Cholim had to develop a clear mission to care for the growing Jewish population on what was to become a national scale, which had implications for health care in Israel after 1948.

The central role of the Jewish workers in establishing Kupat Cholim left them in charge of management and health policy while the doctors, and other health care professionals such as nurses and pharmacists, were seen as salaried employees just like any other. However, Kupat Cholim faced competition from other Jewish agencies. The American Joint Distribution Committee was involved in malaria prevention for a time during the 1920s and Hadassah developed its own arrangement with the Government's Health Office by transferring to it its malaria programme, while providing the Health Office with funds from its own budgets. The first years of the Mandate also saw the formation of a number of other health funds for groups of Jewish workers. While these had coalesced by 1920 into one united Health Fund (the General Health Fund of Hebrew workers in Eretz Israel), the various groups who had come together still maintained a degree of operational independence.

The needs of new immigrants and increasing health care costs placed constraints on what could reasonably be provided. By the mid-1920s Kupat

Cholim was organised on a much better financial footing as members' dues were being supplemented by contributions from employers, while around a third of its budget came from subventions from Hadassah. However, the relationship with Hadassah was not always an easy one as the different organisation developed their own spheres of interest and activity. In addition, financial support from Hadassah came with conditions about the use of its funding. Further, it did not take kindly to the expansion of Kupat Cholim services into new areas, such as hospital provision.

Surviving the downturn in the Palestine economy at the end of the 1920s which stimulated the return of many migrants to Europe, Kupat Cholim began the new decade with a clear determination to form the health insurance framework for the growing Yishuv. One example of the growing confidence of Kupat Cholim was the opening, in April 1930, of the new Emek Hospital in the Jezreel Valley near to Afula, seen at the time as the most modern in the country. However, the planning and construction of the hospital proved to be complex, even controversial. Local Jewish rural communities were at odds over the proposed site and Hadassah, committed themselves to hospital management, were not inclined to give the project their support. However, this proved to be an important initiative, and once the financial problems of the first two years had been settled, partly with help from Hadassah, Kupat Cholim could plan in a way which would keep them at the centre of health care.

During the 1930s Kupat Cholim consolidated its position as the key agency of the Histadrut, the general organisation of Jewish trade unions. In January 1930, Kupat Cholim and the Histadrut presented a detailed proposal to the Mandate government for legislation of a compulsory health insurance law. However, Government subventions during the decade never amount to more than 3% of Kupat Cholim running costs, at a time when the Fund was providing health cover to a quarter of the Jewish population, especially to its most disadvantaged groups. Such laws could not be realised until the emergence of the State.

Hadassah

Hadassah, the organisation of American women Zionists, saw its goal as the creation of a modern welfare state for the Jewish population in British Palestine while also providing services for the Arab population. At the same time, as Hadassah was funded from America it saw itself as an output of both Jewish and American social values. It also set priorities in terms of public health nurses and maternity and child care. Guided by its visionary leader, Henrietta Szold, who arrived in Ottoman Palestine in 1909, Hadassah saw its rationale as the creation of a Jewish social democratic society in Palestine based on universal values while eschewing the fragmented nature of Zionist politics.

One important programme, dating back to the 1920s, was *Tipat Chalav*, literally 'drop of milk'. From her first days in the country Szold had been appalled by the high infant mortality in the country, where around a quarter to a third of new-born babies did not survive to their first birthday. Tipat Halav clinics, beginning in 1921, were based on preventative medicine solely for pregnant women and young infants. The medical staff provided the mothers with health information on hygiene, breastfeeding and exposure to sunlight and supplied milk to mothers who could not nurse their babies. Developmental goals for young infants were monitored closely and further clinics were opened throughout the country. Infant mortality in the Jewish population was halved within ten years and by the time of the establishment of the state it had reached European levels.

Inevitably, there was a power struggle with Kupat Cholim, even though the two organisations shared many aims and worked together in many different locales and formats. With the Government refusal to involve itself

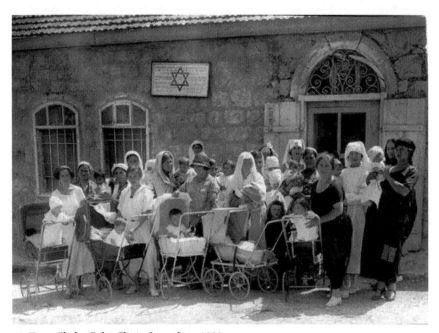

13. Tipat Chalav Baby Clinic, Jerusalem, 1930s.

in running the services that Hadassah was providing there was often no way that Hadassah could ensure the continuing function of their health and welfare activities without direct involvement. The continuing and increasing, American Jewish women's philanthropy had the effect of cementing a deep level of connection with the Jewish community which was sustained after the establishment of the State of Israel in May 1948.

With the rising menace of Nazism after 1933 there was an urgent need to support young, often unaccompanied, refugees arriving in Palestine and Hadassah moved quickly to support the efforts of Youth Aliya in providing help and care for young newcomers to integrate into the Jewish community. Thus, Hadassah was in the forefront of creating the nucleus of what was to become a key element in the care of young people. Hadassah's fund-raising in the United States thus appealed to the maternal instincts of Jewish women seeking to improve health and welfare facilities for women and children in the new Jewish national home.

Around the same time, Hadassah realised one of its long-term goals with the construction of the Hadassah Hospital on Mount Scopus, adjacent to the Hebrew University. The Hospital opened its doors at the end of May 1939, as the Second World War approached. It made practical sense to establish a teaching hospital beside a university but the site was geographically isolated, a factor in the tragic massacre of 78 doctors and nurses on a convoy to Mount Scopus on 13 April 1948. One of the murdered doctors was Haim Yassky, a leading figure in the campaign against trachoma, who had begun his involvement riding a donkey around clinics in rural communities. Yassky had become Director of the Hadassah Medical Organization in 1931 and was one of the major forces behind the establishment of the hospital on Mount Scopus. Yassky was the first non-American based head of the organisation, and he came to New York to spend some time for an orientation on the ethics and practices of Hadassah and American medicine.

Development of Hospital Medicine

The development of hospital specialisation was a gradual process from the beginning of the Mandate, but was much more established by the 1930s. This process coincided with the arrival of significant numbers of Jewish physicians from Germany, experienced in the many medical and surgical disciplines. Among the notable specialists to immigrate to Palestine were the German-born Zondek brothers, sons of physician Max Zondek (1868-1933), who specialised in surgery and the study of renal diseases. In 1913 he was appointed titular professor of surgery in Berlin. Bernhard Zondek (1891-1966) had been a leading obstetrician and gynaecologist in Berlin, where he had developed the first reliable pregnancy test in 1928. He was dismissed from his posts in 1933 and, after a year in Sweden, was appointed Professor of Obstetrics and Gynaecology at the Hebrew University of Jerusalem, and Head of Obstetrics and Gynaecology at the Hadassah Hospital. He was awarded the Israel Prize in Medicine in 1958 and continued his endocrinology studies after retirement as Visiting Professor at the Albert Einstein College of Medicine in New York, where he died in 1966.

Bernhard's medical brothers Hermann (1887-1979) and Samuel Georg also came to Palestine in 1934, frustrated by the regulations for re-qualification in England.[10] In 1951 Hermann was appointed Professor of Endocrinology at the Hebrew University in Jerusalem, where his research on heart, kidney and metabolic diseases had made him a world-recognised figure. Samuel Georg (1894-1970) became a leading internist at the Hadassah Hospital in Tel Aviv, best known for his studies on electrolytes and the therapy of heart diseases.

There was naturally some friction between Hadassah, who saw American medicine as pre-eminent, and the newcomers trained in German medicine.[11] Nevertheless, the influx of German doctors in the 1930s set the parameters for the development of clinical excellence in the years ahead. Haim Yassky, as Director of the Hadassah Medical Organization, now understood the American influence and sent emerging specialists, needed to staff the new departments at the Hadassah Hospital, to America for advanced training. The beginnings of formal medical education in Palestine date back to 1939 when a 'pre-faculty' of medicine was established, with Arye Feigenbaum as Dean, consisting of the University's School of Postgraduate Studies and the Hadassah Hospital. The formal opening of the Hebrew University-Hadassah Medical School, the first in the country, followed soon after the establishment of the State, beginning in May 1949.

Specialisation covers the whole range of clinical practice but here we will look at obstetrics and paediatrics as exemplars of the process. Midwifery practice and birthing conditions in Ottoman times were very poor, as mentioned above, exacerbated by factors such as malnutrition, early age at marriage and child birth and multiple pregnancies and births.

Midwifery

In 1898 there were 22 Jewish 'traditional' midwives in Jerusalem, of whom 13 were Ashkenazi and 9 were Sephardi, who relied on superstition as much as clinical ability. However, the last decades of Ottoman rule saw the arrival of several local women who had been trained abroad as midwives Not only did they sometimes have to overcome mistrust on their return, some of the young women encountered difficulties when expressing their wish to study midwifery abroad.

Two of the midwives, Rachel Deutsch (1867-1965) born in Tzefat, and Elka Godel (1879-?) born in Jerusalem, studied in Vienna. Godel went to England to study medicine and then spent some years in Australia before returning to Palestine in 1919.

Another midwife was Russian-born Olga Belkind (1852-1942), who studied in St. Petersburg at a time when residence in the city was very restricted for Jews. In 1886 she came to Rishon Le-Zion to join other family members there. Gradually these midwives made an important impact and Muslim families too came to prefer the certified Jewish midwives and valued their work.[12] However, the situation for Arab mother and child care, in the poorest sections of the population, remained serious. Dr. Alexandra Belkind, a medical graduate from Geneva specialising in women's medicine, came to the country in 1906. She was highly critical of the traditional Muslim midwives who 'more than anything do them harm, for in their ignorance, they cause them damage and after birth, cause injury to the new-born baby's limbs, leading to deformities and other diseases'. A study, conducted by the Palestinian paediatrician Tawfiq Canaan in 1925, showed a still-birth rate of a fifth of all Arab pregnancies while nearly half of live births died within a short period.[13] The system only improved with a Government training programme for Arab midwives employing British nurses from the Colonial Service who had worked in India, Africa and Iraq. They quickly learned Arabic and worked with mothers both in clinics and in their homes.

The arrival of paediatricians was also of crucial important in raising standards and reducing morbidity and mortality. Leading this was Tashkent-born Helena Kagan (1889-1978). Kagan, a medical graduate from the University of Bern, settled in Jerusalem in 1914 and is recognised as the first paediatrician in the country. She established the Israel Pediatrics Association in 1927 and in 1936, she set up the paediatrics department of the Bikkur Cholim Hospital in Jerusalem, which she headed until 1975. Like many of the other early doctors and midwives she was active in social groups and was a founder of the *Histadrut Nashim Ivriot* (Hebrew Women's Organization).

In 1925 the rate of infant mortality in the Muslim Arab population was 200 per 1,000 births, and 131 in the Jewish community, and improvements continued in the following years. In 1939, for example, the level in the Jewish community had fallen to 54 per 1,000 births, a figure similar to that in Britain and the United States. Birth rates were much higher in the Muslim population during the Mandate at around 50 per 1,000 live births while the figures for Jews and Christian fell, between 1923 and 1942, from around 37 per 1,000 live births to 23 and 29 respectively. The Regulations for the role of midwives, introduced at the beginning of the Mandate, were substantially revised by an Ordinance in 1929, following consultation with British, Arab and Jewish sources. The aim of improving child and maternal health and reducing infant mortality health had to be balanced with an understanding of the role of the midwife in traditional society. The Jewish population came to express a strong preference for hospital care in childbirth and services continued to be supplied by a wide variety of providers.

Mental Health[14]

Psychiatry as a medical field did not exist in Palestine in Ottoman times. Although a law for the mentally ill was passed in 1892, it was poorly implemented and no asylum was established in the country. Only one mental hospital serving the Jewish population, the Ezrat Nashim Hospital for women, was founded in Jerusalem in 1895. However, it was seriously over-crowded and could provide only general medical treatment rather than psychiatric care, and Jewish patients often had recourse to Government or Christian institutions. One of the first steps of the Mandate Government was to establish a mental hospital in Bethlehem. It hoped both to end the Arab villagers' practice of confining the mentally sick or handicapped to home or the urban sick wandering free without recourse to treatment. However, the Bethlehem Mental Hospital was always over-crowded with long waiting-lists. As late as 1942 it was recognised that bed provision for mental illness was only a tenth of what was required, a situation that High Commissioner Sir Harold MacMichael felt 'reflected badly on Government'.

The Zionist aim of creating a society where Jews would be healthier and fitter had to also confront the issue of mental illness. Mental health problems have been a source of shame in many societies and the stigma of mental illness clearly clashed with the imperative of creating the 'new Jew'.[15] This stigma extended to the criteria for immigration to Palestine as most authorities, including the British Mandatory Government in its Immigration Ordinance of 1925, aimed to exclude individuals because of mental or physical illness. People with chronic infectious diseases, epilepsy or mental deficiency were most likely to be excluded. This was not a new measure in the early to mid-twentieth century context. Influenced by eugenic beliefs, most governments around the world before and during the interwar period restricted immigration based upon medical un-fitness, and such concerns extended to Zionist immigration policy in its early years.[16] Such selection processes may have served to minimise rates of Jewish mental illness as fitter and healthier Jews were more likely to be productive and contribute to the growing Zionist enterprise.

Psychiatric hospital provision in British Palestine was exceptionally weak, even by general Middle Eastern standards, and this problem was not solved during the Mandate era. Zionist organisations too placed a low priority on providing the necessary resources for the mentally ill. The situation changed dramatically after 1933 with the arrival of many Jewish psychiatrists fleeing from Nazi Germany. The newcomers brought modern psychiatric techniques to the country, opening private clinics and founding psychiatric and psycho-analytic societies, and provided the basis for developments in the State of Israel.[17]

The Third Aliya brought around 40,000 Jews to Palestine between 1919 and 1923. Mostly young idealistic pioneers from Eastern Europe, they were spurred to leave by antisemitic pogroms and attracted by the opportunities of British rule in Palestine. They took the lead in major infrastructure projects. The psycho-analysts dealt with the issues, often ignored by the Zionist authorities, faced by these pioneers, separated from family and often working in a hostile environment. Dr. David Eder (1865-1936), the first practising psycho-analyst in Britain, had been a member of the Zionist Executive at the beginning of the Mandate but the beginnings of psycho-analytic practice only began with the arrival in 1933 of Max Eitingon (1881-1943), a student of Sigmund Freud. He founded the Palestine Psychoanalytic Association in 1934 but, despite Freud's recommendation, he did not manage to gain a chair in psychoanalysis at the Hebrew University of Jerusalem.

At the beginning of the 1930s an asylum was established in Bnei-Brak, supported by the Tel-Aviv municipality and Jewish charity organisations. In 1944, a third governmental psychiatric hospital, for mainly Jewish patients, was built in Bat-Yam, a town near Tel Aviv, following a campaign by residents of Tel Aviv. Given the focus of the immigrant psychiatrists it was not surprising that mental health of the Jews from Eastern communities was regarded less positively.

Infectious Diseases

The processes of urbanisation put pressure on housing and sanitation leading to problems with several infectious diseases. The last cholera epidemic occurred during the First World War but enteric diseases, which were most common in the Jewish population during the 1920s, increased during the 1930s in the Arab sector. By the end of the 1930s most of the deaths due to enteric diseases were in the Arab population, where there was a higher mortality rate for typhoid, despite the disease being commoner amongst the Jews. Measles, a rare cause of death in the Jewish population, led to over 3,000 deaths among Muslims between 1938 and 1945.[7] Diseases such as schistomsiasis, leishmaniasis and hookworm, all related to poor hygiene, were also much commoner in the Arab population.

There were still some patients with leprosy, Hansen's Disease, during the Mandate, mostly cared for, as we have noted, at the Jesus Hilfe Asylum, subsequently known as Hansen's Hospital in Jerusalem. During the Mandate patients were mainly Muslim and Christian with just a few Jews and inmates were generally free to come and go. The leprosy hospital came to house the most afflicted cases while others came for treatment once the diagnosis had been made.

A study of the prevalence of tuberculosis during the Mandate was conducted in 1935. This indicated a level of disease like that found in England and Wales, although it did not produce the same level of fatalities. Arab patients formed most of the patients at Government TB clinics while Jewish patients were cared for by the Jewish Anti-Tuberculosis League, supported by many Jewish communities abroad, which maintained a sanatorium near Jerusalem. Another sanatorium was situated in Haifa while Hadassah ran a 60-bed TB hospital, supported by some Government funding.

Malaria was also a health scourge from even before the Mandate years. Seen as a scar in the geography of the Land of Israel, as well as in its inhabitants, its eradication was pursued with zeal. In Jerusalem, and other cities and towns, the winter epidemics were blamed on the water cisterns, which collected rainfall during the wet winter but also allowed the anopheles mosquito to breed. There were also reservoirs of the mosquito along the coastal plain and in the Hula Valley marshes. Malaria was a major cause of mortality and morbidity especially during the early years of the Mandate. Patients debilitated by the condition were susceptible to other diseases and were often unable to survive them.

A leading figure in malaria research and management was Dr. Israel Kligler (1888-1944), who arrived in Palestine in 1921.[18] Kligler had been born in Galicia and educated in the United States and he brought skills of public health control and organisation in the fight to eradicate malaria using realistic goals, including the introduction of larva-eating fish and the draining of swamps by planting eucalyptus trees. Therapy with quinine was also introduced and by the end of the mandate the number of malaria cases had dropped by three quarters. The importance of Kligler's work was recognised as early as 1925 with a visit by the League of Nations Malaria Commission. A Research Station was opened in Rosh Pina in 1927, and in 1930 Kligler published his authoritative work on malaria. In 1929, the local doctor, Gideon Mer (1894-1961), became the manager of Kligler's Malaria Research Station, devoting himself to eradicating malaria from the mosquito-infected swamps in the nearby Hula Valley. After Kligler published his authoritative work on malaria in 1930 and collaborated with Mer in further research. Full eradication only came after Kligler's untimely death in 1944 at the age of 56 years.

Another leading figure in the treatment of malaria in the early twentieth century was Hillel Yaffe (1864-1936). Yaffe had studied medicine in Geneva and arrived in Ottoman Palestine in 1891 with a license to practice medicine. Two years later he settled in Zikhron Yaakov, which was then blighted with malaria. He tackled the scourge both as a physician and as a community activist involved in public health measures, gaining an international reputation for his work. His first efforts to eradicate malaria focused on drying the swamps through channel draining or with eucalyptus trees. Later, he focused on household measures to prevent mosquito access to settlers' homes.

There was a high prevalence of the chronic eye disease trachoma in British Palestine, amongst the highest in the world, and its virtual elimination in the Jewish population, in barely 30 years, is a story of the successful integration of health planning and national policy in what was described as a 'war against trachoma'. Trachoma can be passed from person to person through poor personal hygiene, flies or other contaminated material. The obsessive approach to trachoma by the Jewish health organisations led to a higher expenditure for the disease which, before the introduction of modern therapies, would often progress to severe sight loss and blindness, than for such chronic health diseases as tuberculosis. Further, funds which could have ameliorated other eyes diseases, or even paid for the management of refractory eye problems, were diverted into trachoma prevention and treatment. It took resources of hygiene, medicine, education and national ideology to provide a determined framework to defeat this visible scourge but within a generation the task was almost completed.

Facilities for the surgical treatment of eye disease developed rapidly from the last years of the nineteenth century. The St. John's Ophthalmic Hospital in Jerusalem began treating patients in 1883and Jewish hospitals began to deal with eye diseases from 1900. The first Jewish special eye clinic opened in Jerusalem in 1912. The first medical conference in the country, held in spring 1914, brought together 24 doctors involved in treating eye diseases and their practical approach reduced the prevalence of trachoma in the Jewish agricultural villages and schools even before the First World War.[19]

The drive against trachoma began in the schools in Jerusalem in 1918. Early figures indicated that 60 to 95 per cent of school children, depending on locality, could be affected by trachoma and quick action was needed. The Mandate Government concentrated on the treatment of the disease in schoolchildren as most cases of adult infection were due to infection in the first three years of life and the rest were infected in later childhood. By 1924 the Government Department of Health was running six eye-clinics and preventative ophthalmic work reached 60,000 school children.

However, school programmes missed pre-school children and rural Arab children where school enrolments were low. The high levels of trachoma in the Arab population also created an impetus for more active management of the disease.[20] Government initiatives in training nurses and medical personnel and the short-term initiative of a Government Travelling Ophthalmic Hospital helped reduce the over-all rate.

Leading figures in the fight against trachoma were Dr. Arye Feigenbaum (1885-1981), who became Professor of Ophthalmology at the Hebrew University of Jerusalem in 1939, Dr. Haim Yassky, (1896-1946) Director of Hadassah, who was killed in the Hadassah convoy massacre and Dr. Abraham Ticho, (1883-1960) Director of the Lemaan Zion Eye Hospital. Hadassah formed hospital-based ophthalmic services in Jerusalem, Jaffa, Tiberias, Haifa and Tsefat and also in Jewish rural villages from 1924. Besides these patient contacts there was a simultaneous effort to target infected children at home and in school. Treatment was time consuming and labour intensive involving doctors and nurses in daily school visits and careful screening before treatment helped to minimise loss of teaching time! This had major benefits, perhaps most spectacularly in Jaffa, where prevalence fell from 64.8 per cent in 1918-1919 to just 16.1 per cent five years later.

Schools were provided with proper treatments so that they would not contribute to the spread of the disease. Each child had a medical inspection and an individual trachoma schedule. School and clinic nurses administered topical therapy and there was monthly medical supervision. Children with acute eye infections and trachoma granulation were excluded from school till the end of treatment. Separate kindergartens for infected children were established and families were advised on diet and hygiene and prizes were awarded to school children for completing a programme of eye examinations. This activity was supported by the Health Scouts movement sponsored by Hadassah nurses. Members had to take a course in health and hygiene and were required to promote the health ideals within the community to obtain the official uniform and Health Scouts pin. This all supported their ideal of developing the communal responsibility befitting a 'pioneering country'.

By the end of the 1920s Hadassah could claim credit for reducing the prevalence in Jewish schoolchildren to below 10 per cent. However, this figure conceals variations in the different Jewish ethnic communities with the highest prevalence found in Kurdish and Persian Jews. Jews in Yemen experienced little trachoma but once they left Yemen for Palestine the prevalence increased dramatically.[21] The highest prevalence in the Jewish community was found in schools of the eastern communities in the Jewish Quarter of the Old City in Jerusalem and even as late as 1942/3 this had only fallen to 27.9%. Yet there was progress within the poorest, most traditional sections, of the Ashkenazi community of Jerusalem where trachoma prevalence had fallen to only 1.2% in 1938.

During the 1930s the expense of the Jewish public health services became a major issue. In 1936 the Tel Aviv municipality took over school hygiene and eye clinics in the Yemenite districts from Hadassah and the Vaad Leumi assumed responsibility for preventative health care enabling Hadassah to concentrate on specific programmes within disadvantaged groups. Within the Arab population GDH eye clinics and rural mobile units began to tackle the problem, but there was no provision for an intensive daily school and home care service. Nevertheless the levels of trachoma in the Arab population was falling, with an encouraging drop in eye complications and blindness.[22]

While the proportion of Jewish children with trachoma was falling sharply, in absolute terms numbers had changed little during the 1920s and 1930s, partly because of large-scale immigration. This gave a feeling that the trachoma campaign had stalled and that the concentration on one disease had led to the wider range of eye problems, including eye refraction, being virtually neglected.[23]

Trachoma was no longer pandemic but was confined to certain localities and communities and future efforts were concentrated there.[24] In 1937 the introduction of the antibiotic sulphanilamide began to revolutionise the management of the disease.[25] By 1946 the level of trachoma in the Jewish schools of Palestine stood at 2.9% and only 1.6% in Jerusalem, with almost all the 16,000 cases in the Yishuv in the eastern communities.[26] Haim Yassky concluded that it was now time to reduce the scope of the campaign.[27] However, trachoma in the area was not yet over. The major waves of immigration in Israel's first years brought large numbers of Holocaust survivors, many in poor health, and Jewish refugees from other countries in the Middle East and North Africa where trachoma was still endemic.

Conclusions

Jewish health care was part of the fabric of the Zionist movement and the creation of a fit, healthy modern nation was a key goal. Disease ran counter to this vision. The conquest of malaria represented a healing of the land while the veritable war against trachoma aimed to eradicate a disease that by its nature was both uniquely visible and potentially debilitating. In this chapter, trachoma has served as a key example of how Jewish health policy took on national characteristics, in a sometimes obsessive way. We have noted how health disparities developed between Jewish and Arab populations in the Mandate period due to the special emphasis on health funding and provision in the Jewish sector. Ironically, it was in the health field that the two communities came closest together as health staff and patients shared facilities. War, civil unrest and communal strife were also factors in limiting the effectiveness of health care during the three decades of British rule. Nevertheless, by the end of the Mandate, the Jewish bodies, led by Kupat Cholim and Hadassah, were able to provide the emerging state, and its developing institutions, with the fundamental aspects of a modern health service.

Acknowledgements

I would like to thank those who provided help and guidance for the material in this chapter: Professor Efraim Lev, Department of Israel Studies, University of Haifa, provided much appreciated advice on text and references. The staff at the Central Zionist Archives, Jerusalem (CZA) and at Hadassah Archives, New York provided helpful archival information on trachoma. Marcella Simoni and Shifra Shvarts helped with references and Zalman Greenberg shared his extensive bibliography. Rakefet Zalashik retrieved material from German journals which Rosa Sacharin translated.

Select Bibliography

Further details on the topics covered in this chapter can be found in the following articles and books.

1. Collins, K., 'The Torrance Collection at the Archive, Records Management and Museum Services at the University of Dundee, Scotland', *Vesalius: Journal of the International Society for the History of Medicine*, vol. XX, pp.99-102.
2. Collins, K., 'Trachoma in the Jewish Community in British Palestine, 1919-1948', *Korot: the Israel Journal for the History of Medicine and Science*, 21, (2011-2012), Supplement on Infectious Diseases and Epidemics in the land of Israel, pp.89-120. This issue also has articles on polio, cholera, malaria and leprosy.
3. El-Eini, R., *Mandated Landscape: British Imperial Rule in Palestine 1929-1948* (Abingdon: Routledge, 2006).
4. Levin, M., *It Takes a Dream: the Story of Hadassah* (Jerusalem: 2002).
5. Levy, N. and Levy, Y., *Physicians in the Holy Land: 1799-1948* (Hebrew) (Itay Bachur: Zichron Yaakov, 2008); Perry, Y. and Lev, E., *Modern Medicine in the Holy Land: Pioneering British Medical Services in Late Ottoman Palestine* (London: 1999).
6. Reiss, N., *British Public Health Policy in Palestine, 1918-1947* and Waserman, M., 'The Hadassah Medical Organisation: Critical Years, 1928-1951: Oral History Interview with Dr. Eli Davis Manfred Waserman' in Kottek, S.S. (Ed.), *Health and Disease in the Holy Land: Studies in the History and Sociology of Medicine from Ancient Times to the Present*, (Lampeter: 1996).
7. Shehory-Rubin, Z., 'Jewish Midwives in Eretz Israel During the Late Ottoman Period, 1850–1918', *Soc Hist Med* (2011) 24 (2), pp.299-315.
8. Shepherd, N., *Ploughing Sand: British Rule in Palestine 1918-1948* (London: 1999).
9. Shvarts, S., *Health and Zionism: the Israeli Health Care System: 1948-1960* (Rochester: 2008).
10. Shvarts, S., *The Workers Health Fund in Eretz Israel: Kupat Holim*, (Rochester: 2002).
11. Sufian, S.M., *Healing the Land and the Nation Malaria and the Zionist Project in Mandatory Palestine 1920-1947* (Chicago: 2007).
12. Sufian, S.M., 'Arab Health Care during the British Mandate, 1920-1947' in Barnca, T. and Husseini, R. (Eds), *Separate and Cooperate, Cooperate and Separate: The Disengagement of the Palestine Health Care System from Israel and its Emergence as an Independent System* (Westport, CT: 2002).

Notes

1. Livingstone, W. P., *A Galilee Doctor: the Life of Dr. Herbert Torrance of Tiberias* (London, n.d.).

2. Shepherd, N., *Ploughing Sand: British Rule in Palestine 1918-1948*, (London: 1999), p.136. Shepherd points out that the parsimonious attitude to sanitation frequently ended in disaster.
3. See Reiss, N., 'British Public Health Policy in Palestine, 1918-1947' in Waserman, M. and Kottek, S.S. (Eds), *Health and Disease in the Holy Land: Studies in the History and Sociology of Medicine from Ancient Times to the Present*, (Lampeter: 1996), p.311. Reiss considered that the administration's answers to claims for a larger share of the budget were self-serving with regard to the Jews and condescending with regard to the Arabs.
4. Shepherd, *Ploughing Sand,* p.142.
5. Health details can be found in Statistics Palestine Government Department of Statistics, e.g. *Statistical Abstracts of Palestine 1944-5* (1946).
6. Sufian, S.M., 'Arab Health Care during the British Mandate, 1920-1947' in Barnea, T. and Husseini, R. (Eds), *Separate and Cooperate, Cooperate and Separate: The Disengagement of the Palestine Health Care System from Israel and its Emergence as an Independent System.* (Westport, CT.: 2002). Sufian notes the paucity of Arabic sources and refers to Mohammed Karkara's unpublished master thesis (in Hebrew) as the most complete investigation of Arab health before and during the Mandate.
7. Ibid., p.14.
8. Ibid., p.16.
9. Sufian, S.M, *Healing the Land and the Nation Malaria and the Zionist Project in Mandatory Palestine 1920-1947* (Chicago: 2007), pp.315-331.
10. http://aerzte.erez-israel.de/hermann-zondek/, consulted 5/1/2017.
11. Baader, G., 'The impact of German Jewish physicians and German medicine on the origins and development of the medical faculty of the Hebrew University of Jerusalem', *Korot: the Israel Journal for the History of Medicine and Science*, 15 (Jan 2001), pp.9-45.
12. Katvan, E. and Bartal, N., 'The midwives ordinance of Palestine, 1929: historical perspectives and current lessons', *Nurs Inq.* June 2010; 17(2), pp.165-72.
13. Lev, E. and Amar, Z., 'The Turning Point from an Archaic Arab Medical System to an Early Modern European System in Jerusalem according to the Swiss Physician Titus Tobler (1806–77)', *Canadian Bulletin of Medical History*, 21, 2004, pp.159-1.
14. Zalashik, E., 'Psychiatry, ethnicity and migration: The case of Palestine, 1920-1948', *DYNAMIS: Acta Hisp. Med. Sci. Hist. Illus.* 2005, 25, pp.403-422; Sufian, S., 'Mental Hygiene and Disability in the Zionist Project', *Disability Studies Quarterly,* Fall 2007, vol. 27, no.4, http://www.dsq-sds.org/article/view/42/42#endnoteref07, consulted 15/1/2017; Halpern, L., 'Insanity among the Jews in Palestine', *Harefuah.* vol 7, no. 4, 1937; Halpern, L., 'Some Data of the Psychic Morbidity of Jews and Arabs in Palestine', *American Journal of Psychiatry,* March 1938, vol. 94, p.1,215.
15. Rolnik, E., *Freud in Zion: Psychoanalysis and the Making of Modern Jewish Identity* (London: Karnac, 2012), Hebrew edition 2007; Niederland, D., 'The emigration of Jewish academics and professionals from Germany in the first years of Nazi rule', *Leo Baeck Institute Year Book,* 1988, 33, pp.285-286.
16. Shvarts, S., Davidovitch, H., Seidelman, R. and Goldberg, A., 'Medical Selection and the Debate over Mass Immigration in the New State of Israel (1948-1951)', *Canadian Bulletin of Medical History* 22:1 (2005) 8; Davidovitch, N. and Shvarts, S., 'Health and Zionist Ideology: Medical Selection of Jewish European Immigrants to Palestine' in Borowy, I. and Gruner, W.D. (Eds), *Facing Illness in Troubled Times: Health in Europein the Interwar Years, 1918-1939* (Frankfurt: Peter Lang Publishing, 2005), pp.411-18.

17.　*Statistical Abstracts of Palestine 1944-5* (1946).

18.　Greenberg, Z., Alexander, A. and Kligler, I.J., 'The story of "little big man": A Giant in the Field of Public Health Medicine in Israel', *Korot: the Israel Journal for the History of Medicine and Science*, 21, (2011-2012), Supplement on Infectious Diseases and Epidemics in the land of Israel, pp.175-208.

19.　Navot, O. and Gross, A., 'The Campaign Against Trachoma: the Beginnings of Public Health in Eretz Israel' (Hebrew), *Cathedra*, 94 (1999), pp.89-114; Friedenwald, H., 'The Ophthalmias of Palestine', *Transactions of the American Ophthalmologic Society*, vol.14, 1915, p.280; Shimkin, N., 'On the Question of the War Against Trachoma in the Jewish Population in the Land of Israel' (Hebrew), *HaRefuah*, vol.22, 1942, pp.57-59, 70-72.

20.　Navot and Gross, 'The Campaign Against Trachoma', pp.92-93.

21.　Report by His Majesty's Government in the United Kingdom of Great Britain and Northern Ireland to the Council of the League of Nations on the Administration of Palestine and Trans-Jordan, 1928, p.56 and 1936/7.

22.　Sinai, A., Das Trachom unter denyemenitischen (südarabischen) Juden', (German) *Folia Ophthalmologica Orientalia*, 1 (1932), pp.83-89.

23.　A Survey of Palestine, Prepared in December 1945 and January 1946 for the Information of the Anglo-American Committee of Enquiry, 2, pp.623, 701-702.

24.　Yassky, H., 'Ophthalmological Work of Hadassah Medical Organisation in Palestine', Central Zionist Archives (CZA) J113/101, 1934

25.　Dobrzynsjki, N., 'The Fight Against Trachoma in Palestine: its Results and Prospects', *Harefuah*, 28, (1942).

26.　Shimkin, N., 'The Treatment of Trachoma with Sulfanilimide', *Acta Opthalmologica Orientalia*, 1, 4 (1939), pp.251-257; MacCallan, A.A., 'Trachoma', *British Encyclopaedia of Medical Practice*, Ed. Sir Humphrey Rolleston (London: 1939), vol.12, pp.210-221.

27.　Dobrzynski, N., 'The Anti-Trachoma Campaign in Palestine in the Past and in the Future', Lecture at the Jubilee Conference of the Jewish Physicians' Association, Jerusalem, September 1944, p.4; Yasski, H., Director, Hadassah Medical Organisation, HMO#45, periodic letter, 29/1/1947, Hadassah Archives, Box 110/F8.

8

Health Schemes and Health in Israel

Nadav Davidovitch

Background

In January 1995, the National Health Insurance Law of 1994 entered into force, establishing compulsory health insurance for every resident of Israel. The law prohibited health management organisations (HMOs, Kupot Cholim) from denying insurance to anyone, and it established insurance fees based on a resident's income and a specified rate. Unemployed residents are also required to pay health insurance based on a minimum that is periodically updated. The enactment of this law, one of the most important social laws adopted since Israel's founding, marked the end of a struggle for the provision of healthcare services, which had begun even before statehood.

To a large extent, since the British Mandate era Israel's healthcare services can only be characterized as a 'healthcare system'. Until then services were provided primarily by local and voluntary organisations, with almost no planning, management or central coordination. The Ottoman government provided some health services, which focused mainly on public health issues such as quarantine centres, examinations of immigrants and a limited selection of government medical services. During the British Mandate era, an infrastructure of community and hospital-based healthcare services gradually developed, and with the founding of the State this infrastructure steadily expanded, alongside the spread and growth of the population. The main difference was that before Statehood this system had been voluntary and operated in parallel to the British Mandate system, which created tension and redundancy. Nonetheless, the healthcare infrastructure that served the pre-State Jewish population had a very strong community network, including clinics in peripheral locations as well as pre-natal and early childhood healthcare centres (*Tipot Chalav*), among other Services, and this provided an important foundation once Israel achieved statehood.

The Mandatory government invested in public health as well, primarily to prevent the spread of contagious diseases, whereas it invested relatively little in the hospital system. The infrastructure of military hospitals developed by the British during the Second World War provided a foundation for military hospitals after Israel was founded. In the 1950s these were transferred to the Ministry of Health in what was meant to be an interim arrangement prior to their transfer to local authorities, a process that never took place and left the Ministry of Health responsible to this day for many hospitals, some of which are spread across several old facilities – as exemplified by Sheba Medical Centre and Assaf HaRofeh-Shamir Medical Centre. This contrasts with the manner in which the HMO Clalit constructed its hospital network, which began even before Israel's founding and was based on infrastructures of higher quality. Another hospital system that the State of Israel 'inherited' is the Hadassah network of hospitals which, with the exception of Jerusalem, were transferred to other entities. Hadassah Tel Aviv, for example, was transferred to the Tel Aviv municipality as early as the 1930s.

A survey of developments in the healthcare system since the 1920s indicates that to a large extent those years shaped the character and organisation of the healthcare system in Israel prior to passage of the National Health Insurance law, and to some extent to this day. The characteristics of this healthcare system included:

- A pluralistic healthcare network comprising many institutions and organisations.
- Adoption by the pre-State Jewish community leadership of a model based on HMOs in many aspects within the purview of the state-in-the-making, as practised in various European countries. Later the healthcare system adopted certain characteristics of centralized control, on the one hand, and a market economy, on the other, thus making it more of a 'mixed' than a distinct model. Even before statehood, the principles of relatively accessible care for the community, including in remote areas, and the political ideological composition of health organisations constituted unique features of the healthcare system, and they continue to shape its nature today.
- Financial activity characterized by a permanent deficit.
- Direct provision of health services by the Ministry of Health, alongside its ministerial functions.
- Direct provision of health services by the HMOs, alongside their role as an insurer.

After many attempts to enact a national health insurance law, the right political moment eventually arrived. It had first been necessary to separate Histadrut HaOvdim Ha'Clalit (the national trade union association) from Kupat Holim Clalit (the HMO originally affiliated with the Histadrut) at the political level, while also allowing the economy and healthcare policy to mature sufficiently. In the early 1990s the political, economic and professional conditions became ripe for legislation of the law on which Israel's healthcare system is now based.

The guiding principle underpinning the National Health Insurance Law is that medical care in Israel is to be provided on the basis of medical needs, independently of the financial means of the insured. The law also defined a uniform basket of medical services that HMOs must provide, with government oversight over the operations of the HMOs. In addition to compulsory insurance, HMOs were granted the option of offering complementary insurance to the insured, for additional services not included in the public medical services basket. Health insurance fees are paid via the National Insurance Institute, allowing for managed competition among the HMOs, freedom of choice for citizens to select their preferred HMO, focused dues collection as needed, and guaranteed income for the HMOs. At the same time, the responsibility for managing the Ministry of Health's budget was delegated to the Ministry of Finance.

The public sources of funding for the HMOs are determined on the basis of a capitation formula that is, according to the number of insureds in each HMO, weighted by age and other socio-demographic factors. This mechanism is an important means for implementing the system's policy of resource allocation. Its structure and implementation represent the financial expression of the system's structure, management, precedence and concept of social justice. Given that there is variance in the consumption of services across different age groups, allocations are based on the relative weight of each group in relation to its consumption of the medical services covered by the basket of services for which HMOs are responsible. Furthermore, for five 'severe diseases' (end-stage renal failure, Gaucher disease, haemophilia, thalassaemia, AIDS), HMOs receive an additional budgetary allocation based on the actual number of patients because these diseases are highly responsive to treatment. These days, in light of the changing social and economic context, the Ministry of Health is considering a new model for capitation and the designation of severe diseases.

In addition, HMOs are entitled to charge members' co-payments for some of the services in the services basket. The Ministry of Health updates the maximum co-payments that HMOs may charge for services and drugs approved by the Finance Committee of the Knesset (Israeli parliament). The original purpose of the co-payments was to prevent the overuse of services (a market failure termed 'moral hazard'), but in time it became a system for collecting fees from members to cover growing budget deficits. Having a co-payment for some of the services constitutes a heavy burden for patients, undermines equality and increases economic gaps within the population.

The following sections discuss the characteristics of morbidity and health in Israel and their impact on health needs.

Morbidity Characteristics in Israel, with Attention to Demographic Distribution

In the past decade there has been a decline in the mortality rate in Israel for most of the leading causes of death. Most notably, the mortality rate among men and women for all deaths, adjusted by age, declined by 25% during 2000-2015.[1]

In 2016 Israel recorded 43,966 deaths. Since 1999 the leading cause of death in Israel for both men and women has been cancer, and the second leading cause has been heart disease. During 2013-2015, on average, cancer was the leading underlying cause of death for all ages combined, as well as for women aged 15-74 and men aged 25 and above. Heart disease was the leading cause among women aged 75 and above, and the second leading cause among men aged 45 and above and women aged 45-74. Accidents were the leading cause of death among men aged 15-24, and the second leading cause among men aged 25-44 and women aged 15-44. Suicide was the second leading cause among men aged 15-44 and the third leading cause among women age 15-44.

Since the end of the 1990s, cancer has been the leading cause of death and heart disease the second leading cause. Cerebrovascular diseases were the third leading cause and diabetes was the fourth among men and women in most of the years. These four causes accounted for approximately half of all deaths in 2015 (51% for men, 52% for women), compared with higher percentages in 2000 (57% for men, 60% for women).

The age-adjusted mortality rate for heart diseases decreased significantly over the past decade, by 33% for men and 37% for women for the years 2013-2015, on average, relative to 2004-2006.[2] A considerable decrease was also recorded for cerebrovascular diseases (32% for men, 35% for women), diabetes (25% for men, 29% for women), and kidney diseases (40% for men 38% for women). A relatively large decrease was also recorded for deaths caused by accidents (30% for men, 39% for women) and chronic lower respiratory diseases (16 per cent for men, 22 per cent for women).

For some causes of death an increase was recorded during 2013-2015, on average, relative to the previous decade. The highest increase in mortality rate was recorded for dementia, by a factor of 2.5 for women and nearly 3 for men. A considerable increase was also recorded for deaths caused by septicaemia (76% for men, 49% for women) and by Alzheimer's disease (27% for men, 37% for women). The mortality rate for deaths caused by kidney diseases increased until 2006 and has been decreasing in recent years.

Percent of change 2005-2007/2014-2016 (age-adjusted mortality rate per 100,000 persons)[2]

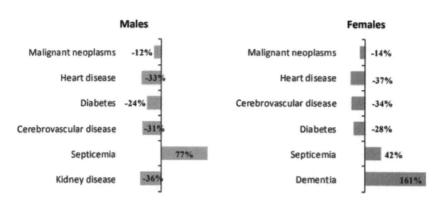

The distribution by sub-districts indicates differences in mortality rates by a factor of up to 1.6. The sub-districts of Be'er Sheva, the Jezreel Valley and Acre had higher mortality rates than the Judea and Samaria Area, Rehovot, Petah Tikva and the Golan Heights.

Cancer Morbidity

The incidence of cancer varies generally by location and specifically across sub-districts, although a number of sub-districts consistently recorded values that differed from what was expected throughout or during most of the periods: The Haifa sub-district recorded a significant excess morbidity rate for most types of cancer examined (excluding prostate cancer in men) during most or all of the periods (excess morbidity varied between 9% and 14%). The Tel Aviv sub-district also recorded a significant excess morbidity rate for some types of cancer during all or most of the periods (3%-6% for women), as did the Ashkelon sub-district among men (6%-9%), the Rehovot sub-district among men (5%), and the Petach Tikva sub-district among women (4%). In contrast, the Jerusalem sub-district recorded a significantly lower than expected cancer morbidity rate among both genders for most types of cancer (excluding non-Hodgkin's lymphoma) during most or all periods. The Jezreel Valley, Sea of Galilee and Acre sub-districts also recorded low morbidity rates for some types of cancer during all or most of the periods.

In 2013 the International Agency for Research on Cancer (IARC) of the World Health Organization classified outdoor air pollution as carcinogenic to humans and noted a positive association with an increased risk of bladder cancer. According to current data on cancer incidence, excess lung cancer rates were recorded among men in the sub-districts of Hadera, Haifa, Jezreel Valley, Sea of Galilee and Acre, and among women in the sub-districts of Haifa and Tel Aviv. The greatest excess during the latest period (2011-2015) was recorded in the Acre sub-district among men (38%) and the Tel Aviv sub-district (24%).

In 2016 Israel recorded a total of 30,569 cases of tumours that required reporting to the cancer registry. Of the reported cancer cases, 88% were malignant – 12,553 (47%) among men and 14,380 (53%) for women. Among both men and women, 84% were Jewish, 10% were Arab and 6% were classified as other.

The main types of cancer, accounting for more than 50% of all the morbidity cases among men in Israel, were the same for Jews and Arabs. They included prostate cancer, lung cancer, colorectal cancer, non-Hodgkin's lymphoma and bladder cancer. Among Jewish men, however, prostate cancer accounted for 17% of all malignant tumours, compared with a figure of 9% for Arab men, and malignant melanoma accounted for 5.5%, whereas among Arabs it is very rare (<1%). In addition, among Arab men lung cancer accounted for 22% of all malignant tumours, compared with 12% among Jewish men.

Among Jewish and Arab women, likewise, there were similarities in the most prevalent types of cancer. For both population groups breast tumours accounted for about one third of all tumours, and colorectal tumours for about 9%-10%. Lung cancer, thyroid cancer, non-Hodgkin's lymphoma and uterine cancer were also prevalent among women.

Heart Diseases

In recent years heart diseases have been the second-leading cause of death in Israel among men aged 45 and above and women aged 45-74. The main behavioural risk factors for heart disease are smoking, nutritional imbalance and lack of physical activity, which result in high blood pressure, high LDL cholesterol levels, overweight and obesity.

All heart diseases: These occur among both Jews and Arabs. Heart disease rates are higher among men, and the highest rate is among Jewish men. The rate among Jewish men is about 29% higher than the rate among Arab men. The rates among women are nearly identical between the two population groups.

Coronary heart disease: The rates are higher among men, with the highest rate among Jewish men. The rate among Jewish men is about a quarter higher than among Arab men. The rate among Jewish women is about two thirds higher than the rate among Arab women.

The incidence of heart disease is higher among men than among women for all age groups. The frequency of heart diseases increases with age for both genders. The rates of incidence of heart disease, diagnosed by a physician, peak at ages 75 and above, with 42% for men and 31% for women. Heart disease rates among young men (up to age 45) are relatively low and are comparable for Jews and Arabs. For ages 45-64, heart disease rates are higher among Arabs, and for age 65 and above the rates are higher among Jews. Among Jewish men the morbidity rates increase sharply at ages 65 and above, whereas they increase moderately among Arabs. Among women, Arabs have higher rates of heart diseases, until age 75. At ages 75 and above, Jewish women have higher rates, although it should be noted that that the rate among Arab women is based on a very small number of cases within this age group. As with the men, among Jewish women there is a sharp increase in morbidity at ages 65 and above, compared with a moderate increase followed by steady rates among Arab women.

The coronary heart disease morbidity rates in Israel are lower than in most states of the Organisation for Economic Co-operation and Development

(OECD), an inter-governmental economic organisation founded in 1961 by developed countries committed to democracy and the market economy, to stimulate economic progress and world trade. Of the 33 OECD member states as of 2010, Israel is ranked 25th for men and 23rd for women.

Stroke: Each year about 15,000 Israelis experience a stroke, which is a manifestation of cerebrovascular disease. The leading risk factors for a stroke are smoking and high blood pressure. Cerebrovascular diseases have been the fourth leading cause of mortality in Israel since 2008. Recent years have seen a decrease in the incidence of strokes in many developed countries, primarily as a result of increased attention to risk factors such as high blood pressure and smoking. At the same time, the absolute number of strokes is rising because the population is aging.

Stroke

The incidence of strokes is higher among the Jewish population than the Arab population for both men and women. In both population groups, the incidence is significantly higher for men, by a factor of 2 for Jewish men compared with Jewish women and 1.5 for Arab men compared with Arab women. The incidence of strokes increases with age for both men and women. In the 55-64 age group there is a sharp increase in strokes among men, which continues at a more moderate rate for ages 65 and above. Among women, in contrast, there is a sharp increase at later ages (65-74), which continues in the age group of 75 and above. Below age 75 the rates among men are significantly higher than among women. The rate among men is higher by a factor of 1.5 than the rate among women at young ages (35-54) and higher by a factor of 3.6 in the 55-64 age group. At ages 65-74 the discrepancy diminishes, and at ages 75 and above the incidence of strokes is nearly identical among men and women (6.8% and 7.1%, respectively).

The mortality rates for strokes in Israel are lower than those of most OECD countries. Israel is ranked 31st among men and 33rd for both men and women.

Diabetes

Diabetes is a chronic disease characterized by a high concentration of glucose in the blood. There are three types of diabetes: Type 1 (juvenile onset) occurs before the age of 30 and characterizes about 10% of diabetes patients. Type 2 diabetes usually occurs after age 30 and its prevalence increases with age. About 90% of diabetes patients have this type. The risk factors for developing Type 2 diabetes include family history, lack of physical activity, overweight, high blood pressure, and previous gestational diabetes, among others. The third type, gestational diabetes, first occurs or first manifests during pregnancy and its symptoms are similar to those of type 2 diabetes.

The incidence of diabetes within the population increases with age (excluding ages 85+) among men and women. In the 65-74 age group there is a sharp increase in diabetes for men as well as women, which continues at a more moderate rate at 75-84 years. The incidence of diabetes is higher among men than women for all ages.[3] The incidence of diabetes is higher among the Arab population than the Jewish population for both men and women.[4]

There has been a dramatic increase in diabetes, particularly among the socio-economically disadvantaged, a status that is based on entitlement to a waiver from payments as determined by the National Insurance Institute. The proportion of diabetics exempted from deductible payments is 4.5 times higher than the number of HMO members who are not exempted. For immigrants from Ethiopia their incidence of diabetes increases every year they are in the country. After ten years in Israel, the diabetes rate for Ethiopian immigrants reaches 17.6%.[5]

The prevalence of controlled diabetes among diabetics of both sexes is lower among people with a low socio-economic status than people with a high socio-economic status.[6] As socio-economic status increases so too does the proportion of diabetics with controlled diabetes, for both sexes. Controlled diabetes was less frequent among diabetics aged 18-24 of both sexes (males: 41.6%, females: 48.5%) than diabetics aged 75-84 (males: 85.8%, females: 86.0%).

Lifestyle Risk Factors

Cigarette smoking is one of the most dangerous behaviour patterns in terms of health, as it causes many types of harm and severe diseases.[7] According to Israel's Central Bureau of Statistics (CBS), as of 2017, 22.1% of people aged 20 and above reported that they smoke at least one cigarette per day – 29.9% of men and 14.7% of women. The highest rate of smoking was found among Arab men (47.5%). This was almost double the rate among Jewish men (25.8%). The lowest rate of smoking was found among Arab women (4.8%), which was significantly lower than the rate among Jewish women (16.2%). In both population groups smoking was found to be more prevalent among men than women, with a larger gender discrepancy in the Arab population. The rate of smoking among Jewish men was 1.3 times higher than the figure for Jewish women, whereas the rate of smoking among Arab men was 5.3 times higher than the figure for Arab women. The percentage of smokers in Israel is relatively high compared with other OECD member states and 20% higher than the average for all OECD states.

For all population groups the prevalence of smoking was found to be lower among interviewees with a high level of education (17.1%) than those with a low or medium level of education (23.2% and 29.1%, respectively). The highest rates of smoking were reported by interviewees with a medium level of education (29.4% for Jewish men, 29.0% for Jewish women, and 10.7% for Arab women), with the exception of Arab men, for whom the highest prevalence of smoking was found among those with a low level of education. For all levels of education, the rate of smoking was higher among Arab men than Jewish men, and higher among Jewish women than Arab women. The rate of smoking among Arab men with a high level of education was greater than double the rate among Jewish men. The rate of smoking among Arab men with a low level of education was higher by a factor of 1.3 than the rate among Arab men with a high level of education. The rate of smoking among Arab women with a high level of education was lower by a factor of 2.2 than the rate among Jewish women with a high level of education.

Obesity is a major public health problem because of its short-term as well as long-term effects. The extent of obesity among the population has increased over time, and there is much evidence linking it to a large number of chronic diseases. It also reduces the lifespan and undermines quality of life. In developed countries obesity is recognized as the second most important cause (after smoking) of preventable death. Obesity also constitutes an economic burden. In a number of developed countries, the economic costs of obesity range between 2% and 7% of healthcare expenditures. The expenditure for an obese adult is significantly higher than the expenditure for an adult of normal weight.[8]

In Israel, as of 2017, about half of those aged 20 and above (48%) are overweight, obese, or morbidly obese: 55% of men compared with 41% of women, 46% of Jews compared with 54% of Arabs, 37% of the 20-44 age group, and 60% of those aged 45 and above. For all age groups the prevalence of overweight is higher among men than women (39% compared with 26%, respectively).[9]

Prevalence (%) of obesity by age, ethnicity and gender, 2017

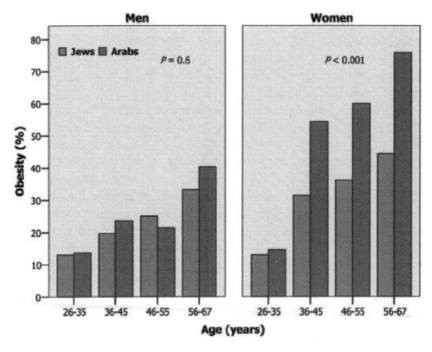

Among diabetics, the lower their socioeconomic status, the higher their rates of obesity and morbid obesity. These discrepancies exist for both sexes but appear to be especially significant among women.

Socio-demographic Trends and their Impact on the Healthcare System

In 2016 the worldwide elderly population (aged 65 and above) reached 626 million, accounting for 9% of the global population. By 2030 the number of elderly people worldwide is expected to reach 997 million and account for 12% of the global population. A majority of the worldwide elderly population (56%) resides in Asia. The continent with the highest percentage of elderly is Europe (about 18% of the total population), where they will constitute about 23% of the population in 2030.

Israel has a relatively young population compared with most OECD states.[10] In 2016 the population aged 65 and above accounted for about 11% of Israel's total population, compared with an OECD average of 17%. In fact, only three states (Chile, Turkey, and Mexico) have a lower percentage of elderly people.[11] According to CBS projections, however, even though the average age in Israel is significantly lower than the average for OECD states, the number of elderly is expected to increase considerably, reaching 1.66 million in 2035. This means that the elderly population will increase by 77% during 2015-2035, and its rate of growth will be 2.2 times greater than that of the general population for this period. The percentage of Arabs within the elderly population is expected to increase from 8% in 2015 to 14% in 2035. This data has dramatic implications for the healthcare system: an increase in the prevalence of chronic diseases (such as diabetes, heart diseases and the like), and a higher number of chronic diseases per person and over the course more years, thus placing a heavier burden on Israel's healthcare system.

Projected Growth of the Elderly Population, 2015-2045 (as % of the total population)

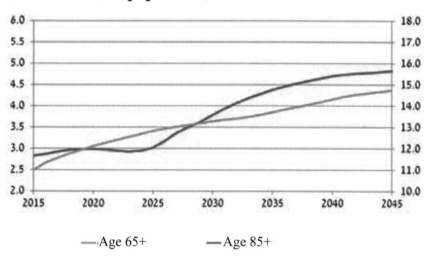

———Age 65+   ——Age 85+

Israel's elderly population increased rapidly as the large numbers of children born after the Second World War aged and the life expectancy increased significantly.[12] An additional and unique characteristic that contributes to the aging of Israel's population is the wave of immigration from the former Soviet Union during the 1990s. The population experienced a sharp increase within a brief period, and immigrants from the former Soviet Union, as a group, were heavily weighted towards older people rather than children and infants. According to current CBS projections, the percentage of elderly is expected to rise gradually from about 11% in 2015 to about 15% in 2045. The percentage of very elderly (ages 80+), which tends to be highly dependent on long-term care, is expected to remain at about 3% until the middle of the next decade, after which it will sharply rise to 4.8% in 2045.[13]

Health has a strong impact on the life and welfare of the elderly. Deteriorating health, and especially the emergence of disabilities, greatly undermines their quality of life. It is therefore important, concurrent with the significant increase in life expectancy, to identify and underscore ways of improving life for the elderly, ensuring not only their longevity but also their quality of life.[14]

Expected Changes in Morbidity: Trends and Implications for the Uptake of Health Services

Chronic diseases (long-term conditions lasting more than three months), with which a person might live for many years, are becoming more prevalent throughout the world and their impact on human health is increasing. Unhealthy lifestyles result in ever-growing numbers of heart diseases, diabetes, and the like. Moreover, thanks to technological developments, diseases that in the past were harbingers of a few months' life expectancy, such as AIDS or even cancer, have become chronic diseases with which patients can live for many years. A chronic patient consumes healthcare services – in the community or through hospitalization – on a scale that is several times higher than the average per person, and this is further multiplied in cases of chronic morbidity involving several diseases simultaneously.[15]

These days, chronic diseases also increasingly affect the younger generation and middle-aged population. For example, a significant percentage of children suffer from chronic diseases of the respiratory system, such as asthma, and about 20% of HMO members in Israel over the age of 45 suffer from two or more chronic conditions. Multiple chronic conditions are the most frequent impairment among several age groups.[16]

Chronic diseases also lead to increased consumption of healthcare services, negative health results and high medical expenditures. It is estimated that about 75% of healthcare expenditures are dedicated to treating chronic patients. Furthermore, chronic diseases undermine an individual's employability and income, and reduce the labour force participation rate and market productivity, while simultaneously accelerating early retirement, high turnover and the incidence of disabilities. Accordingly, chronic patients pose a challenge to healthcare systems and a future threat to their ability to operate effectively.

The main difficulty faced by healthcare systems globally is the gap between demand, on the one hand, and supply as well as the ability to provide services, on the other. The needs of chronic patients are many and varied – their medical care is characterized by numerous medications and examinations, as well as numerous care providers and types of treatment. The patients, who are mostly elderly, undergo a vast and varied array of treatments, and on top being main consumers of healthcare services, the challenge of continuity of care is the most acute for them.

Furthermore, as life expectancy has increased, so too has the number of long-term care patients and the burden of their care. The growing numbers of life-extending medical discoveries contribute to growing costs of long-term care. According to Ministry of Health projections, the number of long-term care patients is expected to double in the next 15 years. The number of people who need long-term care is growing rapidly, and the duration of such care in Israel will continue to increase: their number is expected to reach 233,000 by 2020 and 342,000 by 2030.

These findings underscore the importance of preventing and managing chronic diseases, as well as the importance of adequate numbers of medical staff and primary care providers. Although the balance between primary and specialist physicians in Israel has changed over the past decades, resulting in a proportional increase of specialists, the overall ratio of practicing physicians to the population in Israel has decreased in recent years, whereas in most OECD countries it is increasing. Similarly, the physician-to-population ratio – the number of practising physicians per 1,000 persons – in Israel is lower than the OECD average (3.1, compared with 3.3).[17]

Moreover, the proportion of physicians in Israel over the age of 55 is the largest among OECD states, accounting for approximately half of all physicians, compared with an average of 34% for all OECD member states. The ratio of practicing nurses to the population in Israel is particularly low relative to OECD states – five nurses per 1,000 persons, compared with the OECD average of 9.3. The ratio between practicing nurses and practicing physicians in Israel is also lower than that of most OECD states – 1.3 in Israel compared with an average of 2.8 among member states.[17]

The Expected Compatibility of Medical Staff and Personnel with the Needs of the Healthcare System and Physical Infrastructures

The demand for healthcare services is increasing as a result of population aging, increased awareness on the part of health services consumers, and a rising quality of life. Accordingly, it is necessary to adapt the personnel of the healthcare system to its changing needs. One example along these lines is the establishment of a medical school in Safed in the Galilee region that is affiliated with Bar-Ilan University and aims to train additional physicians in Israel. Currently there are five medical schools operating in Israel: at the Hebrew University, Tel Aviv University, Ben Gurion University, the Technion in Haifa and the Bar-Ilan Faculty of Medicine in the Galilee. In addition, as discussed below, many Israeli students attend medical schools abroad.

Physicians

Many factors have contributed to the imbalance in most OECD countries between the number of physicians and the need for them: the fact that training does not keep pace with the growing demand for healthcare services, a reduction in the number of working hours in the profession, a growing number of specializations, the average age of practising physicians, and retirement rates. The ratio of physicians to 1,000 persons in Israel is lower than the OECD average. In Israel the ratio is 3.1 practising physicians per 1,000 persons, whereas the OECD average is 3.3 per 1,000 persons.

The number of new medical licences rose to 1,184 in 2014, from 721 in 2010 and 547 in 2007.[18] About half (45%) of the licences were issued to graduates of medical schools in Israel and about one third (34%) to physicians trained in Eastern Europe. The number of graduates trained in Israel rose to 536, from 417 the previous year and 344 in 2010. In parallel, the number of Israelis who had trained abroad rose to 437 in 2014, from 188 in 2010 and 111 in 2005. These account for 37%, 26%, and 18% of all new licenses, respectively. In 2014 about half the licences granted to graduates who had trained abroad were issued in Hungary (90), Jordan (70), Romania (69) and Italy (44). The percentage of licences granted to women has been steady in the last three reported years, at 42% (51% of graduates trained in Israel and 23% of Israelis who graduated abroad).

As of the end of 2014, Israel had 34,231 registered physicians, of whom 25,637 were below the age of 65 and 30,683 were below the age of 75.[18] The ratio of physicians below the age of 65 dropped to 3.09 per 1,000 persons, from 3.11 the previous year and 3.39 at the end of 2005 (a 5% decrease). In 2014 a quarter (25%) of registered physicians were aged 65 and above, a 17% increase from 2005 and about one third (30%) were below the age of 45, a 34% decrease from 2005. The percentage of female physicians relative to all licenced physicians below the age of 65 rose to 43% (from 39% in 2000). As of the end of 2014, the percentage of graduates who had trained in Israel rose to 42% of all physicians below the age of 65, compared with 36% in 2000, and to 52% of all physicians below the age of 45, compared with 41% in 2000. A third (30%) had trained in the former Soviet Union, 5% had trained in Romania, 5% in Italy, and the rest (18%) had completed medical school in other countries.

The data indicate that the highest ratio of physicians to 1,000 persons is in the Tel Aviv District, while the lowest ratios are in the Southern and Northern Districts.[18] This fact points to the differences between the centre and the peripheries in terms of accessibility to healthcare services.

Medical Specialties in Crisis

For various reasons, many medical specialties suffer from a shortage of personnel, an infrastructure that cannot meet the needs, an increasing workload, and remuneration that is incommensurate with the crisis. As a consequence, good physicians are deterred from applying for these positions and physicians at all levels – department heads, specialists and residents – 'flee' elsewhere, which raises serious concerns about the future of these specialties. Ultimately the crisis is most evident in personnel shortages and heavy workloads, the direct effects of which are first and foremost an impaired ability on the part of medical staff to provide proper medical care, inferior patient services, frustration, stress and burnout among physicians and an inefficient system.

The characteristics of this crisis vary by specialty. An examination of the medical profession as a single case reveals a number of key characteristics: a shortage of physicians, a workload that impairs the medical staff's ability to provide proper medical care, the percentage of active on-call shifts, a high number of on-duty shifts, an impaired quality of life and a shortage of residents.

The Israel Medical Association (IMA) lists the following as specialties in crisis: neonatology, paediatric oncological haematology, family medicine, surgery, internal medicine, physical and rehabilitative medicine, paediatric intensive care, general intensive care, pathology, child and adolescent psychiatry, emergency medicine, geriatrics and anaesthesia. In addition, the IMA identified a number of fields where the crisis stems from lack of positions: nephrology, oncology, X-ray imaging, medical administration and haematological oncology.

According to the IMA, the following solutions could improve the current situation:

1. Increasing the current economic incentives (specializations that do not currently provide a special bonus would be granted one based on the existing rate) – as a response to the physician shortage.

2. Full-time work – based on specific consideration of each specialty: Currently physicians divide their work across several positions. Full commitment by physicians to the public healthcare system will make senior physicians available at hospitals throughout their working hours and strengthen physician-patient relations, among other things.
3. By agreement between the physician and the employer, the aim would be to have physicians carry out all their work at their principal workplace, rather than work for several employers. In addition, various wage levels should be established on the basis of the current wages.
4. Grants to attract physicians to a specialty (incentives to choose the specialty).
5. Increasing the number of department heads.
6. Increasing on-call shifts so that each specialty has a physician on-call every day of the month.
7. Increasing on-call shifts to ensure a minimal number of specialists per department.
8. Preventing burnout – reducing the number of weekly work hours.
9. Position-specific bonuses.
10. Specialist on-duty shifts – at different rates (multiple working days). (This recommendation applies not only to specialties in crisis).[19]

Forecast of Physician Supply for 2025

Over the years various commissions have been appointed in Israel to address personnel planning in the health professions. A 2010 report by the Committee for Planning Medical and Nursing Human Resources included a long-term projection based on existing data, aimed at forecasting the workforce supply of physicians and nurses in the healthcare system.

After measuring the rate at which personnel are trained in Israel and abroad against physician retirement rates as well as physician-to-patient ratios in various other countries, the Committee decided to recommend a ratio of 2.9 physicians to 1,000 persons as a minimum point of reference.[20] According to its calculations, and assuming that the physician-to-patient ratio in Israel would continue to decline in the coming years, the Committee concluded that absent any intervention aimed at increasing the number of physicians who enter the healthcare system, the physician-to-patient ratio is expected to reach 2.83 physicians per 1,000 residents by 2020 and 2.6 by 2025. To reach the desired ratio, the Committee recommended expanding the capacity of existing training centres as well as establishing a fifth medical school, encouraging physicians trained abroad to return to Israel, and reducing the numbers of foreign students who study in Israel, as needed, in order to train more Israelis.

Nurses

Over the years the nursing profession in Israel has undergone significant changes, foremost among which was that it became an academic profession. Simultaneously, the training track for nurses who are not registered nurse practitioners was scaled back. The decrease in number of nurse practitioners without a commensurate increase in the number of new registered nurses, alongside reduced immigration to Israel, have contributed to a decline in the number of new nurses who join the healthcare system each year. This trend, along with the fact that in most countries the ratio of nurses is on an upward trend, led to a considerable drop in the ratio of nurses in Israel compared with most OECD states, to the extent that Israel is currently experiencing a significant nursing shortage.[21] Not only is the ratio of nurses to 1,000 persons in Israel one of the lowest among OECD states, it is also continuing to fall.[22] In Israel the ratio of nurses to 1,000 persons is 5.0, whereas the OECD average is 9.3 nurses per 1,000 persons.

New licences by year of receipt[21]

New licences, not including recertification of nurse practitioners as registered nurses

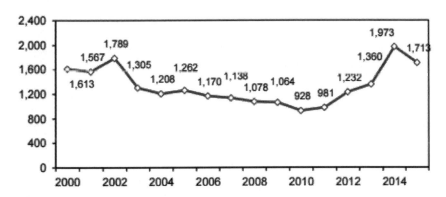

In 2002 a total of 1,789 new licences were issued. After 2002 there was a downward trend until 2012. In 2014 a total of 1,973 new licences were issued, after which there was another downward trend. There are also significant discrepancies among Israel's districts in the ratio of nurses to 1,000 persons. The ratio is higher in Haifa and Tel Aviv, and lowest in the Southern District.

Projected Workforce Supply of Nurses in 2025, Based on an Expansion of Training Programmes[22]

The main basis on which nurses enter the healthcare system is Israel's nursing training programmes. This is supplemented by the entry of new immigrants, who are relatively few in number and whose impact on the total number of nurses in Israel is insignificant.

Using data on the entry of nurses into the healthcare system versus their retirement, the Committee for Planning Medical and Nursing Human Resources estimated that a ratio of 5.8 nurses to 1,000 persons in 2025 was a preliminary and attainable target, the aim of which would be to stop the downward trend, so that the healthcare system could function properly. However, the Committee also recommended examining the possibility of raising financial and other resources that would enable more significant growth, in an effort to reach a ratio of 5.6 nurses to 1,000 persons before 2025.

In addition to this ratio, the Committee recommended a 20% increase in the nursing workforce, including the addition of nursing assistants and skilled support staff. The assistants would contribute to elderly care, among other areas, thereby freeing registered nurses from basic care and enabling them to focus more on providing advanced nursing care to severely ill patients.

Possible Changes in the Structure of Medical Services and its Adaptation to Evolving Needs

The healthcare system faces new challenges, as noted above (an aging population, under-funding, and personnel shortage). This assessment was made before the COVID-19 pandemic caused chaos in health systems around the world, reducing planned hospital admissions, cancelling outpatient clinics and producing excess deaths especially in Western Europe and the Americas. Its impact will be present for some time and it is clear that it will make us rethink our healthcare systems' structures such as the relationship between hospital and the community, continuity of care and the need for strong public health systems.

The first and most important change is to bolster primary medicine throughout the community – by increasing the integration and equality of population groups with varied, complex and changing needs, and concentrating chronic treatment in the hands of the community's primary care physician and support staff. Boult and Wieland (2009) presented a (basic) comprehensive primary care model that could provide continuous, effective managed care for older patients with a complexity of multiple chronic conditions. This model has the most potential to improve the quality of care and quality of life for patients, while also reducing the cost of their care. It is based on team care that includes a primary care physician and at least a nurse and another health specialist who work together with the community. The elements of such care include:

- Comprehensive diagnosis and assessment.
- Developing a comprehensive treatment plan for the specific patient.
- Implementing the treatment plan (and follow-up to ensure its actual implementation).
- Proactive monitoring of the patient's health and adherence to the treatment plan.
- Case management and coordination of the care provided in the community, by consultants, hospitalization, emergency room visits or other urgent care, and other care providers (e.g., dietitian, psychologist, social worker, etc.).
- In cases of patients released from hospital, assistance in reintegrating into the community (and preventing re-hospitalization).
- Assistance for patients in accessing social and other community services, particularly those that will help them remain active and promote their health.

The second change involves prevention and check-ups. The main health problems in the developed world usually include chronic non-communicable diseases such as diabetes, heart diseases, and cancer. These result, among other factors, from the modern lifestyle. In fact, currently available knowledge indicates that individual lifestyle is a major factor in determining the risk of developing a chronic disease during one's lifetime.

Primary prevention is concerned with maintaining a healthy lifestyle before the onset of disease. The aim of primary prevention measures is to reduce exposure to factors that increase the risk of a disease or diseases. These measures include behavioural changes, reducing exposure to harmful factors, policy changes, and a change in the physical and social environment. Although prevention is not usually seen as a core issue for the healthcare system, relative to issues involving patient care at both the provider and system levels, it is of great importance for human health.

Moreover, medical check-ups are an important strategy for detecting an abnormal health condition among asymptomatic members of a specific population group, in order to intervene as soon as possible and prevent the onset of illness, suffering, or death. Early detection has potential advantages and disadvantages. The advantages of early detection are self-evident: the possibility of providing more targeted treatment at an earlier stage of the disease, thus reducing symptoms and costs, improving the chances of a full recovery, and sometimes even reducing mortality. Conversely, check-ups can cause significant harm, such as side effects of the exam itself, anxiety while waiting for results, false-positive results, over-diagnosis and misleading negative results that in turn lead to an unfounded sense of security and potential disregard of future symptoms.

The third change relates to hospital-level care for patients at home. Home care provides an alternative to hospitalization at general hospitals (and to internal medicine wards in particular) or follow-up care facilities. Re-admission, a widespread and frequent phenomenon throughout the world's healthcare systems, can be minimized by 30%. It is possible to reduce re-admission by making treatments available in the community, educating patients at the time of their release from hospital, and improving communication between hospitals and the community so as to maintain continuity of care.

The fourth change involves the integration of digital tools and use of information technologies. In the late 1990s the World Health Organization adopted the concept of telemedicine as the delivery of healthcare services, where distance is a critical factor, by health care professionals using information and communication technologies. These services use current information for purposes of diagnosis, treatment, prevention of disease and injury, research, assessment, and providing health education to patients, as well as promoting the health of individuals and communities. Telemedicine can be seen as a way to bridge the physical distance between a patient and physician or among a patient's various physicians.

The applications of telemedicine comprise five areas in which it is possible to provide consultation and assessment without direct contact with the patient:

- Home/mobile monitoring – the use of telemedicine for long-distance monitoring of health. Data (such as weight, blood pressure, glucose levels) is measured at the patient's home and transmitted to the healthcare provider via the Internet.
- Diagnosis (teleradiology, tele-dermatology, telepathology) – the transmission of medical information such as X-rays, lab results or prescriptions from one health professional to another for consultative or diagnostic purposes.
- Triage medical call centre – urgent preliminary assessment using frontal or audio imaging transmitted by the patient. The information can be transmitted between the patient and healthcare provider or between a provider and a specialist.
- Consultation (e-consultation, e-visit, video visit) – interaction between the patient and healthcare provider or among providers using video-conferencing or other technologies.
- Procedures (telesurgery, healthcare assisting robot) – surgical procedures performed remotely, which require swift and precise transmission of information.

Conclusion

The changing patterns and scope of morbidity pose new challenges to the Israeli healthcare system, which must change accordingly. In the coming years, the healthcare system will face a variety of challenges stemming primarily from the aging of the population and increased morbidity, from chronic diseases. This will increase the already existing burden on the healthcare system in terms of both community healthcare and hospitalization.

A chronically ill person consumes health services – at the community and hospital levels – on a scale that is several times higher than the average per person, and this is further multiplied in cases of chronic morbidity involving several diseases simultaneously. Moreover, chronic morbidity affects not only the elderly. We are already seeing significant percentages of children who suffer from respiratory diseases such as asthma.

Furthermore, differences in the nature of morbidity – and the outcomes of medical treatment – among population groups that vary by ethnic background and socio-economic status will continue to be one of the major challenges of the Israeli healthcare system. For example, the percentage of diabetics with well-controlled diabetes is higher among population groups with a high socio-economic status than among diabetics with a low socio-economic status. Likewise, differences were found in morbidity rates across Israel's various sub-districts, with higher morbidity rates in the peripheries than the central regions.

These growing inequalities are not a 'given' but a result of policies and priorities. While in the last decade the Ministry of Health, as well as other actors within the Israeli medical system, have become much more aware of the need to reduce health inequalities, sustaining a strong healthcare system available for all, as envisioned in the Israeli National Health Insurance Law, is one of the major challenges for Israeli society.

Bibliography

1. Knesset Research and Information Centre. Netunim be-nose ezrahimvatikim, hizdaknutve-zikna be-Israel [Data on senior citizens, aging, and old age in Israel]. Jerusalem (IL): *Knesset Research and Information Centre*; 2017 (Hebrew).
2. Brill, N. and Boiko, A., He'arkhut le-hizdaknut ha-ukhlusiya – skirabatkhum [Preparing for an aging population – a field survey]. Jerusalem (IL): *National Economic Council, Office of the Prime Minister;* 2015 (Hebrew).
3. Ministry of Health (IL). I-shivyon be-bri'utve-hitmodedut 'imo [Inequality in health and the means of coping with it]. Jerusalem (IL): *Ministry of Health;* 2019 (Hebrew).
4. Silverman, B., Dichtiar, R, Fishler, Y. and Keinan-Boker, L., 'Idkunnetunimlegabeihe'ar'utsartan u-tmuta li-shnat 2016 [Statistical update on cancer incidence and mortality, 2016]. Jerusalem (IL): *Ministry of Health;* 2019 (Hebrew).
5. Organization for Economic Co-operation and Development. Death from cancer [Internet]. Paris (FR): OECD. Available at https://data.oecd.org/.
6. Central Bureau of Statistics (IL). Shnaton statisti le-Israel 2018 [Statistical abstract of Israel, 2018]. Jerusalem: *Central Bureau of Statistics;* 2018 (Hebrew).
7. Ministry of Health (IL). Mabat al ha-bri'ut 2011 [A look at health, 2011]. Jerusalem: *Ministry of Health;* 2011 (Hebrew).

Notes

1. Goldberger, N., Aburbeh, M. and Haklai, Z., Sibot ha-mavet ha-movilot be-Israel 2000-2015 [Leading causes of death in Israel, 2000-2015]. Jerusalem (IL): Ministry of Health; 2018, pp.27-28 (Hebrew).
2. Ministry of Health (IL). Bri'ut 2013 [Health 2013]. Jerusalem: Ministry of Health; 2014 (Hebrew).
3. Knesset Research and Information Centre. Rikuz netunim 'al mahalat ha-sukeret be-Israel [Collected data on diabetes in Israel]. Jerusalem (IL): Knesset Research and Information Centre; 2010 (Hebrew).

4.   Tamir O. Tmunat matsav be-Israel ha-shmena, sukeret ve-Hergelei bru'it [State of affairs in the fat Israel, diabetes and health habits]. Ramat Gan (IL): Gertner Institute; 2010 (Hebrew).

5.   Ministry of Health (IL). taktsiv misrad ha-bri'ut li-shnat 2019 u-dgashei pe'ilut merkazi'im [Ministry of Health budget for 2019 and main focuses of activity]. Slideshow presentation to the Knesset Finance Committee; February 2018 (Hebrew).

6.   Ministry of Health (IL). Hatokhnit ha-le'umit le-madadei ikhut lerefu'at ha-Kehila be-Israel dokh lashanim 2015-2017 [National plan for indicators of community healthcare quality in Israel, 2015-2017 report]. Jerusalem: Ministry of Health; 2018 (Hebrew).

7.   Ministry of Health (IL). Dokh sar ha-bri'ut 'al ha-'ishun be-Israel 2018 [2018 report by the minister of health on smoking in Israel]. Jerusalem: Ministry of Health; 2019 (Hebrew).

8.   Gross, R., Ashkenazi, Y., Hemo, B., Ben-Shoham, O., Doron, D. and Nahshon, I.., Hashmanat yeladim: gormei sikun, tahlua nilveit ve-shimush be-sherutim [Childhood obesity: risk factors, associated morbidity and service utilization]. Jerusalem (IL): Brookdale Institute; 2011 (Hebrew).

9.   Central Bureau of Statistics (IL). Ha-seker ha-hevrati 2017: mishkal, dieta, tzuna ve-hergelei akhila [2017 social survey: weight, diet, nutrition, and eating habits]. Jerusalem: Central Bureau of Statistics; 2018. Leket netunim be-nos'ei bri'ut ve-orah ha'im [Collected data on health and lifestyle] (Hebrew).

10. Bruchim. M. and Kinney, D., Ma'arekhet ha-bri'ut be-Israel be-re'I ha-OECD 2018 [The healthcare system in Israel in relation to the OECD, 2018]. Jerusalem (IL): Ministry of Health; July 2018. p.47 (Hebrew).

11. Cohen Kovacs, G., Ramot-Nyska, T. and Haran Rosen, M., Ha-bituakh ha-si'udi be-Israel [Long-term care insurance in Israel]. Jerusalem (IL): Research Department, Bank of Israel; 2017 (Hebrew).

12. Brookdale Institute. Hazkenim be-Israel 2017 [The elderly in Israel, 2017]. Jerusalem (IL): Brookdale Institute; 2018 (Hebrew).

13. Trajtenberg, M., Alterman, R., Ben-David, D., Perry, D., Bechor, S., Lev Ami, S., Han, I., Katz, D. and Elkan, D., Atidtsafuf – Israel 2050 [A crowded future – Israel 2050]. Israeli Population, Environment & Society Forum; 2018, p.38 (Hebrew).

14. 'Itsuv mehadash shel ma'arkhot ha-bri'ut [Restructuring the healthcare systems]. Proceedings of the 15th Dead Sea Conference. Tel Hashomer (IL): Israel National Institute for Health Policy Research; 2015 (Hebrew).

15. Public Commission for Assessing the Future of the Insurance Sector (IL). Dokh ha-va'ada ha-tsiburit li-vhinat 'atid 'anaf ha-bituakh [Report of the Public Commission for Assessing the Future of the Insurance Sector]. Tel Aviv: Bureau of Insurance Agents in Israel; 2017 (Hebrew).

16. Ministry of Health (IL). Koakh adam be-miktso'ot ha-bri'ut 2015 [Manpower in the health professions, 2015]. Jerusalem: Ministry of Health; December 2016 (Hebrew).

17. Israel Medical Association. Miktso'ot be-metsuka [Medical specialties in crisis] [Internet]. Ramat Gan (IL): Israel Medical Association [cited 2019 Aug 2]. Available from: https://www.ima.org.il (Hebrew).

18. Ministry of Health (IL). Dokh ha-va'ada le-tikhnun koakh adam refu'I ve-si'udi be-ma'arekhet ha-bri'ut [Report of the Committee for Planning Medical and Nursing Human Resources]. Jerusalem: Ministry of Health; June 2010 (Hebrew).

19.   Ministry of Health (IL). Koakh adam be-miktso'ot ha-bri'ut 2015 [Manpower in the health professions, 2015]. Jerusalem: Ministry of Health; December 2016 (Hebrew).

20.   Israel Medical Association. Miktso'ot be-metsuka [Medical specialties in crisis] [Internet]. Ramat Gan (IL): Israel Medical Association [cited 2019 Aug 2]. Available from: https://www.ima.org.il (Hebrew).

21.   Ministry of Health (IL). Dokh ha-va'ada le-tikhnun koakh adam refu'I ve-si'udi be-m'arekhet ha-bri'ut [Report of the Committee for Planning Medical and Nursing Human Resources]. Jerusalem: Ministry of Health; June 2010 (Hebrew).

22.   Bruchim, M. and Kinney, D., Ma'arekhet ha-bri'ut be-Israel be-re'i ha-OECD 2018, July 2018, p. 47.

9

Rehabilitation Medicine in Palestine and Israel

Avi Ohry and Nava Blum

'What cannot be cured, must be endured.' Dr. Francois Rabelais (1494 - 1553)

Introduction

This chapter examines the development of physical medicine and rehabilitative health services during the British Mandate and in the first decade of the young state of Israel (1948-1958). Neither the medical establishment during the British Mandate in Palestine, nor the medical care provided during the four centuries of Ottomans rule, could cope with existing medical or psychiatric disabilities. The British Mandate health authorities did not help to establish any purpose-built hospitals or clinics for the disabled. Such facilities as existed during the Mandate Period (1919-1948) included just a few modest physical therapy departments.

During the British Mandate, Arab uprisings caused many injuries and casualties and rising antisemitism in Europe caused significant Jewish immigration to Palestine.

During this period, especially between the Israeli War of Independence and the Operation Kadesh (Sinai Campaign, October 1956), Israel was overwhelmed by the problems of establishing new medical facilities and recruiting new health professionals in order to care for large numbers of disabled or injured people. There was significant Jewish immigration to Israel after the Second World War and especially after the War of Independence (29 November 1947-20 July 1949) and the declaration of the State of Israel (on 14 May 1948). Among these immigrants were many sick people and individuals living with various disabilities.

The development of physical medicine and rehabilitation in Israel occurred during the process of the creation of a new nation-state, and this only increased during and after the Second World War and the War of Independence. Also, among the new immigrants were many trained physicians who developed new medical fields, although few were specialized or expert in physical medicine.[1] Adding to the demand for rehabilitation services were first the large number of handicapped soldiers wounded in the War of Independence and later, an outbreak of polio that plagued the country during its earliest years.[2] The new State would be forced to deal with the issue of rehabilitation as there few such services already in existence.[3] The development of Governmental rehabilitation services in Israel occurred during the creation of a new nation-state.

Some of the new immigrants were trained physicians and nurses but very few were specialized or expert in physical medicine.[4] These new arrivals drew on past training and experience, gained in many different countries, to develop medical services in Israel. These were shaped by new priorities and the exigencies of the time. The demand for adult rehabilitation services had been stimulated by the need to treat soldiers injured in the War of Independence when treatment and rehabilitation of war casualties made Physical Medicine and Rehabilitation (PM&R) an increasingly important field.

Immigration brought new groups of service-users with more diverse needs into the ambit of still limited provision while the polio epidemic added to a significant demand for child rehabilitation centres. Polio was already known to be a dangerous disease that spread quickly and extensively, and required an urgent and comprehensive response.[5] This, more than anything else, provided the impetus for WHO and UNICEF to get involved in the 1950s and help the young country to develop the unfamiliar concept of rehabilitation services for infants and children.

The Development of Physical Medicine and Rehabilitation

Rehabilitation medicine is a medical branch concerned with the diagnosis, treatment and long-term follow-up that aims to enhance and restore, where possible, functional ability and quality of life to people of all ages with disabilities. Disability may be caused by acquired injury, illness or congenital disease. The aim of the rehabilitation process is to enable the patient to live a healthy and productive life and to return, if possible, to mainstream society.

Although physical medicine and rehabilitation in a sense has existed since ancient times this is a relatively young specialty. Many cultures have recognized the healing power of the sun (heliotherapy), the importance of water (hydrotherapy) and the relief gained from rubbing sore muscles (massage). Hippocrates' writings mentioned the principles and practices of physical modalities.[6] After the First World War, when thousands of wounded soldiers filled hospitals in the USA, Europe, Canada and Australia, and the epidemics of the 'Spanish Flu' and poliomyelitis hit the world, the first signs of rehabilitation infrastructure began to emerge. However, even by the mid-twentieth century many physicians regarded physical medicine and rehabilitation as pertaining more to social work and vocational training than to medicine or public health.[7]

In the United States and Europe, physical medicine and rehabilitation began to develop as a branch of medicine during the First and Second World Wars.[8] It is perhaps paradoxical that physical medicine and rehabilitation have developed most strongly in wartime. Through wars – discovering ever more efficient methods to kill and maim people – we have also learned more and better ways to take care of the injured, to nurse and to restore people as much as possible to full functioning after being disabled.[9] The experience of rehabilitating war casualties has supplied valuable principles and practices to rehabilitation medicine, enriching the specialty and magnifying its importance and prominence.[10]

As currently understood, physical medicine and rehabilitation (sometimes called physiatry), is a relatively new branch of medicine that became recognized as a separate medical specialty only in 1947. It provides integrated care of all neurological and musculo-skeletal disabilities from traumatic brain injury to lower back pain.[11] The specialty focuses on the restoration of function to people with simple physical mobility problems up to those whose physical ailments are complicated by complex cognitive issues. The focus of medical rehabilitation is not limited to any one part of the body but emphasizes treating the 'whole person': medically, socially, emotionally and vocationally.[12] This is accomplished with the full cooperation of many experts: nurses, physical therapists, occupational therapists, speech-language pathologists, psychologists, social workers and more; also essential are orthotics and prosthetics in providing rehabilitation aids and appliances.[13]

Formal education had its beginning in 1926 when, after service in the US Army during the First World War, Dr. John Stanley Coulter joined the faculty of Northwestern University Medical School as the first full-time academic physician in physical medicine. Then Frank Krusen, MD, recognized as the 'Father of Physical Medicine'[14] established the Physical Medicine Programme at the Mayo Clinic and in 1936 he initiated the first three-year residency in Physical Medicine and also provided short courses in physical medicine for army physicians.[15] Krusen wrote the first widely-used textbook on Physical Medicine on 1941.

In England, Professor Sir Ludwig Guttmann (1899-1980), a Jewish refugee from Germany, initiated and established the concept and model of treatment of spinal cord injuries. This work was carried out at the National Spinal Injuries Centre at Stoke Mandeville Hospital in Buckinghamshire which opened in 1944. Today he is best known as one of the founding fathers of organised physical activities for people with a disability and the first 'Olympics' for the disabled, now known as the Paralympics, was held at Stoke Mandeville.

As a result of experience in and immediately after the Second World War, physical medicine was broadened from its roots in bed rest followed by physical therapy – helping the disabled to walk and move their limbs – to the far more comprehensive ideas initiated by Dr. Howard A. Rusk.[16] Rusk insisted that each patient should reach the optimal level of his or her physical, mental, emotional, vocational, social and sexual capabilities. Rusk argued that prolonged bed rest was counter-productive; rehabilitation must start as early as possible. The injured must exercise their minds as well as their bodies and, as they improved, must be taught the skills of daily living. They would then need to develop vocational skills that would help them adapt to the world of work and future careers.[17] Social and emotional skills and abilities helped the injured person to become fully functional in the family and in the social arena. These concepts of comprehensive rehabilitation would later be adopted in Israel.

Physical Medicine and Rehabilitation during the British Mandate

In this period, there were few specialized personnel (doctors, physiotherapists and occupational therapists) to help rehabilitate the handicapped. Physicians and nurses who offered physical therapy services simply incorporated these into their regular practice; one nurse would teach another. The first physicians in the field of PM&R were working at the Hadassah Medical Organization, funded by women Zionists in America, offering some physical therapy services. During the Mandate no appropriate treatment was developed by the authorities for those in need of medical rehabilitation, casualties of illnesses and accidents, the handicapped and wounded. because this service was not developed in the country.[18] During this period there were few individual physicians who dealt with the field of physical and rehabilitative medicine such as occupational therapy, communication speech therapy, social work and physiotherapy.[19] In the 1930s and 1940s professional rehabilitation therapy was not possible in cases of spinal cord injuries (quadriplegia, triplegia, paraplegia). Amputation of limbs, brain injuries casualties and other severe disabilities in Israel did not receive any pharmacological or rehabilitative treatment.[20]

In 1923, in Tel Aviv, a society for chronic and convalescent patients was established and in 1935 the Municipality of Tel Aviv opened a rehabilitation institution for, in their words, 'the invalids'. In September 1940 it was totally destroyed by an Italian bomber, deflected from bombing the oil refinery at Haifa, which killed 137 people in a civilian area near the port. During the 1930s Dr. Robert Simon, a German orthopaedic surgeon, opened a therapeutic gymnastics service in Jerusalem with balneotherapy, electrotherapy and other physical methods.

Alyn Hospital, a comprehensive rehabilitation centre for physically challenged and disabled children, adolescents and young adults was founded in 1932 by Dr. Henry Keller, an American orthopaedic surgeon who had dedicated his life to voluntary work amongst the physically challenged children in Jerusalem and spent five years in the city. Keller helped to establish a special clinic for the handicapped in Jerusalem and in 1932-1937 he visited Israel to help treat the patients. As a result of the polio epidemic in Israel in the 1940s and 1950s and the ensuing emergency situation, the Ministry of Health provided Alyn Hospital with a monastery belonging to the St. Simon Orthodox Church to be used as a hospital. The Hospital has been situated on the outskirts of Jerusalem since 1971.

The beginning of physical medicine was mostly to be found in the two main health service providers, the Hadassah medical organisation and the Kupat Holim, the Sick Fund of the Histadrut (Workers' Trade Union). The next significant steps in the field of PM&R in both main organisations emerged in the Hadassah Hospital in Jerusalem and in the Sick Fund in the village of Ramot Hashavim. The Kupat Holim had established a 'committee for the needs of chronic patients' in 1922. It maintained a small hospital, Beit Feinstone, from 1944 for chronically disabled patients at Ramot Hashavim, which later became Beit Lewenstein in Ra'anana, and was directed by Dr. Ludwig Ginsburg from 1945. At the time, no one expected the chronically ill to recover but Dr. Ginsburg decided to rehabilitate his patients. By giving them hope, physical therapy and vocational rehabilitation he succeeded in releasing his patients back to their homes, changing the institute into a rehabilitation centre.[21]

A rehabilitation clinic was opened at Hadassah Mt. Scopus in 1931 by Dr. Abraham Rosenthal (1875-1938) which used physical methods for the treatment of patients with chronic neurological problems. At the Hadassah Hospital a physical therapy outpatient clinic headed by Dr. Helmut Menke was organised in 1938, and when Dr. Emil Adler started to direct this little clinic in 1940, a small collaborative team was added. Adler became associate Professor of Physical Medicine at the Hebrew University and Director of Physical Medicine at the Hadassah University Hospital. He worked with Mrs Erna Viller Kriger, then the only qualified physiotherapist in Palestine, and later also with Ethel Bloom, an occupational therapist from the United States.[22] Nowadays, Adler is widely regarded as the 'father' of physical medicine and rehabilitation in Israel.[23]

One of the forgotten figures of rehabilitation medicine in Israel was Dr. Batia Noseh-Chen, an Israeli pioneer in electro-diagnosis and electrotherapy. She was born as Berthe Neoussikine in Russia in 1897 and studied medicine in Germany and France. Before immigrating to Palestine in 1936, she co-operated in Paris with the leading physiologists at the time. She had published many articles and a basic book on the treatment through 'ion-transfer'. Her outstanding achievements were made despite her own physical disability.[24] She opened an electro-diagnostic service first at Hadassah Hospital and in her private practice in Tel Aviv, and then at Tel Hashomer hospital. She died in Tel Aviv in 1990. Other physicians during the Mandate who ran small-scale private clinics offering physical therapy methods included Dr. Ernst Simon[25], Dr. Pochovsky,[26] Dr. Y. Friedman, Dr. Y. Blumenthal[27] and Dr. M. Buchman.[28]

At this time a few physical therapy methods were used. Hydrotherapy was commonly practised in Tiberias, where peloid (mud packs) were used for local treatments. Moor and peat soils from the Galilee heights and the Hulah Lake were also used for health baths.[29] Other treatments at that time were electrotherapy, diathermy, ultra violet and ultra-red radiation, hot baths, medical gymnastics, massage and a variety of other therapies. These were used to treat rheumatic diseases, spinal cord injuries, peripheral and central nervous system paralysis, painful joints, muscles, tendons and fractures. They were also used to treat venous system problems, and also cholecystitis and vaginitis.[30]

In the 1930s a single room was set aside for physical therapy in some clinics in the main cities.[31] Kupat Holim established a Disability Fund from 1930 to extend treatment and financial aid to workers incapacitated through disability or chronic disease.[32] The disabled workers received medical treatment and effort was made to find them suitable new employment.[33]

Another PM&R expert was Dr. Hans Isidore Weiser. In 1935 he began his career as a young doctor in Tel Aviv and was the director of the Institute of Sporting Medicine at the Strauss Health unit in Tel Aviv. He also worked as a physician at the Herzliya Gymnasium and introduced the importance of physical fitness. In his article, 'Physical Healing in Military Medicine', he brought the essence of rehabilitation into the military medical literature in Hebrew.[34]

Reuth Medical and Rehabilitation Centre, originally named Women's Social Service, was founded in 1937, on the seashore of Tel Aviv, by a group of women immigrants from Germany, under the leadership of Mrs Paula Barth. The aim of the newly-established organisation was to assist new immigrants who were hard put to find a sufficient livelihood in their new land. The women set up a soup kitchen, offering warm meals to the needy, opened a nursery school to enable parents to find employment and built Beit Shalom, a new home in the centre of Tel Aviv for elderly immigrants who had left their world behind.

The founders set the guiding principle that has directed Reuth ever since: filling in the gaps! The mission, in every era, is to respond to the most urgent, yet unaddressed, needs of Israeli society, to lend a helping hand to those whom no one else will help. Thus, in every period and every situation, Reuth has met the changing social challenges, assisting those who are weak and helpless: the old, the sick, the poor and the disabled.

As the needs changed with time, Reuth's services changed and grew to address them. After the Holocaust, when survivors flooded in from the ravaged continent of Europe, the organisation built Beit Bracha and Beit Achva, subsidized housing complexes offering 300 residential units for elderly immigrants. During the economic slump of the early 1950s, the women of Reuth handed out clothes and basic food products to needy families. And at the beginning of the 1960s they established two retirement homes for immigrants looking for a traditional lifestyle – Beit Gila in Tel Aviv's Yad Eliyahu neighbourhood and Beit Barth in Jerusalem.

In 1961 Reuth opened the Lichtenstaedter Hospital for the disabled and chronically ill. The facility, which offered 44 beds, was the only one of its kind in Israel at the time, and the demand for its services grew very rapidly: in 1966 two more storeys were added, and the number of beds rose to 120, and later to 160. In the 1970s the organisation established the current campus of what is today the Reuth Medical and Rehabilitation Centre, offering more than 300 beds.[35]

Following the War of Independence and the establishment of the State of Israel, there were large numbers of wounded and disabled soldiers and civilians. This situation forced the State of Israel to develop temporary rehabilitation centres. Rehabilitation centres for disabled patients to attend following hospital release were non-existent at the time in civilian hospitals. Gradually, the old departments of physical medicine were replaced by new updated rehabilitation centres.[36]

PM&R at the War of Independence

On 29 November 1947 the United Nations voted to end the British Mandate and to partition Palestine into two independent states, one Jewish and the other Arab. The War of Independence broke out on 30 November 1947 and continued until 20 July 1949; on 15 May 1948, one day after Israel's declaration of independence, five Arab armies invaded the new-born State.[37]

The War of Independence created a new stressful situation. About 6,000 lives were lost, and of the 4,000 injured soldiers, many were left crippled for life requiring long-term if not life-time care.[38] The newly-established State had to deal with a great number of handicapped people who needed medical care and rehabilitation but, with few structures in place, this required improvisation and often temporary and partial solutions.[39]

On 22 February 1948 Dr. Joseph Meir, senior officer of health services,[40] asked to open a rehabilitation centre for the handicapped. He expressed his distress and anxiety explaining the urgent need for such a facility, as he estimated that within a period of six to eight weeks the hospitals would be filled with the newly wounded, and under these circumstances hospitals would be forced to release existing patients before their rehabilitation and healing process was accomplished.[41] Dr. Meir requested to establish a rehabilitation centre with 100-150 beds designed to fulfil three goals:

1. Easing and assisting the hospitals, by releasing casualties who had completed their urgent treatment and to allow the removal of beds for new casualties.
2. The centre should enable full rehabilitation (as far as possible (for the handicapped until they will be able to go back to productive life.
3. The rehabilitation centre should be staffed by professionals and supervised by medical and educational specialists who would also provide vocational rehabilitation.

The war created acute demand for medical services in the new State. Despite the war, the development of army medical rehabilitation services was very slow. The directors of the medical civilian and military institutions did not realize the enormity of the changes happening in the country and failed to provide immediately the right medical treatment for the thousands of severely wounded soldiers and civilians who had been injured within a short period of time.[42]

Conscious of the need to be seen to be developing facilities for the rehabilitation of casualties who had suffered neurological injuries in the War of Independence, in December 1949 the Government of Israel invited Sir Ludwig Guttmann to visit and advise. Guttman's pioneering work in England, and his Europe-wide reputation, was well-known based on comprehensive care of spinal patients at Stoke Mandeville. This work is mentioned in his correspondence with Prime Minister David Ben Gurion and is noted as well as in the Prime Minister's diaries. This episode offers a unique insight into Guttmann's approach to rehabilitation in his early years.[43]

Establishing Three Rehabilitation Centres

It took about six more months following the urgent proposal of Dr. Meir to establish three temporary rehabilitation centres in Israel. The explanations for the delay were absence of financial resources, absence of professional knowledge and lack of medical staff.[44] Finally, three rehabilitation centres were established in August 1948 under the conditions of the war, despite the lack of knowledge and resources.

Rehabilitation Centre Number 1 was opened in Jaffa on 14 August 1948, near hospital Number 4 (Dajani later known as Tzahalon). The commander of the rehabilitation centre was the social worker David Reifen, while Dr. Hans Isidore Weiser was the medical director. This centre handled mainly the wounded who suffered from amputated limbs and had 120 beds. In May 1949 this rehabilitation centre was closed.

The rehabilitation centre was opened by Dr. Haim Sheba, head of the medical services of the Israeli Defence Force. David Ben Gurion, then Prime Minister, provided the financing. The medical treatments were given in two school buildings to the soldiers, all of them amputees. It was organised like the American rehabilitation centres with comprehensive medical, vocational and educational services. The centre faced many problems with so many amputees to cater for and patients had had to wait a long time for artificial limbs. Many became upset and frustrated while the medical staff (led by Dr. Weiser and Dr. Ernest Spira) struggled with their own lack of experience with such injuries. It was difficult to provide artificial limbs to so many soldiers and while they were waiting many months for their new limbs, they became frustrated, upset and disappointed.[45] These soldiers had originally come from 25 different countries and cultures and some of them, newly-arrived in Israel, had been sent immediately to the battlefield without speaking or understanding Hebrew. Then they had suffered serious injuries and were left in the centre without homes, work, family or limbs.[46] Weiser and Spira and their staff were trying their best despite the lack of relevant experience with this kind of injury. Dr. Sheba wrote that their first attempts to produce artificial limbs failed miserably. Some of the attempted surgery was unsuccessful, resulting in soldiers being sent for repeated operations, thus delaying even more their lengthy rehabilitation.[47]

One group of soldiers at this centre formed a 'Disabled Veterans' Organization' to assist all disabled veterans to obtain their rights to comprehensive rehabilitation and compensation from the state following their injuries.[48] In May 1949, Rehabilitation Centre Number 1 was closed, and the patients transferred to an army hospital (number 5) in Tel Hashomer.[49]

Rehabilitation Centre Number 2, 'Beit Ha-Yod Daled', was officially opened on 27 August 1948 in Ness-Ziona and served exclusively the 'Palmach' disabled (the Palmach was the strike force of the Haganah, the pre-State underground defence organisation)[50] and had 60 beds. In September 1949 the rehabilitation centre was closed, and the facility became a government psychiatric institution. Surprisingly, it was organised by a group of women friends, headed by a 23-year-old woman, Esther Avni Kantor, a soldier of the Palmach. Together with her best friends Yonina Talmon, Hanna Lieberman-Bazam, Hannah Talmi, Tamar Duvdevani-Yeshuvi, Esther Ram, Dvora Lieberman-Erez and Shoshana Hazor, they succeeded in organising and managing the rehabilitation centre.[51] They found the grand house of Abdul Rahman al-Taji, on a hill near Ness-Ziona, which had been destroyed during the war and together rebuilt it.[52]

They then gathered all the furniture and equipment needed. Esther Avni Kantor stayed many days and nights in the site taking care of the renovation and of all the materials that were needed, including beds and mattresses. She also found the medical staff needed to treat the wounded soldiers. She brought in Dr. Ogen Heyman who treated his patients in an unconventional manner, using orgone therapy and homeopathic methods.[53] The rehabilitation centre provided also physical therapy, occupational therapy, vocational rehabilitation, horticultural therapy and zootherapy (therapy using animals). Esther Avni thought that animals would promote healing and would help rehabilitate the soldiers. She brought in a deer and other animals, which was in those days a most unusual treatment-admittedly, yet one that proved very successful.[54]

Rehabilitation Centre Number 3 was opened during war time and was the only one that was not a military but a civilian centre. Three months before the end of the war, the centre was closed due to lack of financial support and for political reasons.[55]

It had been the most modern rehabilitation centre in Israel and the army sent their wounded soldiers from the area of Jerusalem to the facility. It had taken Dr. Emil Adler and his colleagues six months to find a suitable building and organise the rehabilitation centre which had 70 beds.[56] Adler was disappointed when the centre was closed just three months before the end of the war because of lack of financial support and because Dr. Haim Sheba, head of the medical services of the Israeli Defence Force, decided to move all wounded soldiers to one military hospital (number 5) at Tel-Hashomer.[57]

In August 1948 the Hadassah Medical Organisation opened the first civilian rehabilitation centre in Jerusalem as a result of financial help from the Hadassah organisation in the United States.[58] Rehabilitating the disabled soldiers during the war was a very tough mission but it was considered a high priority. Providing comprehensive physical, mental and social rehabilitation services for all who needed them was beyond the capabilities of the young state during the war, but the Hadassah rehabilitation facility managed, although only for a brief time, to provide conventional comprehensive high-quality care to its patients after Dr. Emil Adler did a short fellowship at Dr. Rusk's rehabilitation centre at the USA.[59]

We have seen that following the War of Independence and the establishment of the State of Israel (November 1947-July 1949), the country faced the need to take care of a large number of wounded and handicapped soldiers and civilians. Because of the necessity of taking care of a large population without the right means, there was a lot of improvisation. The three rehabilitation centres built during the war were closed by war's end and the handicapped were transferred to Military Hospital No. 5 (Tel-Hashomer), where continuing attempts were made to rehabilitate the disabled.[60] The military hospital provided physical therapy but no comprehensive state-of-the-art rehabilitation services.[61]

In addition to the restoration of rehabilitation centres, handicapped and injured persons were treated with physical healing methods in other places around the country, such as nursing homes, clinics and other military hospitals. In Tel-Hashomer the rehabilitation services were given to severe handicapped, among them wounded who suffered from paralysis due to a spinal cord injury.[62] The medical staff consisted of volunteers from all over the world. According to David Ben Gurion's archive, in August 1949 there were 3,160 handicapped of whom 1,460 were disabled due to military service. Among Palmach fighters at the time, in February-November 1948, 604 reported wounded of whom approximately 67 were disabled. In August it was reported that there were 250-350 amputees in the Israel Defence Forces (IDF), who required prostheses and rehabilitation.[63]

All three rehabilitation centres were established by force of circumstances during the war, despite the lack of knowledge and resources. Rehabilitating the disabled soldiers during the war was a very difficult mission but it was considered a high priority. Providing comprehensive physical, mental, and social rehabilitation services for all who needed them was beyond the capabilities of the young State during the war, but the Hadassah rehabilitation facility managed, although only for a brief time, to provide comprehensive high-quality care to its patients.[64]

The First Decade PM&R: A Medical Specialty is Born (1949-1958)

By the end of the war at least 2,500 to 3,000 disabled and injured people needed medical attention and rehabilitation. The State and the medical organisations were forced to find some solution to the problem.[65] The injured and handicapped had great expectations for adequate and professional rehabilitation programmes, but the new State of Israel lacked the knowledge, ability and financial means to meet these needs. Prime Minister David Ben Gurion supported and in 1949 approved the 'Law of the Physically Impaired', which provided a scale of the degree of impairment – a measuring stick for the needs of those claiming the privileges and rights of the handicapped. This law stated that every handicapped person would have the right to free full medical treatment, that the paralyzed would be provided with suitable transportation, that amputees would be provided with artificial limbs and the blind with guide dogs. The aim was to improve the quality of life for those injured by providing safe mobility, independence and self-confidence.[66]

In 1950, Israel's 'Law of Return' was passed, stating that every Jew had the right to enter the country and become citizens. The Jewish population in 1948 was approximately 650,000. The new immigrants – Holocaust survivors from Europe, others from Islamic countries and Jews from almost every nation – almost tripled the population by 1956.[67] The American Jewish Joint Distribution Committee provided the funds to treat physically or mentally disabled immigrants. It established 'Malben', a complete system of health services for the immigrant population.[68] The Israeli government was itself unable to provide these services for the physically and mentally disabled because of economic difficulties.[69]

Then, on top of other problems, came the polio epidemic. This, more than anything else, provided the impetus for the World Health Organization and UNICEF to get involved and help the young country to develop rehabilitation services.[70]

The polio epidemic struck Israel in the early 1950s and created an urgent need for immunization against the disease. By 1956 there were 5,835 cases of poliomyelitis, 85% to 90% of whom were children aged 5 years and younger. This pandemic began in part as a result of the massive immigration of Jews from post-war Europe and Middle Eastern and North African countries and it is possible that the virus was imported from these countries. In addition, the crowded, insanitary conditions in the immigrant temporary camps facilitated the fast spread of the virus among the population.

Israeli health authorities asked Dr. Natan Goldblum, director of the Ministry of Health's virology laboratory, and his colleagues to develop and produce the vaccine and work began in the winter of 1955-1956.[71] In 1957 Israel became only the third country in the world (after the United States and Denmark) to produce the Salk vaccine independently when Goldblum and his colleagues prepared the vaccine at the Ministry of Health Central Virus Laboratories, at that time located in Jaffa. Children were then immunized with the new vaccine as part of the routine infant immunization programme (together with Diphtheria-Pertussis-Tetanus). Almost immediately the vaccinations had an impact. The number of poliomyelitis cases in Israel dropped to 57 in 1957. The number of cases increased to 573 in 1958, but then decreased again, to 36 in 1959 and 38 in 1960.

The United Nations organisations (WHO and UNICEF) named their joint plan the 'Plan of Operation for the Rehabilitation of Handicapped Children, Israel'. The plan was to build a general rehabilitation centre to

Table 1 Polio cases in Israel 1950-1956[72]

Years	1950	1951	1952	1953	1954	1955	1956	Total
Cases	1,621	918	874	636	785	468	533	5,835

take care of handicapped children, provide modern methods of physiotherapy and build a national school of physiotherapy.[73] In December 1953 they opened the first school for physiotherapy at the Assaf Harofe Hospital in Zerifin (Sarafand). A trained teacher of physiotherapy from England, Diana Kidd, came for two years to organise the school.[74] Applicants had to have completed high school and understand English well because the teaching was all in English. Along with the school, a general rehabilitation centre was created which was at this time the only comprehensive governmental rehabilitation centre in Israel.[75] In July 1954 the children's rehabilitation centre at the Assaf Harofe government hospital was ready to serve polio patients. 'Beit Feinstone', the institute for chronically ill patients that had been established in 1944, now expanded its medical staff and gave special attention to rehabilitate children by opening a special department with 25 beds for children suffering from polio.[76]

The field of physical medicine further developed at Hadassah Hospital in Jerusalem. In 1949 physical medicine and rehabilitation became an integral part of the first medical school in Israel, and in 1950 Dr. Emil Adler was invited to head an association of Physical Medicine and Rehabilitation.[77] But it took time to reopen a new rehabilitation centre in Jerusalem after the closing at the end of war time. Just in 1956 Adler reopened one and headed up a small department of physical medicine and rehabilitation with only nine beds. Here, he created the first residency in the field.[78] As the first professor of the subject in Israel, Adler insisted on high standards of academic excellence and research in field of PM&R.

Conclusion

In developed countries, physical medicine and rehabilitation, health care specialties focused on restoring the health and functional abilities of injured people, were created during and in the aftermath of war. The concepts of comprehensive rehabilitation medicine were developed in the United States, primarily by Howard Rusk. The young State of Israel, facing the problem of thousands of handicapped people following the War of Independence, and thousands of injured or handicapped immigrants, also had to deal with a polio epidemic, mainly affecting children. Dr. Emil Adler was the main leader of efforts to introduce comprehensive rehabilitation services into Israel. Finally, the first government rehabilitation centre and the first school of physical therapy were opened, thanks to the generous support of WHO and UNICEF. Physical medicine and rehabilitation in Israel developed from this firm foundation.

Notes

1. Niederland, D., 'The Influence of the German Immigrant on the Development of Israeli Medicine', MA thesis, Hebrew University, Jerusalem, 1982; Baader, G., 'The Impact of German Jewish Physicians and German Medicine on the Origins and Development of the Medical Faculty of the Hebrew University', *Korot*, 15 (2001), pp.9-45.

2. Blum, N. and Fee, E., 'The Polio Epidemic in Israel in the 1950s', *American Journal of Public Health*, 97 (2007), p.218.

3. Blum, N., *Ha-Shikum Asah Historia: Maarakhot Shikum Refu'i be-Yisrael 1940-1956* (Haifa: Ha-Michlalah ha-akademit Tsefat, 2006), pp.58-60.

4. Niederland, *The Influence of the German Immigrant on the Development of Israeli Medicine*; Baader, 'The Impact of German Jewish Physicians and German Medicine on the Origins and Development of the Medical Faculty of the Hebrew University'.

5. Tamar Novick, T., 'Jump-Starting Society: Polio in Israel in 1950', *Korot*, 21, 2011-2012, pp.149-174.pp.149-174 .

6. Coulter, J.S., *Physical Therapy* (New York: Paul B. Hoeber, 1932), pp.1-21.

7. Robinson, L.R., *Trauma Rehabilitation* (Philadelphia: Lippincott Williams and Wilkins, 2006), pp.2-3.

8. Whittaker, V.B., 'Rehabilitation in the Services. II. The Army', *Rheumatology and Physical Medicine*, 10 (1970), pp.428-430; Cope, R., 'Robert Jones: Father of Modern Orthopedic Surgery', *Bulletin (Hospital for Joint Diseases (New York)*, 54, 2 (1995), pp.115-123; Guttmann, L., *Textbook of Sport for the Disabled* (Aylesbury: H M and M Publishers, 1976), pp.21-22; Lowman, E.W., 'Symposium on Rehabilitation', *The Medical Clinics of North America*, 53 (1969), pp.485-487; [Anon.] 'Report of the Committee on the Present Status of Physical Therapy', *Journal of the American Medical Association*, 107 (1936), pp.584-587.

9. Rusk, H.A., 'The Growth and Development of Rehabilitation Medicine,' *Archives of Physical Medicine and Rehabilitation*, 50 (1969), pp.463-466.

10. Eldar, R. and Jelić, M., 'The Association of Rehabilitation and War', *Disability and Rehabilitation*, 25 (2003), pp.1,019–1,023.

11. Licht, S., 'Rehabilitation Medicine: Definition and Origin', Twentieth John Stanley Coulter Memorial Lecture', *Archives of Physical Medicine and Rehabilitation*, 51 (1970), pp.619-624.

12. Rusk, H.A., 'Total Rehabilitation', *Journal of the National Medical Association*, 45 (1953), pp.1-16.

13. *American Academy of Physical Medicine and Rehabilitation, Frequently Asked Questions About PM&R*. 2003. Available at: http://www.aapmr.org/condtreat/faq.htm

14. https://www.aiu.edu/publications/student/english/Physical-medicine-and-Rehabilitation.htm, *The History of Physiatry* (27/1/2018).

15. Opitz, J.L., Folz, T.J., Gelfman, R. and Peters, D.J., 'The History of Physical Medicine and Rehabilitation as Recorded in the Diary of Dr. Frank Krusen: Part 1. Gathering Momentum (The Years Before 1942)', *Archives of Physical Medicine and Rehabilitation*, 78 (1997), pp.442-445.

16. Blum, N. and Fee, E., 'Howard A. Rusk (1901-1989) from Military Medicine to Comprehensive Rehabilitation', *American Journal of Public Health*, 98 (2008), pp.256-257.

17. Blum, N, and Fee, E., Excerpted from Rusk, H.A., *A World to Care For: The Autobiography of Howard A. Rusk* (New York, NY: Random House, 1972), pp.3-291. *American Journal of Public Health*, 98 (2008), pp.254-255, 257.

18. Blum, N., *Ha-Shikum Asah Historia: Maarakhot Shikum Refu'i be-Yisrael 1940-1956*, (Nofit: Ha-Michlalah ha-akademit Tsefat, 2006), pp.37-60.

19. Ibid., pp.58-60.

20. Ohry, A., 'Medical and rehabilitation aspects of the treatment of disabled people during the British Mandate in Palestine and the War of Independence 1920-1949', *Harefuah*, 1989, 10;116 (10), pp.549-51.

21. Gottfried, W., 'Dr. Ludwig Ginsburg, In Memoriam', *Meida Larofe*, 9 (1977), pp.66-67.

22. Adler, E., 'Remarks on the New Physiotherapy', *Harefuah*, 20, 1-2 (1940), pp.8-10; Ibid., 'Remarks on the New Physiotherapy', *Harefuah*, 20, 3-4 (1940), pp.23-24.

23. [Anon.] 'In Memoriam, Emil Adler, Chairman of the Executive Board of the Israel Journal of Medical Sciences', *Israel Journal of Medical Sciences*, 7, 2 (1971), p.326; Ohry, A., *Introduction to the Development of Rehabilitation Medicine in Israel/Mevo' le-toldot ha-refu'ah ha-shiqqumit be-Israel* (Tel Aviv, 1999), p.11.

24. Ohry A, 'Dr. Batia Nose-Chen (Berthe Neoussikine) (1897–1990): a Forgotten Israeli Pioneer in Rehabilitation', *Korot*, 24 (2017–2018), pp.103-114.

25. Stein, J., *Health resorts in Erez-Israel (Palestine)*, Ha-histadrut ha-refu'it ha-ivrit be–Eretz Israel, 1928/1927, p.50.

26. Ibid., p.57.

27. Ibid., p.59.

28. Ibid., pp.49; 53.

29. Buchman, M., 'The Tiberias Baths at the Present Time', *Harofe Haivri*, 21 (1948), pp.159-162 (English), pp.48-55 (Hebrew).

30. Ibid., p.134.

31. Yaski, H., 'Pe'ulot Ha-histadrut Ha-medizinit Hadassah Be-Eretz Israel', *Harofe Haivri*, 10 (1933), pp.62-76. Hadassah health care organisation was founded in 1912 by Henrietta Szold and the Women's Zionist Organization of America.

32. Kanev, I., *Mutual Aid and Organized Medicine in Israel; Forty Years of the Workers' Health Services Kupat Holim* (Tel Aviv: Central Kupat Holim, 1953), p.66. The 'Sick Fund' was founded in 1911 by a small group of agricultural workers who joined together to form a mutual aid health care association, and it was taken over by the Histadrut (General Federation of Labor) in 1920.

33. [Anon.] *Pe'ulot Kupat Holim ve-hitpatutah ke-shanot 1935-1936* (Tel Aviv: Central Kupat Holim, 1937), pp.24, 16, 21, 44-46.

34. Weiser, H., 'Physical Treatment in Army Medicine', *HaRefuah*, 24, 1 (1942), p.7.

35. Today, Reuth is one of Israel's leading non-profits in the fields of health, welfare and old age and the Reuth Medical and Rehabilitation Centre is today one of the country's most advanced facilities for rehabilitation and long-term care. Details of the facilities available through Reuth can be found at http://reuth.org/index.asp?id=2338

36. Koven, B., 'Medical rehabilitation in Israel', *N Y State J Med.* (1955), 15; 55 (14), pp.2,064-7; Adler, E., Eliakim, C. and Magora, A., 'Poliomyelitis in Jerusalem in 1953', *Acta Med Orient* (1955),14 (6), pp.147-63; Ohry, A., Shemesh, Y., Meltzer, M. and Rozin, R., 'Treatment of Yom Kippur War Spinal Cord Injuries', *Harefuah* (1976), 91(8), pp.215-8 (Hebrew); Bergman, M., Najenson, T., Hirsch, S. and Solzi, P., 'Auditory Perception in Patients with CVA without Aphasia', *Scand J Rehabil Med Suppl.*

(1985),12, pp.84-7; Ring, H., Schwartz, J., Elazar, B., Berghaus, N., Luz, Y., Solzi, P and Najenson, T., 'Criteria for Referral of CVA patients for rehabilitation', *Scand J Rehabil Med Suppl.* (1985),12, pp.143-7; Nadav, D., *Way of Rehabilitation: the Rehabilitation department of MOD*, (Ministry of Defence), 1948-2005 (MOD Publishing House, 2008); Nadav, D., *White and Khaki: the History of the Israeli Medical Corps, 1949-1967* (MOD Publishing House, 2000); Makin, M. and Winter, S.T., 'Henry Keller MD of New York and the Alyn Hospital in Jerusalem', *N Y State J Med* (April 1990), (4), pp.201-205; Ohry, A., 'Medical and rehabilitation aspects of the treatment of disabled people during the British Mandate in Palestine and the War of Independence, 1920-1949', *Harefuah* (1989), 116(10), pp.549-51.

37. Ben Zion Netanyahu (Ed.), 'Eretz Israel', *Hebrew Encyclopedia*, vol. 6, Jerusalem, p.594.

38. P. Yasoor to Matcal Aka, Social Department (7.16.1951), Ministry of Defence Archive, 702/60/1320); Blum, *Ha–Shikum* (cit. n. 15), pp.117-119.

39. Full Diary of David Ben Gurion (31. 8. 1949), Ben Gurion Archives (6315). Available at http://bgarchives.bgu.ac.il/archives/archion/

40. Blum, N., 'Beit Ha-Yud-Dalet of the Palmach: the First Rehabilitation Centre', pp.151-172 in Dr. Nir Man (Ed.), *Military Medicine*, (Modan: Misrad HaBitachon, The Centre for Defence Studies, 2018).

41. Ibid., p.153.

42. Hurwich, B., *The Fifth Front*: The History of Military Medicine in Palestine and through Israel's War of Independence, *1911-1949* (Tel Aviv: Ministry of Defence Press, 2000), p. 51.

43. Ohry, A., 'Professor Ludwig Guttmann (1899-1980)', *Harefuah* (1999), pp.137 (1-2):79-80. Guttmann's recommendations were 'hidden' by Spira and Sheba, and David Ben Gurion never received them. It was not until 1973 that Prof Raphael Rozin 'revived' the Guttmann's Model, see Ohry, A. and Silver, J.R., 'Ludwig Guttmann (1899-1980) and David Ben Gurion (1886-1973): an early account of the rehabilitation facilities in Israel', *Journal of Medical Biogra*phy (2006), 14 (4), pp.201-209.

44. Zalmanovich, Y., 'The struggle to apply central authority: Public medicine in Israel' in Pilowski, V. (Ed.), '*Moving from a Settlement to State 1947 – '*, *Continuity and Permutations*, (Haaifa: The Herzl Institute for Research of Zionism', 19), pp. 144.

45. Spira, E., 'The Medical Rehabilitation of War Amputees', *Acta Medica Orientalia*, 9 (1950): p.69

46. Reifen, 'Some Observations' (cit. n. 38), p.3

47. Ibid.

48. Memorandum to the Prime Minister, Ministry of Defence Archives, 129/51/282, (30.12.1948).

49. Nadav, D., *White and Khaki; The History of the Israel Medical Corp, 1949-1967* (Tel Aviv: Ministry of Defence, 2000), p.35.

50. See http://www.us- Israel.org/jsource/Society_&_Culture/palmachmuseum. html/ http://www.palmach.org.il/show_item.asp?itemId=8096&levelId=42798&itemType=0.

51. Blum, *Ha–Shikum*, p. 76.

52. Blum, *Beit Ha-Yud- Dalet*, pp.151-172.

53. Blum, *Ha–Shikum*, p.79. Orgone therapy was developed by Dr. Wilhelm Reich (1897-1957). Dr. Heyman used a box (accumulator) constructed of alternating layers of organic and metallic materials. The soldiers (his patients) would sit inside the accumulator for about 20 minutes and absorb orgone energy.

54. Ben-Zvi, Z., *Interview of Palmach Women* (9.11.1990), Yad Tabenkin Archives (25/25/34/1), p.3. In January 1949 the Centre was transferred to the army services and was renamed 'Rehabilitation Centre, Number 2'. In September 1949 it was closed.

55. Blum, N., Shvarts, S. and Ohry, A., 'The foundation of the first civil rehabilitation centre by the Hadassah Organization during the War of Independence', *Harefuah* (2006), 145 (10), pp.773-6, 780 (Hebrew). PubMed PMID: 17111717.

56. Ibid.

57. Ibid.

58. Blum, Shvarts and Ohry, 'The Foundation of the First Civil Rehabilitation Centre by the Hadassah Organization during the War of Independence', pp.773-776, 780.

59. Ibid.

60. Dr. Haim Sheba to Uri Brenner (3.2.1969), Yad Tabenkin Archives (25/25/34/1), file 1, p. 4.

61. Blum, *Ha–Shikum* (cit. n. 15), pp.101-107, 123-132.

62. Nadav, D., 'Hospital 5 (Tel-Hashomer) until his transfer to the Ministry of Health at 1953', *Studies in Israel's resurrection*, 7, Be'er Sheva: Ben Gurion University Negev, 1997, pp.442-439.

63. Record 6315 (31. 8. 1949), Full diary Division Ben Gurion, Archive for Ben Gurion.

64. Ibid.

65. P. Yasoor to Matcal Aka, Social Department (7.16.1951), Ministry of Defence Archive, 702/60/1320); Blum, *Ha–Shikum* (cit. n. 15), pp.117-119.

66. *Full Diary of David Ben Gurion* 29.8.19)), Ben Gurion Archive (6313, cit. n. 31).

67. Ben Zion Netanyahu (Ed.), *'Eretz Yisrael'*, p.674.

68. Ibid., p.720.

69. Grushka, T. (Ed.), *Health Services of Israel* (Jerusalem: The Ministry of Health, 1952), pp.100-101.

70. Blum and Fee, *The Polio*.

71. Blum, N., Katz, E. and Fee, E. 'Professor Natan Goldblum: the pioneer producer of the inactivated poliomyelitis vaccine in Israel', *American Journal of Public Health*, 100 (11), (2010), pp. 2,074-5.

72. Davies, A.M., Marberg, K., Goldblum, N., Levine, S. and Yekutiel, P., 'Epidemiology of Poliomyelitis in Israel, 1952-59, with Evaluation of Salk Vaccination during a Three-Year Period', *Bulletin of the World Health Organisation*, 23 (1960), pp.53-72.

73. Blum and Fee, *The Polio*.

74. Miss Diana Kidd had trained at King's College School of Physiotherapy in London, England. In 1950 she helped to open a physiotherapy school in Greece.

75. Grushka, T. (Ed.), *Health Services of Israel* (Jerusalem: Ministry of Health, 1968), p.330.

76. Solsi, P., 'Dr. Ludwig Ginsburg', *Meida Larofe*, 46 (1987), pp.60-61.

77. Adler, E., 'Thumei ha-refuah ha-fisiqalit' ('The Discipline of Physical Medicine'), *Harefuah*, 39, 4 (1950), pp.45-47.

78. Grushka (Ed.), *Health Services* (cit. n. 59), p. 261.

10

Emergency Services in Israel and Abroad

Roman Sonkin, Uriel Goldberg and Eli Jaffe

A. Magen David Adom

The Israeli Emergency Pre-Hospital Medical Services, Magen David Adom (MDA – colloquially named Mada, thanks to its Hebrew acronym), established in 1930, is a national, statutory non-governmental organisation. It is not funded by the government but is supervised by the Ministry of Health. In 1950 MDA was entrusted by the Israeli Parliament (the Knesset) to be the national ambulance service, blood bank and the Israeli Red Cross organisation. In accordance with the law MDA, has a fleet of over 1,100 ambulances, both Basic Life Support (BLS) and advanced mobile intensive care units, in addition to over 750 first response Medi-Cycles, electric bicycles, mini electric vehicles, 4x4 vehicles, 2 helicopters, a Jet-ski and a rescue boat which are used on the Sea of Galilee. They are stationed across the country at over 160 stations to allow for an average response time of less than 5 minutes for first responders and less than 8.7 minutes for ambulances and Mobile Intensive Care Units.

MDA covers a population approximately the same size as London, over a geographical area the size of Wales, spanning over three climate regions and various topographies from the Red Sea resorts, through mountainous regions, desert and even a snow-capped mountain. It is the largest volunteer organisation in Israel with over 24,000 volunteers serving as paramedics, Emergency Medical Technicians (EMTs) and First Aiders. The MDA First Responder unit, with over 7,000 volunteers is fully equipped and units are dispatched automatically by the most advanced emergency medical services command and control system in the world. It all makes for a very diverse ambulance service – the patients, the equipment, the geography, transport distances, even the medical conditions can vary by location. Irrespective of where you may be in Israel, however, or, for that matter in crises around the world, professional MDA

EMTs, Paramedics and First Responders of all types will be ready to help those in their hour of need.

History

Magen David Adom (MDA) began in 1919 concomitantly in New York (USA) and (Yafo) Jaffa, (Israel) to provide medical and nursing aid to Jewish soldiers serving in the 'Jewish Legion' of the British Army. This organisation was disbanded together with the Jewish Legion in 1921. In the 1920s there were attempts to establish an international organisation parallel to the Red Cross. MDA was finally formally established in 1930 as a volunteer association by a committee of volunteer physicians – 'The Society for Rapid Assistance during a Disaster – Magen David Adom'. They immediately began with volunteer recruitment and first aid training as well as fundraising activities which yielded the first ambulance vehicle before the end of the year. The first official station was opened in Tel Aviv in 1936. Different cities began establishing MDA local associations for their cities.[1]

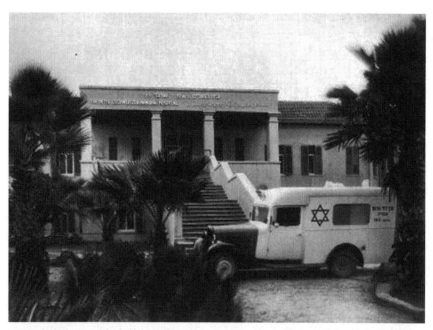

14. Ambulance outside the hospital in Tiberias, 1938 (from *MDA and the State: the History of Magen David Adom in Israel*, 2018)

Ever since its earliest days, MDA has provided care to all those in need, irrespective of their background, religion, race or gender.[2] Today this is entirely a non-issue in most places around the world, but in the Middle East it stands out as a bastion of equal rights. This is true both of those that the crews treat, and of the crews themselves.[3] In 1946 it began operating what became Israel's National Blood Bank, collecting, processing and providing almost all of Israel's blood supplies, both in peace and war time.[4]

The State of Israel gained independence in 1948, and two years later the MDA Law was passed by the Israeli Parliament – The Knesset. MDA law united the various MDA associations which existed in different cities under one national umbrella organisation while keeping their separate autonomy and budgets. The law provided MDA with the status of the national Red Cross organisation and assigned it the duties defined by the Geneva Conventions.[5] The law also assigned MDA with the duty to aid the Israeli Defence Forces (IDF) at times of war, provide first aid services to the residents of the country, provide blood banking services and any other roles as defined in the organisation's statute. In 1952 the MDA statute was approved by the Knesset,[6] over the time adding the responsibility to educate and train the public in first aid and pre-hospital emergency medicine among other roles.[7]

In 1979 the separate MDA organisations began working under a unified budget, combining them into one organisation. Since then and until 1991 the branches were separate entities but working under one budget, In 1991 The *Revah* committee of the Knesset, set up to assess MDA services, concluded that the organisation must be reformed and begin working as one organisation divided into regions with an hierarchical management.[8] Nowadays MDA is a leader organisation and a professional authority in the field of pre-hospital emergency medicine and is part of the health committees setting of standards of care.[9]

Medical Services

Since it was established in 1930 MDA has served as the national Emergency Medical Service (EMS) and provided first aid and ambulance transport services which had BLS capabilities. In addition, there were also 24-hour first aid services provided in the stations and a night time physician service in various stations.[10]

The first paramedic course was run during 1979, when the world of EMS was growing exponentially both in terms of numbers as well as medical knowledge and skill. MDA made an extensive leap away from being merely an emergency transport system, into a system of professional pre-hospital care providers incorporating a two-tier system with BLS ambulances and Mobile Intensive Care Units (MICUs).[11] Since then, over 3,000 paramedics have been trained, and today, some 400 paramedics qualify annually via the various courses that are held by MDA.[12] Every paramedic in Israel is trained by MDA at some point during their qualification. They include those in National Service, the military, combined degrees with nursing, clinical training of university degree paramedic students, as well as direct intake courses within MDA. Simultaneously with the expansion of the MICUs and paramedic training, the night physician service and station first aid services were discontinued.[13]

In 1996, 23 MICUs were already operating in Israel staffed by an Emergency Medical Technician (EMT) driver, a paramedic and a physician. In the same year the first MICU staffed solely by paramedics, without the presence of a physician, was opened in Karmiel.[14] Since May 2012, MDA Paramedics are trusted by the Ministry of Health to declare and document death, a qualification which until then was reserved to physicians solely. This decision was proven to improve MICU availability and Return of Spontaneous Circulation (ROSC) in Cardio-Pulmonary Resuscitation (CPR) patients.[15]

Presently, MDA serves over 9 million people over an area of 22,000 square miles with an extent of over 677,000 yearly incidents in 2018 and over 988,000 responses.[16] In the 1980s and 1990s MDA initiated its First Responders programme initially running through the Hatzalah (Hebrew, meaning Rescue) organisations counting more than 30 organisations such as the Rehovot city branch founded in 1989,[17] one of the Jerusalem branches founded in 1992 and Hatzalah Israel founded in 1994 among many other organisations.[18] In July 2000, MDA's organic First Responder Unit was founded and the Hatzalah organisations became its subordinates. The unit had over 1,800 MDA volunteers on top of those already co-serving in the Hatzalah organisations. MDA founded a unique system where an EMS organisation provides First Responder volunteers free of charge on top of ambulance services.[19] In 2011 the volunteer First Responder Unit was awarded the President of the State of Israel honour for volunteering, for its unique activity as a pioneer of the nation's emergency medical services.[18] Initially, the First Responders received car kits for their personal vehicles until 2002 when the first Medi-Cycles (Medical Motorcycles)were brought into service. Nowadays, MDAs First Responder unit has over 7,000 volunteers operating over 700 Medi-Cycles, 50 Mobile Electric Response Vehicles (MERVs), 200 bicycles and 7,275 personal cars.[19] The Life

Guardians programme incorporates professional bystanders using the MDA Teams' Smartphone Application for response to nearby emergencies such as cardiac arrest, haemorrhage, suffocation and more. These professional bystanders are physicians, nurses, military EMTs and many other people who have undergone BLS training.[20]

Human Resources

MDA began as a volunteer organisation and to this day volunteers are the major human resource of the organisation which continues to grow, incorporating over 2,250 employees and, amazingly, over 24,000 volunteers, who donate over one million hours of their time annually, making it Israel's largest volunteer organisation.[21] Every four years, the volunteers elect their representatives in the branch committee and national committees including the MDA council and board.[22] Over 13,000 of the volunteers are part of the MDA youth organisation, who participate in humanitarian aid, educational activities, leadership training and when they turn 15 and finish the basic first aid class spanning 60 hours they begin volunteering on the ambulances and MICUs.[23]

Training

Throughout the year, MDA provides not only EMS and blood services, but also provides education to many cross-sections of society. This begins with education of the young, the youth volunteers through EMT and Paramedic courses, as well as external courses to the general public and advanced courses to medical professionals. Approximately 6,000 courses are taught each year, with over 100,000 people being taught annually by MDA's instructors. All training courses are offered to both volunteer and employed staff without any discrimination; both are required to meet the same standards in training and in the exams. The EMT course spans 200 hours and is required in order to receive an ambulance driving permit from the Ministry of Transportation. The Training Department has state-of-the-art, online Continuing Medical Education (CME) and video channels with educational videos filmed in cooperation with the Bar-Ilan University. MDA training programmes extend beyond the borders of the State of Israel, as trainings are held for foreign organisations, citizens and communities around the world. Many international training programmes are also held in Israel and trainees specially arrive for this purpose.[24]

Red Cross National Society

After decades of wishing and attempting, in 2006, Magen David Adom was finally admitted as a full member of the International Committee of the Red Cross and Red Crescent Societies (ICRC). MDA is recognized for its humanitarian aid across the world, having attended scenes of natural disasters and major terror attacks as far and wide as Haiti (2010), Nepal (2015), Turkey (2016), the USA (2017) and many others. MDA brought with it not only medical assistance, but also their expertise in mass-casualty incidents (MCIs). Israel has faced several wars and ongoing terror attacks, with major waves of terror in the early 2000s leading to incidents with multiple scenes and large numbers of casualties. All of which led to MDA developing advanced management and treatment protocols and methods that are now recognized and taught around the globe.[25]

Funding, Budget and Friends Societies

Although MDA is a national, statutory organisation and is supervised by the Ministry of Health, it is non-governmental and is therefore not funded by the government. In 2017, the MDA budget was 750 million Israeli Shekels (ILS).[26]

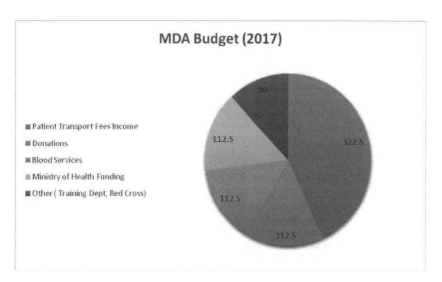

In 1940 the American Friends of MDA (AFMDA) society was founded and began donating ambulances, funds and other supplies to MDA in Israel. Today over 20 MDA Friends' societies exist, the youngest of which is in

Hong Kong and the veteran is in the USA (AFMDA) which is also the largest.[27] Additional Friends societies include United Kingdom, Australia, Uruguay, Italy, Argentina, Belgium, Germany, South Africa, Holland, Israeli Christian friends of MDA, Israeli friends of MDA, Mexico, France, Columbia, Canada, Switzerland and Sweden. MDA friend societies also aid in building new MDA stations, service centres and technological advances.

Technology

Technological advances allowed MDA in 2009 to finally develop and implement cutting edge technology in the new National Medical Dispatch Centre (NMDC). Since then, there have been multiple improvements to the technologies of the command and control systems that are developed in-house. The systems allow for advanced call management, resource management, decision-making support, dispatch and MCI management.[28] Emergency calls are received every 15 seconds and are answered within an average of less than 3.2 seconds in the nearest available dispatch centre around the country while skipping busy dispatch centres, the dispatcher in the relevant regional dispatch centre that receives the information while the nearby available Life Guardians,[29] First Responders, ambulances and MICUs are already activated by the automatic response system.[30] An ambulance is dispatched every 38 seconds. A smartphone application MDA was developed, which allows calling the emergency dispatch centre using one click from the app automatically sending the location of the caller and personal and medical information which is stored in the app beforehand. The app also allows for direct video streaming from the scene of an incident or sending pictures directly to the dispatch centre.[31] Another way to shorten response times is integration with social media navigation apps which allows for accurate locations of car accidents and navigation to the scene and hospitals.[32]

Blood Bank Services

Even before the establishment of the national blood bank in 1946 by MDA, in the era when blood preservation was yet to be, blood donors were transported by MDA ambulances to the hospitals for donations. The donor organisation was established in 1936 in order to contact with donors quickly in times of need and today 12,000 volunteers are part of it.[33] During September 1936, blood products were scarce and much needed due to the extensive amount of wounded. Dr. Levontin, one of MDA's founders, established the blood bank based on volunteers collecting blood from donors and distributing it to the hospitals.[34] During the 1950s, MDA blood services began fractioning whole blood to its products to produce plasma for infusion.[35] In 2002 the national umbilical blood bank was founded in order to keep stem cells from umbilical blood for future needs in case of cancer, hematologic disease or genetic disease – this blood can be kept for 25 years and over 6,000 units have been collected. The amount of blood needed in Israel is about 300,000 (4% of the Israeli population) blood donations per year, 96% of which is collected by the MDA blood services crews. A special app was created to update the public and regular blood bank volunteers about blood 'levels' and needs.[36]

MDA in Times of War

When the State of Israel was founded, MDA was already experienced both in treating civilians and wounded soldiers. After it was established, the young state and MDA signed the three Geneva Convention treaties that existed at the time. Beginning with the War of Independence and continuing through the following wars, MDA gained more experience as the national EMS organisation, national blood bank and as the national Red Cross Society. With the beginning of the war the ICRC sent a letter requesting both MDA and the Red Crescent to uphold the treaties during the war. MDA responded with a positive response to the letter. The ICRC also notified the Arab counties fighting that the MDA symbol will be recognized as a symbol equal to the Red Cross although it is not an official symbol. During the War of Independence, the AFMDA society shipped dozens of ambulances to allow MDA to treat the increasing amount of wounded in the battles. A number of these ambulances were transferred to the newly-founded IDF medical corps.

In the following wars and military operations such as Kadesh, the Sinai Campaign of 1956, the Six-Day War in 1967 and the Yom-Kippur War in 1973, MDA, through its branches and crews, both volunteer and employed, fulfilled its duties and roles as a national organisation. Before the Kadesh military operation, the blood bank quietly collected over 3,000 blood units. In the following wars and operations MDA held first aid trainings for the public, training thousands of people. MDA also fulfilled its duties as the National Red Cross society. In October 1973, the Yom Kippur War took the country and the IDF by surprise, but not MDA. MDA had already accustomed itself to always be prepared. As soon as a state of emergency was declared all MDA personnel, both employed and volunteers, reported for duty and increased the level of preparedness. The collaboration between MDA and the IDF medical corps was extraordinary.

The 1982 Lebanon War, to eradicate the missile threats over northern Israel, found MDA in a highly trained and efficient working state prepared for any scenario. During the war, over 1,000 soldiers were transported from the frontlines to Israeli hospitals by MDA ambulances and MICUs. Red Cross activities also commenced from the beginning and medical aid in the front lines by MDA crews was used. The Gulf War in 1990 put MDA in a constant state of awareness from rocket attacks. MDA was prepared to treat various scenarios including chemical weapon injuries. The Second Intifada was characterized by suicide bombers and extensive MCIs, and MDA treated and evacuated all casualties. MDA ambulances continued to provide care for all people regardless of their nationality while even being attacked by rocks or Molotov cocktails. The Second Lebanon war in July 2006 caused Northern Israel to become a front with high rates of missile fire and almost 3,000 casualties were treated by MDA. MDA entered the highest level of alert and all emergency vehicles were staffed; crews were working twelve-hour cycles of shifts and rest. During the 33 harsh days of battle, MDA crews responded to 1,479 incidents. During operations 'Cast Lead' and 'Protective Edge' to protect the Southern population of Israel from the missile threats of Gaza, MDA stations, crews and vehicles in the affected areas were in the range of missiles and operated bravely under fire. Unfortunately, MDA lost some of its best people during the wars, both in MDA duty and IDF service.[37]

Emergency Medicine Abroad

Since its foundation in 1930, MDA has been providing humanitarian aid around the world in times of disaster. The first such mission departed Israel in 1939 following a large earthquake in Turkey. MDA supplied medical supplies and blankets. However, the outbreak of the Second World War forced MDA to cease the mission earlier than planned. However, that war did not stop MDA's humanitarian aid activities. During the war, MDA provided continuous aid to Jewish soldiers on all fronts and their families. Immediately following the war and the devastation of the Holocaust, MDA sent emergency aid to the displaced persons camps to assist in recovery efforts. In addition to the aid sent to the displaced persons camps, MDA sent supplies to survivors living in Poland, Romania, Germany, France and Italy to assist them in their efforts to rebuild their lives. The humanitarian aid sent both to Europe and distributed around Palestine not only included supplies and equipment, but also taught the general public about hygiene, health and first aid.

In the years immediately following the establishment of the State of Israel MDA did not have much in the way of resources. Despite the minimal resources available, MDA continued to distribute aid around the world.

The 1960s saw a great famine in Biafra, Nigeria. As usual, MDA was at the forefront of support and sent several tonnes of food to those in need. In addition, at this time, MDA hosted a wide variety of first aid courses for developing countries, allowing them to improve their own emergency services. An additional example of MDA's aid to foreign countries in times of crisis is a shipment of plasma to Cuba in the last days of the Revolution.

An additional major function of MDA's humanitarian aid has been training teams from around the world in first aid and as first aid instructors. As determined by the MDA Law of 1950, MDA serves to provide first aid training to the public and increase the number of lives saved in the time it takes an ambulance to arrive. As such, MDA places great emphasis on sharing its knowledge and experience as one of the world leaders in emergency medical services (EMS) around the world.

During the wars in Israel in the 1970s and 80s, MDA provided evacuation and medical services to wounded soldiers, as well as what is known as the 'White Caravan' which provided clothing and medical care to refugees of the Lebanon War. The Caravan was made up of 20 ambulances which were able to navigate the difficult terrain and to provide medical care to those wounded in the battles. During the Second Lebanon War in 2006, MDA once again provided aid to the victims of the war. During the war, MDA distributed first aid kits and held training sessions in the bomb shelters for those effected by the many rocket attacks on the north of Israel.

One of the lesser-known humanitarian activities that MDA holds to date is the assistance provided to the Palestinian Red Crescent. Due to MDA's prominent position in EMS, often EMS organisations from around the world would turn to MDA's expertise and experience for guidance. One such example is the Palestinian Red Crescent, for whom MDA holds periodic training on pertinent medical topics. An additional such example of MDA's expertise is in the area of refugee care. Over the years, Israel and Europe both have seen an influx of refugees from Africa and Syria respectively. These refugees are often in need of medical care, and MDA is there to provide it. As part of providing medical care to Syrian refugees off the shores of Europe, MDA sent medical professionals to join the teams of the Migrant Offshore Aid Station programme, as well as funding and staffing a clinic in the Tel Aviv Central Bus Station for African migrants.

Following the terror attacks of 11 September 2011, the citizens of Israel banded together to provide assistance to their brothers and sisters in the United States who fell victim to one of the largest terror attacks in history. MDA sent an emergency shipment of blood and blood products to the United States to assist in treating the victims of the attacks and mitigate the blood shortage that came as a result. Most recently, MDA has sent aid missions to Nepal, Haiti and Texas following earthquakes and hurricanes to assist local populations in recovery efforts, and MDA hopes to continue to provide aid wherever needed, whenever disaster should strike.

In 2010, over two million people were wounded in an earthquake on Haiti. There were many injured and dead, and many others with no access to food or water. MDA in conjunction with other international Red Cross societies immediately sent medical and logistical teams to assist. In conjunction with the Norwegian and Canadian Red Cross Societies, MDA set up a large field hospital which was staffed for over three years by Red Cross and local emergency and medical personnel. In addition to providing

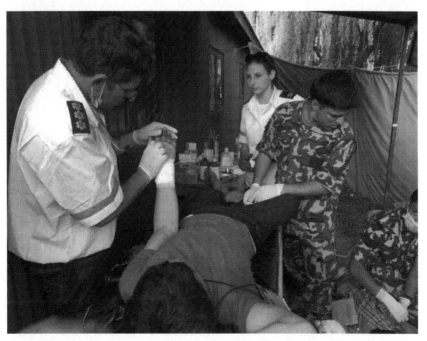

15. Nepal Earthquake 2015: Treating a wounded child. (from *MDA and the State*, p.294)

emergency medical care, MDA in conjunction with the Lands Aid organisation established a rehabilitation hospital for those who had suffered amputations and were in need of prosthetics.

In April 2013, a large-scale earthquake hit Nepal leaving thousands homeless and without access to basic resources. Within 24 hours of the quake MDA teams were on the ground providing emergency services for those in need. MDA teams were responsible for assisting in building shelters, distributing water and sleeping bags and of course, providing medical care to the wounded. During the earthquake, there were four premature infants born to Nepali surrogates on behalf of Israeli families. There was no word on their condition following the earthquake and there were fears that their lives were in danger. MDA called up their best Paramedics for the mission. The mission, to bring them home to Israel to their parents, was exactly what happened. MDA teams loaded incubators and other equipment on to airplanes at Ben-Gurion airport and took off for Katmandu. The infants and their parents were brought home safely.

At the present time, MDA is holding a seminar called 'First Seven Minutes' to teach communities how to act in the first minutes following disasters of various scales. Seven Minutes is the average time in which ambulances arrive in developed countries. 'First Seven Minutes' can be

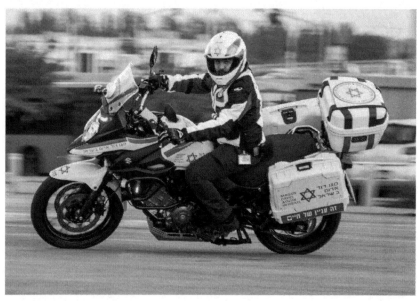

16. MDA Medicycle, 2019. (Shachar Hezkelevich, MDA)

shown around the world to improve community resilience. These events are a very small cross-section of the humanitarian activities going on at MDA daily. In addition to the international activities, MDA operates several projects locally for the citizens of Israel and is always ready for the next humanitarian mission.

Notes

1. A detailed history of Magen David Adom was published by the organisation in 2016: M Dayan, M., Jaffe, E. and Gvirtzman, B., *Magen David Adom of the State: History of Magen David Adom in Israel*. 1st ed. (Magen David Adom, 2016).
2. Ben-Avi, I., 'Announcements: Magen David Adom Association' *(Doar Hayom) Palestine Daily Mail*. Accessed at http://jpress.org.il/olive/apa/nli_heb/?href=DHY%2F1932%2F01%2F01&page=4&entityId=Ar00403#panel=document. on 6/6/2019. (Published 1/1/ 1932).
3. Jaffe, E., Cohen, S.-Y. and Derweesh, A.N. et al, 'The Value of Saving Lives as Seen by the Three Religions'. 2007:1. Published in the history of MDA (see Reference 1), pp.150-151.
4. Levy, N. and Michlin, A., 'The beginnings of Magen David Adom', *Harefuah* (1991), 120 (3), pp.157-161. http://www.ncbi.nlm.nih.gov/pubmed/2032650. Accessed 6/6/2019.
5. *The Geneva Conventions and Their Additional Protocols*. International Committee of the Red Cross https://www.icrc.org/en/war-and-law/treaties-customary-law/geneva-conventions.
6. The Knesset. *Magen David Adom Law* (Israel: Israeli Legislation, 1950). https://he.wikisource.org/wiki/חוק_מגן_דוד_אדום. Accessed 6 June 2019.
7. Revah, M., *Revah Committee Report: The MDA Services Assessment Committee*, 1991.
8. Ibid. See also Shapira, Y.H., *MDA Operational Array in Routine and in Emergency Times and Organization of the Pre-hospital Emergency Medicine in Israel*. 803.; 2019. Accessed on 18/2/2020 at https://www.mevaker.gov.il/(X(1)S(bbwkdn0q4otb051w4h0glu04))/sites/DigitalLibrary/Pages/Reports/1427-15.aspx?AspxAutoDetectCookieSupport=1.
9. Abramovich, I., Hevroni, Y. and Azoulay, D., *Standards of Care: Qualifications and First Aid Equipment in Public Places*, 2016 https://www.health.gov.il/PublicationsFiles/first_aid_equipmen_public_places.pdf. Accessed 24.6.2019.
10. Dayan, Jaffe and Gvirtzman, *Magen David Adom of the State*. See also Revah, *Revah Committee Report*.
11. Jaffe, E. and Bin, E., *Israeli National Prehospital Emergency Medical Services Annual Report*.; 2018. https://www.mdais.org/about/sikumshana.
12. Meeting of the Work and Wellbeing Committee of the Israeli Knesset. 1995. Accessed on 20/2/2020 at https://knesset.org/meetings/2/0/2053477.html.
13. Katz, I., Meeting of the Work and Wellbeing Committee of the Israeli Knesset. 1995. https://knesset.org/meetings/2/0/2053477.html; Jaffe, E., Herbst, R. and Sonkin, R., 'Paramedics declare death: A lifesaving decision', *Health Policy Technology* (July 2017)

doi:10.1016/j.hlpt.2017.07.005; Wacht, O., Schwartz, D. and Miller, R., 'The development and history of the paramedic profession in Israel' *International Paramedic Practice* (2015), 5 (2), pp.31-34. https://www.magonlinelibrary.com/journal/ippr34. https://www.magonlinelibrary.com/journal/ippr

14. Dayan, Jaffe and Gvirtzman, *Magen David Adom of the State.*
15. Jaffe, Sonkin, Goldberg and Strugo, 'Paramedics declare death – A lifesaving decision'.
16. Jaffe, E., Herbst, R. and Sonkin, R., 'Lifesaving Vacation: EMS Overseas Volunteers Willingness to Assist during Disasters', *International Preparedness and Response for Emergency and Disaster (IPRED) 5 Abstr B.* (2018), p.234. http://www.ipred.co.il/wp-content/uploads/2018/01/IPRED-V-eBook.pdf. Accessed 6 June 2019; Yafe, E., Walker, B.B. and Amram, O. et al, 'Volunteer First Responders for Optimizing Management of Mass Casualty Incidents', *Disaster Med Public Health Prep.* (2019);13(02): pp.287-294. doi:10.1017/dmp.2018.56; Israel NGO Registry - 'Nativ Hahesed - Refua ve Revaha.' 1989. https://www.guidestar.org.il/organization/580057628.
17. Israel NGO Registry, '*Nativ Hahesed: Refua ve Revaha*', 1989. https://www.guidestar.org.il/organization/580057628.
18. Israel NGO Registry, 'Hatzalah Israel', 1994. https://www.guidestar.org.il/organization/580246486.
19. See reference 8.
20. Khalemsky, M., Schwartz, D.G., Silberg, T., Khalemsky, A., Jaffe, E. and Herbst, R., 'Childrens' and Parents' Willingness to Join a Smartphone-Based Emergency Response Community for Anaphylaxis: Survey', *Journal of Medical Internet Research JMIR* (2019), 7(8), e13892. doi:10.2196/13892; https://mhealth.jmir.org/; Jaffe, E., Blustein, O., Rosenblat, I. and Sonkin, T., 'Call for Help,Better Before than After: 'Life Guardians.'*IPRED 5 Abstr B.*:232. http://www.ipred.co.il/wp-content/uploads/2018/01/IPRED- V-eBook.pdf. Accessed 6 June 2019.
21. See reference 10.
22. Revah, *Revah Committee Report*; Shapira, Y.H., *MDA Operational Array in Routine and in Emergency Times.*
23. Jaffe, E. and Nave, M., *Volunteer Management: Theory and Practice in Magen David Adom* (Tel Aviv: Magen David Adom, 2011); Ellis, D.Y. and Sorene, E., 'Magen David Adom: The EMS in Israel', *Resuscitation* (2008), 76 (1), pp.5-10. doi:10.1016/j.resuscitation.2007.07.014; Jaffe, E., Alpert, E.A. and Lipsky, A.M., 'A Unique Program to Incorporate Volunteers Into a Nationwide Emergency Medical System', *Journal of the American Medical Association (Surg)*, 2017;152 (11), p.1,088. doi:10.1001/jamasurg.2017.2232; Dadon, Z., Alpert, E.A. and Jaffe, E., 'Enhancing early response to out-of-hospital cardiac arrest', *Am J Emerg Med.* (May 2019) doi:10.1016/J.AJEM.2019.05.055
24. Dadon, Z, Alpert, E.A. and Jaffe, E., 'Enhancing early response to out-of-hospital cardiac arrest', *Am J Emerg Med.* (May 2019). doi:10.1016/J.AJEM.2019.05.055; *Training of Professional Drivers.* Israel: Ministry of Transportation and Road Safety https://www.gov.il/he/service/training_of_professional_drivers; Alutin, A., *First Aid Guide.* 15th edn. (Magen David Adom, 1971); M Raviolo, M., Jaffe, E. and Herbst, E., 'Practicing What You Preach', *Prehosp Disaster Med.* 2019;34(s1):s159-s159. doi:10.1017/S1049023X19003601; Israeli EMS System Trains Hatzalah Medics from Around the Globe | EMS World. https://www.emsworld.com/press-

release/1222774/israeli-ems-system-trains-hatzalah-medics-around-globe. Published 2019. Accessed 6 June 2019; R Herbst, E Jaffe, Seven First Minutes – Community Emergency Response Training. *Prehosp Disaster Med.* 2019;34(s1):s18-s18. doi:10.1017/S1049023X19000542; Jaffe, E., Aviel, E., Kodinsky,N., Knobler, H. and Aharonson-Daniel, L., The dual benefit of first aid training among Civilians in a time of war. *Inj Prev.* 2010, 16 (Suppl 1):A256 LP-A256. doi:10.1136/ip.2010.029215.911; Jaffe, E., Aviel, E., Aharonson-Daniel, L., Kodinsky, N. and Knobler, H., 'First Aid Training among Civilians in a Time of War: Gaining Necessary Skills for Coping with Anxiety', *Prehosp Disaster Med.* 2010;25 (S1):S72-S73. doi:10.1017/s1049023x 00023633; Jaffe, E., Sonkin, R. and Klein, I., 'Effectively Sustaining an International Medical Volunteer Unit for Emergency Times. *IPRED 4 Abstr B.* 2016:323 http://ipred4.pwizard.com/wp-content/themes/eventor/eventor/ipred2016.pdf. Accessed 6 June 6, 2019;

Jaffe, E., Abramovich, I. and Sonkin, R., 'Seeing is better than Reading – Training by Video Saves Time while Improving Comprehension', *IPRED 5 Abstr B.* 2018:235. http://www.ipred.co.il/wp-content/uploads/2018/01/IPRED-V-eBook.pdf. Accessed 6 June 2019; Jaffe, E., Parush, A., Solomon, T., Herbst, R. and Sonkin, R., 'Early Simulation, Like Early Defibrillation -Using MCI Simulators to Improve Preparedness', *IPRED 5 Abstr B.* 2018:233. http://www.ipred.co.il/wp-content/uploads/2018/01/ IPRED-V-eBook.pdf. Accessed 6 June 6, 2019. Eli Jaffe. Virtual reality technology used to teach MCI scene command. 2017. https://www.ems1.com/technology/articles/ 195127048-virtual-reality-technology-used-to-teach-mci-scene-command/. Accessed 6/6/2019.

25. *The Geneva Conventions and Their Additional Protocols.* International Committee of the Red Cross
     https://www.icrc.org/en/war-and-law/treaties-customary-law/geneva-conventions.
     ICRC. Israel's Magen David
     Adom society: key facts on ICRC support - ICRC. 22-02-2005. Accessed on 6/6/2019
     at: https://www.icrc.org/en/doc/resources/documents/misc/israel_mda_040204.htm.
     (2005).
     R Herbst, R., Sonkin, R., Klein, A. and Jaffe, E., 'Seven Minutes – Life Saving Becomes Contagious', *IPRED 6 Abstr B* (Accepted for publication).

26. Alutin A. and Shazar, Z., 'Magen David Adom' - Front of the Shield. *Davar.* 20/1/1948.
     Accsessed on 6/6/2019 at http://jpress.org.il/Olive/APA/NLI_heb/?action=tab&tab=
     browse&pub=DAV&_ga=2.21806395.1812309505.15615 69158-675326289.1560688888#
     panel=document; Shapira, Y.H., *MDA Operational Array in Routine and in Emergency Times;* Jaffe, E. and Bin, E., *Israeli National Prehospital Emergency Medical Services Annual Report.*

27. AFMDA. American Friends of Magen David Adom History. https://afmda.org/
     history/. Accessed 16/6/2019.

28. Blustein, O., Rosenblat, I., Sonkin, R. and Jaffe, E., 'Multi Casualty Incident Management Module', *IPRED 6, Abstract* (Accepted for publication, 2020); Jaffe, E., Blustein, O., Rosenblat, I. and Sonkin, R., 'Building the Infrastructure for the 'EMS-to-Balloon' Era of STEMI Treatment', *Journal of Emergency Medical Serv*ices, 2016. Accessed at https://www.jems.com/articles/2016/08/building-the-infrastructure-for-the-ems-to-balloon-era-of-stemi-treatment.html. Accessed 18/6/2019; Jaffe, E., Strugo, R. and Wacht, O., 'Magen David Adom Provides Nationwide EMS Response in Israel.

*Journal of Emergency Medical Ser*vices, 2018. https://www.jems.com/articles/print/volume-43/issue-6/features/magen-david-atom-provides-nationwide-ems-response-in-israel.html. Accessed22/6/2019.

29. Jaffe, E., Alpert, E.A. and Lipsky, A.M., 'A Unique Program', *JAMA Surg.* 2017;152 (11):1088.

30. Khalemsky, M., Schwartz, D.G., Silberg, T., Khalemsky, A., Jaffe, E. and Herbst, R., 'Childrens' and Parents' Willingness' (see Ref. 20); Dadon, Z., Alpert, E.A. and Jaffe, E., 'Enhancing early response to out-of-hospital cardiac arrest' (see Ref 23).

31. Jaffe, E., Blustein, O., Rosenblat, I., Caspi, G., Raphael, H. and Sonkin, R, 'My Location, My MDA - Locating Victims of Disaster', *IPRED 5 Abstr B.* 2018:176. http://www.ipred.co.il/wp-content/uploads/2018/01/IPRED-V-eBook.pdf. Accessed 6 June 2019.

32. Peleg, K. and Pliskin, J.S., 'A geographic information system simulation model of EMS: reducing ambulance response time', *American Journal of Emergency Med*icine, 2004; 22 (3), pp.164-170. doi:10.1016/J.AJEM.2004.02.003

33. Dayan, M., Jaffe, R. and Gvirtzman, B., *History of Magen David Adom in Israel.*

34. Levontin, M., *Report of MDA Activities in Israel.*; 1946. doi:KH4\9034-1t

35. Alutin and Shazar, 'Magen David Adom' (see reference 26).

36. Shinar, E., Yahalom, V. and Silverman, B.G., 'Meeting blood requirements following terrorist attacks: the Israeli experience', *Current Opinions in Hematology,* 2006;13(6):452-456. doi:10.1097/01.moh.0000245691.32085.66; E Shinar, E., 'The Israeli National Blood Response Program', *IPRED 4 Abstr B.* 2016:99. http://ipred4.pwizard.com/wp-content/themes/eventor/eventor/ipred2016.pdf. Accessed 6 June 2019; Kot, Y., 'Insurance of Blood for times of need', *Voluneers - Magen David Adom Israel News (Lamitnadev - Yediot Magen David Adom be Isr.* 1955: pp.4-5.
doi:SPA2995, 1983, pp.220-355. Plasma Fractioning Facility. *Volunteers - Magen David Adom Israel News (Lamitnadev - Yediot Magen David Adom be Isr.* 1955:8-9. doi:SPA2995, 1983, pp.220-355; Rubin, Y., 'MDA Services Expansion', *HaMashkif.* (published 23/7/1947):
http://jpress.org.il/olive/apa/nli_heb/?href=HMF%2F1947%2F07%2F23&page=4&entityId=Ar00418.

37 Agranat, S., Landoy, M., Neventza, Y., Yadin, Y. and Laskov, H., *Agranat Comission Report - IDF Function During the Yom Kippur War Investigation.*; 1975. http://www.archives.mod.gov.il/docs/agranat/Pages/default.aspx; Winograd, E., *Homefront Prepardness and Function during the Second Lebanon War.*; 2007. doi:0793-1948; Jaffe, E., Strugo, R. and Wacht, O., 'Operation Protective Edge – A Unique Challenge for a Civilian EMS Agency', *Prehospital Disaster Med*icine, 2015;30(5): pp.539-542. doi:10.1017/S1049023X15005026; 21 MDA Ambulances from the USA were festively handed to MDA center. *HaMashkif.* http://jpress.org.il/olive/apa/nli_heb/?href=HMF%2F1948%2F08%2F31&page=4&entityId=Ar00415#panel=document. Published 31 August 1948.

B. United Hatzalah

The story of United Hatzalah of Israel dates back over 30 years to the time that its founder, Eli Beer, then a self-described poor student, 16 years old, signed up as an Emergency Medical Technician (EMT) near his home in the Jerusalem neighbourhood of Bayit V'gan. As an EMT he could perform many of the functions of a paramedic. While paramedics offer more sophisticated procedures than EMTs, such as advanced life support, giving medicines and intubation, an EMT can do anything external, such as administer Cardio-Pulmonary Resuscitation (CPR), use a defibrillator and set up intravenous therapy. To his great distress the slowness of the ambulance response time meant that there was no genuine opportunity for lifesaving. At the time Jerusalem had only nine ambulances to service over 500,000 residents. The ambulances were dispatched from a single location near the entrance to the city and, depending on traffic conditions, it could take anywhere from 10-25 minutes for help to arrive.[1] Aware that brain damage sets in after only four minutes of oxygen deprivation, Beer felt that this response time was simply unacceptable. Simply put, the ambulances always arrived too late. In one case he arrived in the ambulance too late to save a young boy who had literally choked to death on a hot dog. He quickly realized that people with training can save lives – the important factor was getting them to the scene of the emergency as quickly as possible.

Frustrated with the futility and death surrounding him, Beer decided to take matters into his own hands. He began illegally 'listening in' on the ambulance's bandwidths with police scanners, hoping to be able to respond more quickly to distress calls that were nearby. He recruited a small band of 15 EMTs to help him and each day he would go to work in his father's bookstore with the scanner on, intently listening for any nearby emergency calls. One day in 1989, the breakthrough came when the scanner showed that a 70-year-old man had been struck by a vehicle just a 25 second dash from the bookstore. Applying firm pressure to bleeding from a life-threatening neck-wound the patient, who was taking anti-coagulant therapy, was safely transferred to hospital when the ambulance eventually arrived.

After that initial watershed moment, Beer obtained more 'listening devices' and began forming volunteer EMT groups in other Jerusalem neighbourhoods. He was also aware of the work of American Hatzalah.

From these beginnings, a volunteer-based response has changed the way emergency care is both viewed and delivered. From the elation that saved the first life has developed a network with over 5,000 volunteers who answer two or three emergency calls every day of the week. There is a surprisingly low drop-out rate of volunteers as the excitement of delivering immediate life-saving care has been the impetus for volunteers to remain committed. The use of ambucycles, two-wheeled ambulance-motorcycle hybrids, which have the fastest response times, because they can weave in and out of heavy traffic has also revolutionized emergency care. Ambucycles, which now number around 850, are by far Hatzalah's greatest assets. These motorcycles are lightweight, equipped with all of the tools that a typical ambulance has, other than transport capabilities, including defibrillators, and can reach emergencies quickly even in the heaviest traffic. They cost a fraction of a typical ambulance – \$36,000 vs. \$126,000. Each ambucycle responds to an average of 720 emergencies per year. The system's annual budget is \$20 million and the organisation also has 35 standard ambulances.

Today, Hatzalah volunteers, with an average response time of fewer than 3 minutes, cover every single city in Israel. Compared to other developed countries, which average 10 minutes or more for EMTs to arrive and begin

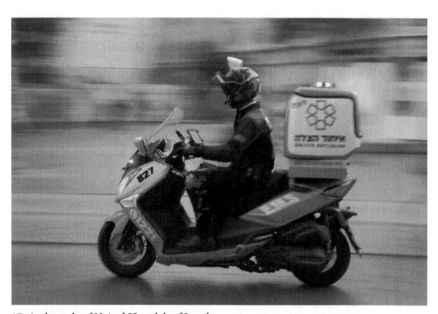

17. Ambucycle of United Hatzalah of Israel.

administering care, Hatzalah's lightning response time is remarkable. Beer has been invited to visit communities from Argentina to China, India to Brazil, and teach his lifesaving methods. Around 20 countries are working on aspects of the United Hatzalah model. Among other awards, he was recently given the prestigious Young Global Leader Award at the World Economic Forum, which pays tribute to leaders under the age of 40 who have made dramatic, global contributions to society. He also has Israel's Social Entrepreneur of the Year Award and the President's Award for Volunteerism and has even addressed the World Economic Forum at Davos.

Advances in technology have also helped. With generous funding from Irving and Cherna Moskowitz, Hatzalah was able to develop the Moskowitz Life Compass System in 2009, some time before smartphones with built-in GPS devices were available. This breakthrough technology allows the Hatzalah call-centre to monitor constantly the location of every Hatzalah volunteer in the country and to send them out based on four criteria:

1) Who is closest, geographically, to the scene?
2) Who has the highest level of training, based on the emergency at hand? (many Hatzalah volunteers are qualified doctors and specialists in addition to being trained EMTs).
3) Who has the best equipment for that particular emergency? (for example, a defibrillator for a heart attack victim or a burn kit for a burn victim).
4) How is the volunteer travelling? (by foot, by car or ambucycle,).

The spur to improving response time further was providing volunteers with GPS systems. A 10-year-old boy had died in Eilat after a heart attack in a hotel where a Hatzalah paramedic was also staying but was unaware of the emergency. The new phone system can be set to walking mode indicating the closest volunteer within walking distance. The Life Compass System also acts as a two-way GPS system, enabling dispatchers to locate victims with incredible accuracy. Even in a dark alleyway, it can pinpoint their location to within two metres.

Following the national emergency situation following the Second Lebanese War in 2006, the informal network of groups around the country agreed to come together to form United Hatzalah as a national organisation. From only having religious volunteers in its initial phase the organisation now has volunteers from all sections of Israeli society. There are now many Arab volunteers, some Druze after army service but the numbers include

Muslims also. Besides providing a rapid response in Arab communities they also deal with urgent cases on Shabbat. All new volunteers, who must be over the age of 21 years, are fully trained for 200 hours with a further 100 hours of ambulance time.

The IDF's elite search and rescue unit, known as 669, has held an active drill in cooperation with United Hatzalah EMS personnel and Israel's Search and Rescue Units with volunteers from the towns of Beit Shemesh, Rehovot, Ramle and Lod. Together with the helicopter evacuation unit of 669 they practised emergency evacuations under a variety of conditions in the field.[2] A further innovation has been the Psychotrauma Unit whose aim is to stabilize the patient at the location of the trauma, whether it be a terror attack or a cot death, to help the patient deal with the realities of their new situation and prevent or manage the onset of psychological shock.[3]

This Unit is comprised of volunteers, many of whom are psychologists and social workers. Volunteers must complete a specialized course on how to best approach and stabilize a patient in the immediate aftermath of a traumatic event. The unit is divided into a two-tiered system of care. The first tier consists of trained psychological professionals who provide a higher level of treatment, akin to a psychological version of amyotrophic lateral sclerosis (ALS). At the second tier, EMTs who have taken a basic course, treat patients at traumatic scenes, similar to BLS medical treatment. Currently, the unit has a goal of training an additional 150 volunteer responders to be able to provide coverage on a national basis. The Unit has been able to provide guidance to other services such as police, fire and rescue services, as well as the various EMS services in Israel.[4]

Innovative developments in Israel which have enhanced the scope of its emergency responses include an emergency bandage which is used to stop bleeding from hemorrhagic wounds caused by traumatic injuries and the Nowforce smartphone application, developed in 2007. The bandage was invented by an Israeli military medic, Bernard Bar-Natan, and was first used to save lives during NATO peacekeeping operations in Bosnia and Herzegovina. The Nowforce application is used by United Hatzalah to locate and dispatch the responders in closest proximity, and with the proper level of EMS training, to a medical emergency. The app has allowed United Hatzalah volunteer responders to cut their response time down from approximately to 3 minutes which represents the current national average for EMS response time. In cities where there are a large number of volunteer responders, the average response time is now 90 seconds. Other similar applications include PulsePoint, which locates the precise location of every nearby defibrillator, and Reporty, which shortens emergency response times by using the community to report emergencies, no matter their location.

United Hatzalah now answers an average of 1,000 calls per day, totaling well over 360,000 calls per year, of which about 25% are life threatening. It operates out of a single call centre near Jerusalem's bus station and has the ability to operate under conditions of direct rocket attacks from a concrete basement bunker. This means that more than 90,000 lives are saved each year in Israel due to the heroic efforts of Hatzalah volunteers.

Notes

1. Peleg, K. and Pliskin, J.S., 'A geographic information system simulation model of EMS: reducing ambulance response time', *American Journal of Emergency Medicine*, 22 (3) (2004), pp.164-170.
2. *Journal of Emergency Medical Services*, October 2017. Accessed at https://www.jems.com/articles/news/2017/10/united-hatzalah-and-idf-669-unit-hold-collaborative-training-drill-in-multiple-locations.html.
3. New 'psycho-trauma response unit' unveiled during bus bombing, EMS1com, April 2016, accessed at https://www.ems1.com/ems-education/articles/84158048-New-psycho-trauma-response-unit-unveiled-during-bus-bombing/.
4. Meisel, D., 'United Hatzalah and Israeli Innovations', *Journal of Emergency Medical Services,* January 2018. Accessed at https://www.jems.com/articles/print/volume-43/issue-1/features/israeli-ems-innovations.html; Kluger, Y., Mayo, A., Soffer, D., Aladgem, D. and Halperin, P., 'Functions and principles in the management of bombing mass casualty incidents: lessons learned at the Tel Aviv Souraski Medical Center', *European Journal of Emergency Medicine*, 11 (6) (2004), pp.329-334; Singer, A.J., Singer, A.H., Halperin, P., Kaspi, G. and Assaf, J., 'Medical lessons from terror attacks in Israel', *Journal of Emergency Medicine, 32* (1) (2007), pp.87-92.

11

Medical Ethics in Israel

Shimon Glick

Within the 'Babylon to Israel' time span of this book, the period of the modern State of Israel represents a relatively minimal fraction and one that may be viewed as an era in formation, perhaps even as a unique, as yet unfinished, experiment.

While Israel's population consists of about 25% non-Jews (Muslims, Christians, Druze and others) their impact on bioethics in Israel is relatively limited, and for the most part the present discussion will largely reflect the Jewish ethos. Although in all areas of public debate on bioethical issues an effort is made to receive and include input from the non-Jewish population, this contribution has a relatively minor influence on the practice. In addition, the Muslim position on many bioethical issues is quite close to that of the Jewish view. The major differences of opinion in many bioethical issues in Israel are rather between religious and secular viewpoints.

Medicine in Israel today essentially reflects Western medicine. It is modern, up-to-date and advanced technologically and scientifically. The leadership in the field sees itself as an integral part of Western medicine, sharing many of its values. Nevertheless, there are important unique features of Israeli bioethics, which will be the focus of the present discussion.

Jewish Medical Ethics

The term 'Jewish medical ethics' was introduced for the first time in the mid-twentieth century by the late Rabbi Lord Immanuel Jakobovits, then Chief Rabbi of Ireland, in his doctoral thesis by that name.[1] In his position in Ireland he was exposed to the detailed and well-organised views of the Roman Catholic Church, and he felt the need to summarize and present the positions of the Jewish tradition, which had not yet been formalized in a modern form. Yet bioethical issues had not been foreign to Judaism and

Jews for millennia. The late former Israeli Chief Justice and Talmudic scholar, Menachem Elon, pointed out many years ago that there are over 300,000 Jewish rabbinic legal responsa, which form the largest and most extensive continuous legal and religious case tradition in non-interrupted daily application over several millennia.[2] These cases include many that can readily be classified as falling under the heading of medical ethics. Rabbi Jakobovits screened these myriad sources for their relevance, organised the materials and created the basis for what has developed into the field of Jewish medical ethics. The field has flourished since, stimulated both by the emergence of the academic and practical field of bioethics in the West during the second half of the twentieth century and by the explosion of scientific advances posing many new ethical dilemmas. The notorious Nazi medical experiments have also stimulated and influenced the field, particularly in Israel but elsewhere in the world as well.[3] Israeli society, while far from a theocracy, nevertheless draws extensively from its cultural roots which, for most of the millennia since Babylon, are religious in origin. Israel is very much a pluralistic society; one example of this is the number of political parties in the Knesset, the Israeli legislature, thirteen in the last election held in 2020.

In order to understand the Israeli situation better it is important to be aware of some of the unique cultural emphases impacting on the local practices. Western bioethics, since its flowering over the past half century, has been, with a few recent exceptions, based on four principles: autonomy, beneficence, non-maleficence and justice. This quartet, as proposed and elaborated by Beauchamp and Childress, still remains the bedrock of Western bioethics.[4] The latter three principles can be said to be fully compatible with the traditional values of medicine, as well with the Jewish culture, but the major innovation and the dominant, almost revolutionary, feature among these principles has been the emphasis on autonomy. This prioritization of autonomy is part of the growth of the civil rights movements in the West, and it represents a clear break with the dominant spirit of paternalism on the part of the physician harking back to the days of Hippocrates. The concept of 'sanctity of human life' as a specific ethical principle is not included in the current secular Western list of values but is indeed a central value in the Jewish tradition. This value, although clearly religious in origin (man being created in 'the image of God'), has its strong impact on Israeli society and culture, influencing as well even those segments of society that are totally secular.[5] The strong emphasis on the unique value of human life has important impact on Israeli legal and ethical decisions, as will be discussed further on in this chapter.

Interestingly enough, as pointed out by the late Israeli Chief Justice Haim Cohen, while much of the origin of the human rights concepts is based on the Jewish Bible and Talmud, the Jewish tradition does not express these rights in the modern terms of 'entitlement'.[6] Instead these values are expressed in a mirror image form, one of duties. For example, in the Jewish sources a child is not said to have a right to an education, but the parents and the community have a duty to provide an education.

This difference, pointed out in Rabbi Jakobovits' classic text and in his other writings, was elaborated by the Jewish legal theoretician Robert Cover.[7]

> Every legal culture has its fundamental words...The word 'rights' is a highly evocative one for those of us who have grown up in the post-enlightenment secular society of the West; Judaism is, itself, a legal culture of great antiquity. When I am asked to reflect upon Judaism and human rights, therefore, the first thought that comes to mind is that the categories are wrong. I do not mean, of course, that basic ideas of human dignity and worth are not powerfully expressed in the Jewish legal and literary traditions. Rather, I mean that because it is a legal tradition, Judaism has its own categories for expressing through law the worth and dignity of each human being. The principal word in Jewish law, which occupies a place equivalent in evocative force to the American legal system's 'rights', is the word 'mitzvah', which literally means commandment but has a general meaning closer to 'incumbent obligation'. All law was given at Sinai, and therefore all law is related back to the ultimate.

This seemingly minor difference in the presentation of the issues has significant implications in the field of medical ethics. For example, in keeping with one of the tenets of Judaism, the Knesset passed a law in 1996 whose title is the biblical sentence 'Do not stand idly by the blood of your fellow man.'[8] The law requires any individual (not just physicians) to come to the aid of any other person in serious acute danger. This requirement contrasts with Anglo-Saxon law, which has no such obligation. In the United States of America there are many 'Good Samaritan' laws protecting from liability those who do come to another's assistance, but almost no laws requiring such assistance. More interesting and unique than the law mandating assistance, however, is the converse; the obligation of a patient to seek medical help. In the Jewish tradition an individual is not the full possessor of their body but is merely a caretaker of the body for the

Almighty and has the responsibility to ensure its integrity and good condition. Therefore, there exists a <u>duty</u> to seek health care and to act in a way to preserve one's health and to prevent harm. In the era of the Sanhedrin, the Jewish court system, people could be punished for neglecting to pursue medical treatment for their illnesses or for acting in a manner endangering their health!

The relationship of Jews and medicine is a long and positive one in every generation and in every culture in which the Jews found themselves. Jews have always been, and still are, relatively over-represented in the medical profession. A dramatic modern example is the events of the day of the infamous *Anschluss* in Austria in 1938, in which all Jewish members of the medical faculty at the University of Vienna were fired overnight, resulting in dismissal of 70% of the staff.[9] The attraction of Jews to medicine has many reasons, but to a major extent may be related to the value placed by the tradition on human life. Because of the high representation of Jews in the medical profession, Israel has for most of its existence had an abundance of physicians, benefitting to a large extent from repeated and continuous waves of immigrant physicians. Recently, however, experts predict an impending shortage of physicians in Israel, largely because of the aging of many immigrant physicians and the limited number of students in Israel's medical schools.

Let us now examine some aspects of Israeli medicine as affected by some of the above principles.

Ethical Principles in Israeli Medicine

National Health Insurance: The foundations of health care in modern Israel were laid by Zionist pioneers, decades prior to the creation of the State of Israel. Beginning in 1912 workers joined together to form a 'sick fund' for mutual assistance and health care insurance. This modest beginning developed into the nongovernmental Histadrut Labour Union sick fund that covered most, but not all, of Israel's citizens. In 1994 the government enacted a national health insurance law covering all of Israel's citizens based on the expressed principles of justice, equality, and mutual assistance.[10] As a result there are virtually no out-of-pocket expenses for patients in hospitals, and many components of preventive medicine too are provided universally free of charge to the patients.

Unfortunately, over the years this excellent service has suffered from continuing under-funding. Israel's current government expenditure on health is only about 7.5% of its gross national product, significantly below the average in the OECD countries.[11] This under-funding has led to long waiting lists for surgical procedures and to the proliferation of private practice, undermining the principle of universal provision of excellent services to all irrespective of income. The government is currently considering several proposals to reverse the trend towards the proliferation of private medicine.

Patients' Rights Legislation: After an incubation period of several decades, the Knesset in 1996 passed a bill mandating a series of patients' rights.[12] The law goes into great detail about the rights of patients to empathic and competent medical care, fully in consonance with the almost axiomatic expectations from a democratic humanistic society. The right to a second opinion and the right to information about the identity of their physicians are included in the legislation. In keeping with the current Western norms of patient autonomy there is insistence on obtaining detailed informed consent before any treatment. So too is there a clear insistence on provision of full and detailed information to patients about their condition in order to allow patient decision making, but several features of the law deviate from the strict Western norms that give full reign to autonomy over all other possibly conflicting values.

One clause in the original proposal created considerable debate. What was a physician to do when a competent patient refuses a treatment that is clearly lifesaving? In the commonly accepted practice in Western bioethics no coercion is ever permitted even at the cost of the patient's life. The government's then chief legal advisor convened a meeting of about 30 physicians, ethicists, philosophers, lawyers and clergy to discuss the issue. The civil libertarians in the group, of course, took the standard Western position: namely that under no circumstances could therapy be rendered against the will of a competent patient, unless the patient's illness threatened the welfare of others, as in the case of certain communicable diseases.

There were others, particularly the rabbis, who invoked the sanctity of human life in the Jewish tradition to support the possibility under certain circumstances of coercion of competent refusing patients. A vigorous debate ensued, resulting in a compromise, which I believe is unique to Israel. Treatment may be imposed on a non-consenting competent patient if an institutional ethics committee, after discussion with the patient, concludes that, if coerced, the patient will give retroactive consent after imposition of treatment. While this clause would seem to be in clear violation of patient autonomy, it is not intended to do so. Rather the clause wishes to take into account the emotional component of the patient's decision, which may limit their ability to reach a fully autonomous rational decision and may harm the patient. This position confirmed a previous Israeli Supreme Court decision permitting abdominal surgery on a prisoner who had swallowed bags of heroin in order to destroy evidence incriminating him.[13] The prisoner's physicians felt that unless the bags were removed surgically they were likely to burst and cause the prisoner's death. The court supported the physicians' actions in performing surgery, overruling the prisoner's objections. Judge M. Beiski stated in his decision:

> I believe that the principle of sanctity of life and its rescue as a lofty value justifies not to follow those rules that support almost rigidly the admonition against interference in a person's body without his consent, without considering the consequences of that policy...when an individual is in immediate and certain danger of death or there is the likelihood of severe and certain danger to his health, one is definitely permitted to do surgery or other invasive procedures even without his consent.[14]

In a related area, that of feeding fasting hunger-striking prisoners, the subject has provoked vigorous discussion and debate. An Israeli district court in Beer-Sheva ordered the forced feeding of a hunger-striking prisoner, basing its decision in part on the Beiski Supreme Court ruling and stating:

> Both legislators and the Supreme Court have decided that in the competition between two rights, the right to life on the one hand and to dignity on the other, the right to life and health takes precedence.[15]

In contrast to above rulings, the Israel Medical Association and its ethics council have unequivocally and repeatedly endorsed the position of the World Medical Association forbidding force-feeding of prisoners. The Association has even threatened with disciplinary actions any physician who engaged in such forced feeding. The Association's position has been opposed by a large number of Israeli ethicists and physicians who argued that when the prolonged fast presents an immediate danger to the hunger-striker's life coercion is legitimate. In spite of the position of the Israel Medical Association the Knesset passed a bill in 2016 permitting such feeding at a stage of a hunger strike that reaches the point of clear and present danger to the prisoner's life.[16] The Israel Medical Association's appeal against the law was turned down unanimously by the Israeli

Supreme Court.[17] In practice, although there have been many cases of Palestinian hunger-striking prisoners, none have died and the strikes have been settled by lengthy and sensitive negotiations between physicians and prisoners rather than by force feeding.

Another clause in Israel's patients' rights law that requires provision of full detailed information to the patient prior to treatment again provides for a loophole. If an institutional ethics committee feels that such information may endanger the patient's life or health, the information may be withheld. Both of these loopholes indicate that in cases in which a conflict exists between autonomy and beneficence the priority is not always given unequivocally to autonomy, as in the West.

Historic Controversies

In the relatively short time of Israel's existence several bioethical issues have caused significant societal conflict. The first issue was that of postmortem examinations. The Jewish ethos historically has been deeply concerned with respect for the human body, not just during lifetime, but requiring early burial and intactness of the corpse after death. This attitude is based on the Biblical admonition of respect for the body of even a convicted criminal.

With the planning of Israel's first medical school in 1948 discussions took place between the physicians and the rabbinic authorities in order to reach a *modus vivendi* with regard to the use of human bodies in the teaching of anatomy and pathology. An agreement was reached in which the rabbis consented to allow postmortem examinations under several conditions: in forensic cases, in cases of infectious diseases, in cases of genetic diseases and, most controversially, if three physicians attested to the fact that the cause of death was not known. This agreement, which gave no standing to the desires of the family or to those of the deceased prior to death, needs to be understood in the context of the reigning culture in Israel at the time. Most of the leading physicians in Israel had been trained in Central or Eastern Europe in which the paternalistic medical culture dating back to Hippocrates predominated. Israel was also governed at the time by a socialist government in which centralized decision-making in many areas of life predominated.

As a result of this agreement, which became part of Israeli law, autopsies were performed in a large percentage of deaths even over the express objections of the families and often in clear violation of the agreement.[18] The issue of autopsies became a *cause celebre* over the next several decades with protest demonstrations in Israel and elsewhere, and even numerous episodes of violence against physicians and hospitals. In spite of recommendations by a Knesset committee for some reasonable compromise, none was reached, and the conflict continued unabated. In the heat of the controversy extreme views on both sides were exacerbated and exaggerated. The disagreements between the medical and the religious establishments over this subject created much mutual distrust, with unfortunate consequences well beyond the particular issue of autopsies. With a change in government in 1977 and the need for the religious parties to form a workable coalition, the law was changed, and no autopsies could now be performed without family consent. Even more restrictions were placed into the law. The issue has subsided, in part because of the law change but also because autopsy rates have plummeted all over the West for a variety of reasons. The changes in Israeli law also reflected a decline in medical paternalism and recognition of the rights of the families of the deceased to have a voice in the disposal of the bodies of their relatives.

A second area of controversy has been the issue of abortions. Under the British Mandate abortions were forbidden, as they were in many Western countries during the mid-twentieth century. With the creation of the State of Israel the laws existing under the mandate were continued, but for many years by unwritten policy the government did not prosecute the many illegal abortions that took place. The attempted revision of the laws about abortion created the expected controversy between the liberal women's rights views and that of the religious establishment.

The first version of the Abortion Law permitted abortions under five different situations, if prior approval was obtained from a hospital committee composed of two physicians and a social worker.[19] The five conditions included foetal birth defects, pregnancies in women older than forty or younger than eighteen, pregnancies that endanger the mother's physical or mental health, out of wedlock pregnancies (including rape and incest), and serious social and economic problems of the mother. The clause most objected to by the religious parties was the one that permitted abortion for social and economic situations. After a heated public battle this clause was removed, but surprisingly there was no fall in the number of abortions; those abortions previously categorized under the social clause were simply re-classified under one of the four other clauses.

The situation has now stabilized with minimal public controversy. About 19,000 legal abortions are performed annually compared to about 160,000 live births. The hospital abortion committees approve about 98% of all requests, making the appearance before them almost a formality. Nevertheless, a significant number of illegal abortions are still performed, with estimates varying from 10,000 to 40,000 annually. Many women do not want to undergo the necessity of appearing before a committee to obtain approval for abortion. The government, in principle, makes no effort to prosecute illegal abortions unless there is malpractice or a serious complication. There is constant pressure by women's groups to eliminate the need for approval by hospital committees, but in general the *status quo* seems to be preferred by the legislature. Unlike the situation in the United States of America, where the abortion controversy is very active and occasionally violent, all sides in Israel seem to have learned to live with the current situation and a change in any direction does not seem to be a high priority for any group.

In comparison to the situation in other Western countries, Israel has a high number of abortions performed for relatively minor foetal defects, because of a widespread desire for a 'perfect baby'.[20] There is also a relatively high incidence of testing of the foetus for various diseases or deformities. Israel also permits late abortions in rare cases if approved by a special national committee.

There has been a fascinating and effective effort to eliminate Tay Sachs disease, and some other genetic diseases, among ultra orthodox Jews who are unwilling to perform amniocentesis and abortion of affected foetuses. In their culture marriages are arranged. There is an organisation, *Dor Yeshorim*, operating in both Israel and the United States that promotes confidential screening of young men and women before they become potential husband and wife to prevent carriers from marrying each other.[21] This organisation's effort has virtually eliminated cases of Tay Sachs disease in this population without violating their religious ethical principles.

Organ Transplantation

The rancour and often vituperative nature of the disputes between the medical and rabbinic establishments, largely over the autopsy issue, created an atmosphere of distrust that had repercussions in other areas as well. For instance, a small but significant number of ultra orthodox Israelis occasionally went abroad for treatment in spite of its ready availability in Israel because of a mistrust of the Israeli health system; more serious was the impact of the distrust on the performance of organ transplants, specifically those requiring the death of the donor prior to organ retrieval. The religio-ethical issue was the use of brain death as an acceptable definition of death. After years of deliberation and detailed investigation, the Israeli Chief Rabbinate accepted brain death, thereby permitting removal of organs from brain dead individuals for transplantation, but they conditioned this approval on the participation of individuals certified by them as members on the committees that determined that such death had indeed occurred, because they were concerned that some of the determinations might not have fully met the necessary criteria. They also insisted on some objective confirmatory test of brain death before granting approval. Now, even after years of further negotiations and full agreement between medical and rabbinic authorities, Israel still has one of the lowest rates of consent on the part of families to remove organs from brain dead individuals for transplantation. Among the reasons for this low rate may indeed be the residual mutual mistrust between physicians and rabbis.

It is important to point out that a significant percentage of the Orthodox rabbinate, the so called ultra orthodox, do not recognize brain death as death and insist on cardio-respiratory death as a criterion for death, thereby rendering almost impossible the use of most organs for transplants. Israeli law, while recognizing brain death, nevertheless respects the position of those families who do not accept brain death, and mandates continuing supportive therapy of a patient who has been determined to have undergone brain death until cardio-respiratory death ensues. This 'pluralistic' law is similar to those in New York and New Jersey, both states with large ultra orthodox populations. In the present socio-cultural climate in Israel it is most unlikely that a law for 'opting out', rather than 'opting in' could pass. Indeed, there is almost no discussion in that direction.

Unlike most other bodily organs, kidney transplantation does not necessitate removal from a dead individual, but indeed it is preferentially desired from a live donor. Kidney donation from live donors is encouraged by all religious authorities as a magnanimous and highly meritorious, but not obligatory, act. Nevertheless, as in most Western countries the demand far exceeds the supply, and with the aging of the population the demand will certainly grow further. Priority for receipt of a kidney is centrally controlled, with detailed criteria worked out by the medical establishment. Commercialization of the kidney transplantation enterprise is strictly illegal in Israel, and many Israelis travel overseas to purchase kidneys in spite of the illegalities involved. The Israeli government has taken some controversial steps to encourage kidney donors. Donors are given some compensation for their loss of income as a result of surgery, and a few other minor benefits. In addition, families of donors are given some preference for them and for their families in receiving organ donations in the future. Even both of these relatively minor inducements have been controversial. In the last few years there has arisen in Israel a movement led by a recipient of a kidney transplant to encourage truly altruistic kidney donations, and several hundred such donations have taken place.

Euthanasia and End of Life

The issue of euthanasia is one of the most contentious ones in medical ethics and is the subject of constant controversy in almost every Western country. Although the issue has been active for millennia it has been exacerbated greatly in the twentieth century by medical and technological advances, which have dramatically increased the survival of individuals at both ends of life expectancy. A clear conflict often arises between the value of human life and that of the quality of that life. Simultaneously, conflicts arise between the value of autonomy and that of beneficence.

In the Israeli culture the value of sanctity of human life is especially high. This evaluation is expressed most eloquently in the Talmudic statement:

> Therefore was man created as a single individual to teach us that he who saves a single life is as if he saved an entire universe, and he who causes the death of a single individual is as if he destroyed an entire universe.[22]

An almost identical statement is expressed by Islamist ethicists. Yet the prolonged and intense human suffering engendered by keeping seriously disabled individuals alive sorely tests the insistence of preserving life at all costs. Israeli courts have on occasion permitted the withdrawal of life-preserving treatment in the face of intense suffering, even in a non-terminal state, as in amyotrophic lateral sclerosis in its late stages.

In 2000 the Israeli government appointed a 59-member commission to recommend policy of treatment at the end of life. This committee had broad representation from all parts of Israeli society. There were four sub-committees: medical, legal, ethical and religious. The committees met over several years, and their proposed legislation was debated over several more years in the Knesset before ultimate passage in 2005.[23] In spite of the broad spectrum of opinions on the committee, it succeeded in obtaining virtually unanimous agreement on all but one issue.

The law expressly prohibits active euthanasia as well as physician assisted suicide in all situations, but in the case of suffering patients with an incurable disease and a life expectancy of less than six months it permits withholding of therapy if the patient requests this. In patients who seem to be in the last two weeks of life it is even more permissive in permitting abandonment of all diagnostic and therapeutic procedures. For the first time, Israeli law grants recognition to the validity of advance directives for some forms of non-treatment, but it does not permit the omission of food and fluids. Palliative medicine is strongly endorsed as is relief of pain by medications, even at the risk of life-shortening. At present the number of patients with advance directives is still quite small.

The one major area of disagreement on the committee relates to the issue of differentiation between withholding therapy and withdrawing it. Most Western countries have come to equate withdrawal of therapy with withholding it.[24] Israeli law, while permitting withholding therapy under specific conditions, does not readily accept withdrawal of therapy. Israeli law uniquely differentiates between two kinds of withdrawal. Withdrawal of 'periodic' treatment such as dialysis may be permitted under certain circumstances, but withdrawal of 'continuous' treatment, such as artificial ventilation, is regarded as similar to active euthanasia and is forbidden.[25] Because of this differentiation the termination of artificial ventilation is not permitted. There is an ongoing attempt to introduce an apparatus whereby artificial ventilation may be 'converted' to a discontinuous form of therapy, thereby making possible cessation of artificial ventilation in certain cases.

The current law, while representing an important advance, is limited to patients with an incurable illness with a prognosis of only six months of life. Other ill and suffering patients, like those with progressive and incurable disease who have a longer life expectancy, are not covered. There is considerable public pressure to extend the coverage. As in most Western countries there is also pressure to permit physician assisted suicide and/or active euthanasia. Aside from the usual arguments against euthanasia, the history of involuntary euthanasia in Nazi Germany makes the subject particularly sensitive in Israel, arousing much emotional reaction.

Reproductive Medicine

In contrast to some of the previous areas discussed, in which the medical establishment and the rabbinic establishment have often had serious differences of position that led to public clashes, the area of reproduction has witnessed close cooperation between the two groups. This cooperation and ongoing dialogue have improved the overall relationship in other areas as well. There are several reasons for this relative harmony. Firstly, the Jewish culture has a traditionally strong pro-natal position dating back throughout its history. The first commandment in the Bible is 'Be fruitful and multiply'.[26] In addition, the creation of the State of Israel closely followed the Holocaust, with the eradication of a third of world Jewry. This tragedy stimulated the almost inevitable reaction of the public to make up for these losses. Israel has the highest birth rate of any of the members of the OECD, and this is due not only to the high birth rate of the orthodox Jewish population. Often heard in conversation is an underlying fear of losing a son in one of the repeated armed conflicts in the area, expressed as 'We cannot afford to have just one child'.

The area of assisted reproduction is highly developed in the country, with more centres per unit population than any country in the Western world. In addition, the Israeli National Health Service covers the full cost for all women citizens (regardless of religion and marital status) of multiple attempts to produce at least two live babies for each woman, again unique in the Western world. In 2016 the number of treatment cycles was over 37,000 leading to about 7,000 live births. The increase in the number of treatment cycles seems to have levelled off now after many years of annual increase.

Among the other evidences for an unusually positive approach to innovations in the area of reproduction are the laws permitting surrogate motherhood. In 1996 the Israeli Knesset became the first country in the world to legalize surrogate mother agreements.[27] There are also the liberal attitude towards the possibilities of research on cloning and on stem cells, the positive attitude towards self-donation of ova by a woman for possible use later in life, consideration of use of sperm from a deceased individual, and the relatively liberal attitude towards pre-implantation genetic diagnosis (PGD).

Legislation introduced in 2010 for the first time permitted ovum donation for *in vitro* fertilization (IVF) from women who were not themselves undergoing IVF.[28] Previous to that time ova could only be obtained as surplus from women undergoing IVF, thereby considerably limiting the number of ova available for IVF. Because of the shortage of ova many Israeli women travelled abroad in order to obtain ova. The law was passed after extensive debate because of the small, but significant, risk to the donor in obtaining ova, and because of the reluctance to contribute to 'commodification' of the woman. The law did include a few restrictions, to accommodate some concerns by the religious establishment, forbidding using ova from married women and ova from a woman from a different religion from the recipient.

PGD has been widely accepted in Israel, almost exclusively for elimination of embryos affected by a variety of genetic diseases. Such activity has met with virtually full approval by rabbinic authorities, but its use for sex selection is forbidden except in unusual circumstances, requiring approval by a special committee. For example, if a couple has had several consecutive births of the same sex and desires one of the opposite sex approval has occasionally been granted.

The issue of the use of sperm from a deceased individual for fertilization of an ovum from his widow, his girlfriend or even a surrogate, continues to be an issue of controversy. If the deceased had left instructions to do so the courts have been liberal in permitting such an act, but the issue is much less clear if the wife or the parents of the deceased desire to ensure an offspring who bears the genetics of the deceased. The subject is one with very high emotional manifestations, especially in cases of young men killed in military combat.

The subject of stem cell research, cloning, and the implications thereof, provide a dramatic example of the uniqueness of the Israeli approach to the issue. The Israeli attitude is the result of a combination of several religious and cultural factors. Perhaps the major difference in Israel's approach to the subject results from the Jewish approach to the fertilized ovum *in vitro* in striking contrast to the attitude of much of Christianity to the fertilized ovum. The status of the fertilized ovum *in vitro* in Judaism is not the same as its status once it has been implanted into a woman's uterus. The fertilized ovum *in vitro* is treated with some respect as living tissue but not as a living embryo deserving total protection against destruction even for positive and useful reasons. The Islamic view is quite similar to that of Judaism.

In 1999, following the creation of Dolly the sheep, Israel became one of the first countries to forbid cloning for the purpose of human reproduction, but it permitted research using human stem cells.[29] The permissiveness of the Jewish faith in this area, in contrast to some Christian groups, is the result of several factors. As mentioned, Judaism has a clearly different attitude towards the pre-embryo *in vitro* compared to that once implanted into the uterus. In addition, the Jewish culture is strongly in favour of the advances of science and technology. Israel's status as a 'start-up nation' is an example of this. The frequently expressed fear in some religious cultures of 'playing God', as a hesitation to move forward, is not part of the mainstream of the Jewish tradition. Rather the opposite view prevails: Man is commanded to be a partner of God in creativity. In addition, as mentioned earlier, the strongly pro-natal attitude provides an impetus for experimentation and progress in the area of reproduction.

The moratorium on cloning was limited to a five-year period because of the feeling that the developments in the field were so rapid that it was advisable to reexamine the situation periodically. The moratorium was renewed in 2004 for another five years, and again in 2009 for a seven-year period. The permission to continue research on stem cells for medical purposes has resulted in a great expansion of research in this area in Israel and has placed Israel as a world leader and innovator in this field.

Major Court Decisions

There have been a number of court decisions in areas of difficult dilemmas that cast some light on the reigning mode of thinking in Israeli society, at least in the courts. A particularly tragic case was that of an elderly man on chronic dialysis who required a kidney transplant.[30] His 39-year-old son, who had a learning disability, was an appropriate match, but was considered not competent to give informed consent. The father had been extraordinarily devoted to the care of his son for many years, and in all likelihood were he to die, the care of the son would suffer seriously. In spite of the fairly certain probability that with improvement in the health of the father the son's welfare too would be benefitted, the Israeli Supreme Court nevertheless refused to allow the donation from an individual who was not competent to give consent. Clearly in this heart-breaking dilemma between autonomy and beneficence the court favoured autonomy.

Another difficult case, and one which attracted much public attention and debate, was the Nachmani case. The couple, who had difficulty in conceiving naturally because of the woman's permanent sterility, had decided on *in vitro* fertilization using the husband's sperm and the wife's ova with the fertilized ovum to be implanted into a surrogate woman, as permitted by Israeli law. The ova were fertilized and were kept in storage for future use until a suitable surrogate could be located, but before some of the fertilized ova could be implanted into the woman the couple separated, the husband took on another partner and had a child with her. The fate of the fertilized ova became a source of intense dispute between the couple; the man refused to allow the ova fertilized with his sperm to be implanted into a surrogate to enable his former wife to be a mother. The woman insisted on having the ovum previously fertilized with her former partner's consent implanted. The case went before a District Court which ruled in favour of the woman, permitting implantation, but the decision was reversed on appeal by the Supreme Court by a four to one margin. Because of the importance of the issue the Supreme Court took the unusual step to have the case reviewed again by an eleven-member court. This time the Court by a seven to four margin reversed the earlier decision by the smaller number of justices and decided that the strong desire of the woman to have a child took precedence over the unwillingness of the man to have the child born with his sperm.[31] The final decision by several of the judges emphasized the strong pro-natal culture of Israeli society.

Bioethical Decision-Making

There are numerous committees and councils of all types in Israel dealing with bioethical issues, some on a national level and others at individual institutions focused on activities at the local level. All institutions have local institutional review boards (called Helsinki Committees) to oversee research ethics involving humans; these meet regularly, and their approval is required before any research project involving human subjects is initiated. There is also a national review board to rule in unusual and precedent-making issues. Animal welfare committees function both locally and nationally. In addition, there are clinical ethics committees at each institution, but they seem to be remarkably underused.[32] There are also institutional committees that deal specifically with end of life issues under the end of life law. There are governmental *ad hoc* committees appointed to recommend policies on specific issues that arise. There are permanent committees dealing with specific issues, such as genetics. There is also a Council of Bioethics jointly representing the ministries of health and justice that meets periodically to recommend on major public issues that arise. The profusion of committees often results in overlap and lack of clarity about jurisdiction in specific issues. The media in Israel are free and active and take an interest in bioethical issues, particularly if they are controversial.

The bioethics scene in Israel is a fascinating and unique one. There is a blend of three vectors, with the influence of each one varying with passage of time. The country is in many ways a continuum of a Jewish culture, largely religious, several millennia in extent. This provides a religious vector. The large influx of Jews and Jewish physicians, largely from middle Europe and beginning in the nineteenth century, was accompanied by a paternalistic view of the physician's role. The socialist culture of centralized authority also influenced medicine. These provided a second vector. Finally, the twentieth century brought with it the powerful and impressive influence of Western, and particularly American, medicine and its values. The dynamic interaction between these three vectors provides a unique mixture of values and practices that characterizes Israeli society in the field of bioethics.

Notes

1. Jakobovits, I., *Jewish Medical Ethics: A Comparative and Historical Study of the Jewish Religious Attitude to Medicine and its Practice* (New York: Bloch, 1959).
2. Elon, M., *Jewish Law: History, Sources, Principles* [Hebrew] trans. Auerbach, B. and Sykes, M.J. (Philadelphia: Jewish Publication Society, 1994).
3. Alexander, L., 'Medical science under dictatorship', *New England Journal of Medicine* (1949), 241, (2), pp.239-247.
4. Beauchamp, T.L. and Childress, J.F., *Principles of Biomedical Ethics*, seventh edn (Oxford University Press, 2013).
5. *Genesis*, Chapter 1, verse 27.
6. Cohen, H.H., *Human Rights in the Bible and Talmud* [Hebrew]. trans. Himelstein, S. (Tel Aviv: MOD Books, 1989).
7. Cover, R., 'Obligation: A Jewish jurisprudence of the social order', *Journal of Law and Religion*, 1998, 5, pp.65-74.
8. Do not stand idly by your neighbor's blood. *Laws of the State of Israel*. (Jerusalem: Government Printing Office, 1998); *Leviticus*, Chapter 19, verse 16.
9. Ernst, E., 'A leading medical school seriously damaged: Vienna 1938', *Annals of Internal Medicine*, 1995, 128 (10), pp.789-792.
10. *National Health Insurance Law*, Laws of the State of Israel (Jerusalem: Government Printing Office, 1994).
11. Weiss, A. and Chernichovsky, D., *A Picture of the Nation* Jerusalem: Taub Centre, 2017).
12. *Patient's Rights Law*, Laws of the State of Israel Jerusalem: Government Printing Office, 1996), p.327.
13. Kurtam v State of Israel, Appeal 527/85 Israel Supreme Court, 19/8/1986.
14. State of Israel v Rahamim Gibli et al., Originating motion, 829/96A, 1996.
15. State of Israel v Rahamim Gibli et al., Originating motion, 829/96A, 1996.
16. A bill to the Prison Ordinance (No. 48), (Prevention of Hunger Strike), 2014, Bill 870.
17. HCJ 5304/15; Israel Medical Association -v- Knesset Israel (Nevo, 11.09. 2016).
18. Law of Anatomy and Pathology. Laws of the State of Israel. (Jerusalem: Israel: Government Printing Office, 1953).
19. Penal Law, 5737-1977, ss 212-321, Chapter 10, article 2.
20. Jotkowitz, A., Raz, A., Glick, S. and Zivotofsky, A.Z., 'Abortions for fetuses with mild abnormalities', *Israel Medical Association Journal*, 2010, 12, pp.5-9.
21. The Dor Yeshorim story: community-based screening for Tay-Sachs Disease, *Advances in Genetics*, 2001, 44, pp.297-310.
22. Babylonian Talmud, *Sanhedrin* 37a.
23. *End of Life Law*, Laws of the State of Israel (Jerusalem: Government Printing Office, 2005).
24. Meisel, A., Snyder, L., Quill, T. et al., 'Seven legal barriers to end of life care: myths, realities and grains of truth', *JAMA*, 2000, 284, pp.2451-2459.
25. Ravitsky, V., 'Timers on ventilators', *BMJ*, 2005, 330 (488), pp.415-417.
26. *Genesis*, Chapter 1, verse 28.
27. *Embryo Carrying Agreements Law*, Laws of the State of Israel (Jerusalem: Government Printing Office, 1996).
28. *Ova Donation Law*, Laws of the State of Israel (Jerusalem: Government Printing Office, 2010), SH#2242, p520.

29. *The Prohibition of Genetic Intervention (Human Cloning and Genetic Manipulation of Reproductive Cells) Law*, Laws of the State of Israel (Jerusalem: Government Printing Office, 1999).

30. Legal Advisor to the Government v Anonymous, Supreme Court Judgements, 1988, 42 (2), p.661.

31. CFH 2401/95, Daniel Nachmani v Ruth Nachmani, *Israel Supreme Court*, 50 (4) 66.

32. Wenger, N.S., Golan, O., Shalev, C. and Glick, S., 'Hospital Ethics Committees in Israel: Structure, Function and Heterogeneity in the Settings of Statutory Ethics Committees', *Journal of Medical Ethics*, 2002, 28, (3), pp.177-180.

12

Complementary and Alternative Medicine in Israel

Menachem Oberbaum

'The opposite of a correct statement is a false statement.
But the opposite of a profound truth may well be another profound truth.'

Niels Bohr

Introduction

Complementary and alternative medicine (CAM) is an elusive term. It includes several hundred therapeutic modalities that have nothing in common other than the fact that they are rejected by biomedicine. Even here, there are no sharp dividing lines. In India, for example, ayurveda, yoga and naturopathy, unani, siddha and homeopathy are part of mainstream medicine, and are directed by a special ministry, whereas in most European countries they are either rejected or unknown.[1]

CAM modalities are both ancient (for example, acupuncture) and modern (biofeedback). Some provide more fundamental curative treatment (naturopathy), while others can, at times, be highly symptomatic (chiropractic). Some shun any artificial aid (nature cure), while others use extensive medicinal intervention (herbalism).[2] The decision as to what is or is not a CAM modality is not based solely on science. Social, political and national factors also play a role. Methods which are part of standard medicine among, say, the Chinese or Japanese will be regarded by Europeans as CAM modalities. Chiropractic, acupuncture and massage therapy are licenced in most North American states, naturopathy and homeopathy are licenced in fewer states. Nor is there any consensus regarding the formal definition of CAM, with more than a half dozen classifications found in the literature.[3]

Complementary and alternative medicine is a fairly new name for the discipline, arrived at after many changes. Until the 1980s, it was known in the literature as 'alternative medicine', signifying therapies alternative to the mainstream. The name then changed to 'complementary medicine', reflecting a more modest position, treatment that was additional or supplementary to conventional medicine. It was only some 20 years ago that the name 'complementary and alternative medicine (CAM)', entered the literature. In recent years, the term 'integrative medicine' is being used with increasing frequency, denoting the integration of two equal paradigms for the benefit of the patient. In this chapter the term CAM is used for all modalities which are not a part of the biomedical paradigm in Israel and are not taught in any Israeli medical school.

Three broad periods can be distinguished in the history of CAM in Palestine/Israel. The first ended with the establishment of mainstream, biomedical medicine in Palestine in the mid-twentieth century. The second, which lasted for about a generation, was practised by a group of 'celebrity' CAM therapists and their followers. The third period, which began in the 1980s and continues into the present, is one in which CAM is struggling for recognition, legalization and integration into the mainstream of conventional medicine.

The First Period: Until the Mid-Twentieth Century

Until the 1840s Palestine had no academically educated physicians, no hospitals and no pharmacies. The local population, mostly Muslim, was treated by folk-healers or so-called 'pharmacists', most of them uneducated, or by barbers, sorcerers and amulet-makers. These traditional healers continued to treat the rural poor through the nineteenth and early twentieth centuries. Medical therapy usually included blood-letting from different parts of the body and in varying amounts, a treatment considered effective for a wide variety of diseases. Medications were based mainly on herbs, adapted to the type of disease. The Ottoman administration (1516 to 1917) provided no medical care, its public health services limited to land and sea closures during time of epidemic.[4] Geopolitical change increased the efforts of contemporary European powers to establish and extend their influence in the lands of the dying Ottoman Empire. Over time, the creation of hospitals in Palestine diminished both the value and social position of natural healers, nudging them to become practitioners of alternative medicine.

The institutionalization of conventional medicine and the increasing exclusion of CAM occurred in parallel and continued into the twentieth century. The Israel Medical Association (IMA) was created in 1912, and quickly developed a compass of what was part of medicine and what was not. A year earlier, the Clalit Health Services had been established as a mutual health-care association: today, it is the largest of the four influential State-mandated, non-profit Health Funds which are responsible for insuring all Israeli citizens. Some of the Funds also own hospitals affiliated with medical schools and are thus deeply involved in medical education. Together with the IMA, they define what qualifies as medicine in Israel, and what does not. CAM was not among the medical disciplines which they accepted and was seen as a competing medical paradigm.

Five 'Celebrity' Healers

It was at this point that CAM emerged from the shadows. It did so in a way that can only happen in a small country with a small population: namely, the appearance of five personalities, who developed unique therapeutic methods, some of which spilled beyond the boundaries of Israel and are used in Western countries to this day.

The first was Moshe Feldenkrais (1904-1984), a physicist, whose conventional background was as an engineer working on the development of rockets. He created a therapeutic method based on an awareness of movement, soft touch and imagination. Over the years, he claimed, people become accustomed to bad and harmful movement habits. This can be rectified by developing a practice which corrects these movements, using minimal effort while maintaining proper breathing. When an individual consciously controls his movements, he improves his health and reaches a balance between mind and body.

The second was Paula Garbourg (1907-2004), a ballet dancer and opera singer, who developed the so-called 'ring muscle method', based on contracting and relaxing the body's ring muscles: eyelids, lips, anus, urethra, vagina, etc. Her system, she asserted, was applicable to everyone, according to their needs. Exercise stimulates self-awareness and the self-healing inherent in each individual, leading to a thorough and comprehensive improvement in the health of the patient.

Mordechai Netzach (1902-1971), an accountant, developed a unique method based on fasts, enemas, hydrotherapy, sun, mud, osteopathy, chiropractic, magnets, massage and special exercises. Walter Hoppe (1917-1986) was a psychiatrist and psychoanalyst, who based his method on physician Wilhelm Reich's ideas that the earth is enveloped in life-energy, which he called 'orgone'. Hoppe sat his patients inside Reich's 'orgone accumulators' to recharge the body with energy.[5] Tzvi 'Nails', a kibbutz member whose family name is unknown, diagnosed his patients by observing changes in their nails, and treating them accordingly with homeopathic remedies. The information which he harvested from nails amazed and astonished his patients, giving him a reputation among them for impressive therapeutic success.

Most of these healers suffered chronic conditions, and developed their methods searching for cures — testing, observing and experimenting. None made any separation between their private and professional lives, treating their patients either in their living rooms or in those of their sponsors and followers. Their personalities, charisma and success were such, however, that they were able to build stable therapeutic methods which met the needs of many thousands of patients and followers, even after their death.[6]

The Struggle for Recognition

The Legal Situation:

Despite increased use of CAM in Israel, its legal status has never been regulated and remains somewhat muddled. On one hand, the right of therapists to practise complementary and alternative medicine is guaranteed through the Basic Law: Freedom of Occupation (1994), under which 'every citizen or resident of the State of Israel has the right to practise any occupation'. A second Basic Law: Human Dignity and Liberty (1992) allows every individual to choose the treatment he desires: conventional, complementary and/or alternative.[7] On the other hand, the Physicians Ordinance (1976) restricts freedom of occupation by permitting only authorized physicians to practise medicine. Paradoxically, this law, which restricts the practice of medicine to physicians, allows non-physicians, acting 'under the direct personal supervision of a licenced physician to practice, as well, a caveat which allows CAM therapists to work, provided they do so under physician supervision.[8] More inconsistent still is a legal interpretation of this law: handed down by the Court in what is known as the Shalchin case, it allows physicians to refer patients to CAM practitioners, whom they know and trust, with a referral and follow-up instructions. All this, without direct physician supervision.[9]

There is, in the current situation, a huge potential for harm to public health. With no law that specifically addresses CAM, and no legal status for CAM practitioners, there is no legal obligation for authorities to supervise their professional training or their methods. Nor are therapists legally obliged to obtain either professional training or Health Ministry approval in order to work. At the other end of the spectrum, serious, well-educated, knowledgeable and efficient therapists have to practise on the borders of the law, at risk of being denounced as criminal.

Increase in the Distribution of CAM

With the discovery of antibiotics, the apparent vanquishing of infectious disease and the introduction of vaccination programmes, conventional medicine experienced a surge of success. This widened the existing gap between biomedicine and CAM for decades. By the 1980s, however, as so often in history, the pendulum had swung back. This led to renewed interest in CAM, and its steadily increasing use. This trend mirrored that seen in other Western countries, reflecting, in part, growing disillusion with the technology and bureaucracy of biomedicine, growing doubt about its excessive invasiveness, heightened consumer awareness of its iatrogenic effects, greater expectation of quality services, and widespread demystification – all of which have considerably eroded confidence in modern medicine.[10] Whereas in 1993 only 6% of Israel's population used CAM, by 2000, that proportion had grown to 10% and in 2007 to 12%, with 2.7 million CAM consultations in 2009 alone, a mean annual increase of some 5%.[11]

This development did not escape institutional Israeli medicine. In 1991, the Assaf Ha'rofe Medical Centre became the first conventional hospital in Israel to open a CAM outpatient clinic, offering a wide variety of CAM practices. While outpatients had to pay out-of-pocket for these services, hospitalized patients received CAM treatment, if requested, free of charge. Patient demand and Israel's competitive medical market ensured that other conventional medical centres followed suit and opened outpatient CAM clinics, which also offered services to hospitalized patients. Today, all the country's major hospitals have such centres.

At around the same time, all four Health Funds, through which every Israeli citizen is insured for conventional medical treatment, opened their own CAM clinics, for which supplementary health insurance must be paid. The CAM treatments used are jointly decided by patient and an 'allocation' (essentially, triage) doctor, who is a conventional physician, who helps patients find appropriate treatment among the clinic's CAM therapies.

The 'Elon' Committee

In 1988, a Committee was established by then-Health Minister Shoshana Arbeli-Almozlino to examine the status of CAM in Israel. Headed by Israel's

Supreme Court deputy president Professor Menachem Elon, the Committee's letter of appointment determined that its role was to investigate CAM 'in all its aspects and its implications, including natural healing methods, homeopathy, acupuncture, reflexology, chiropractic, etc.'[12] The Committee was asked to recommend, *inter alia*, 'whether recognition can be given to treatment by these methods and whom will be authorized to deal with it'. The Committee concluded its deliberations three years later in 1991, submitting a detailed report which determined that the legal status of complementary medicine in Israel was 'far from satisfactory'. Most CAM healers, it said, have no legal status, and there is no supervision of either their practice or their professional training. The Committee recommended changing the law to establish appropriate licencing of CAM practitioners in order to safeguard two basic principles: first, the right of the individual to select the health practitioner of his choice; and, second, to guard against incorrect diagnosis or treatment that could pose a risk to health or harm the patient. In view of this, the Committee recommended permitting CAM practitioners to offer therapies that neither cause harm nor violate the law. CAM practitioners should adopt the ethical code of the medical profession, it continued, but only licenced physicians would be entitled call themselves 'doctor' and certain treatments would remain solely in the hands of qualified physicians.[13]

State Comptroller's Report, the Israel Parliamentary Initiative and the Zaides Committee

The Committee's conclusions were effectively ignored. Four years later, the 1995 State Comptroller's Report (No. 46) harshly criticized the Health Ministry for its inaction, saying:

> The actions taken by the Ministry of Health in the period that passed from the date of submission of the recommendations of the 'Elon' Committee until the date of the audit are insufficient. The Ministry should discuss the issue of complementary medicine, examine it in all its complexity, and formulate rules and legal arrangements that will regulate it in every aspect.[14]

The Report firmly recommended that the Health Ministry act to change the existing legal situation, gain control over medical treatments provided by unauthorized persons, and take appropriate measures to supervise and audit CAM practitioners. It also suggested that the

Ministry consider, after due investigation, whether there is a basis in law for recognizing certain CAM treatments and to establish conditions to protect patients and the public. As with the findings of the 'Elon' Committee, the recommendations of the State Comptroller were largely disregarded.

The number of CAM practitioners, however, was steadily increasing, reaching a size sufficient to lobby Israel's parliament, the Knesset. A decade later, in 2002, the lobby's pressure bore fruit, and another attempt was made to regulate the use of CAM. It started as an initiative of the Knesset's Labour, Welfare and Health Committee, in cooperation with the Health Ministry and other involved organisations.[15] The aim was to enact a law that would eliminate the juridical chaos. A bill was drawn up, dealing solely with the regulation of acupuncture, and passed its first reading in the Knesset in 2003. It then went to Committee, where it was decided that the new law should regulate all CAM disciplines, not simply acupuncture. Proceedings were halted, and the initiative died.[16]

A new committee, with a wider brief, was convened by the Health Ministry the following year under Dr. Itzhak Zaides to examine 'the various aspects of advancing recognition in complementary medicine fields' and formulate a licencing procedure. The Health Ministry proposed that CAM be regulated by the State, and its practitioners be trained in Israel's academic institutions, under supervision of the Council for Higher Education (CHE), which guides Israel's higher education policy. The withholding of Council approval (see below) ensured that this latest attempt to regulate CAM met with failure.

Academization: Yes or No?

In December 2004, the College of Management of Academic Studies in Rishon le-Zion submitted a request to the CHE for the opening an undergraduate programme in Alternative Medicine, in cooperation with Ben Gurion University. To evaluate the application, the CHE appointed an Examining Committee. The Committee's deliberations, concluded three and a half years later, were discussed by the CHE, who decided to establish a Professional Committee to consider the issues raised in their discussions. The Professional Committee was instructed to examine the advantages and disadvantages of different alternatives to determine a comprehensive policy in the field of CAM, as well as to discuss specific questions. These included: Is there a scientific basis for this field? Is it desirable for studies to be within an academic framework, and merit an academic degree? What framework is appropriate for such a programme or specialization track? Should such studies earn a BSc, MSc or other qualification?

The Professional Committee recommended approval of a BSc study track, separate from conventional medicine programmes, to be taught at academic institutions accredited by the CHE. According to Committee recommendations, studies should be general, and include a basis for understanding the human body (Anatomy, Physiology, the Immune System), as well as courses in Scientific Thinking, Research Methods and Ethics. The Committee noted that the issue of alternative medicine's scientific basis remained controversial, but that its non-regulation and lack of supervision and control were serious concerns. This lukewarm vindication was supported by the Health Ministry, which had recommended that CAM be taught in academic frameworks by qualified teachers, according to standardized curricula, as a supervised study programme, and that therapists with academic backgrounds in CAM be permitted to pursue research.

For the purpose of licencing in alternative medical professions, said the Committee, the Health Ministry should require applicants to complete BSc studies in the new track and take an internship under recognized supervision. The Committee was divided over what to call the programme. A minority wanted to see 'Complementary Medicine' as part of its name. The majority objected, arguing that this lacked an academic-scientific basis and was somewhat controversial. They proposed calling it: 'Introductory Studies for Human Therapists'. The name, however, proved irrelevant. Despite the Committee's clear and positive position, in December 2009 the CHE rejected its recommendations. Their reason: there was no scientific basis for CAM.[17]

CAM in Israel Today

In 1995, Israel's National Health Insurance (NHI) Law was introduced, under which every resident has comprehensive health insurance. Individuals can select their provider from among the four competing, non-profit Health Funds, Clalit, Maccabi, Me'uchedet and Le'umit, regardless of age, pre-existing conditions or state of health. Patients have considerable freedom in choosing their community-based physicians, both primary and specialist, from those affiliated with their Health Fund. Health Fund contributions are exclusively income-linked, irrespective of health status, with emergency medical services provided unconditionally. All four Health Funds provide an identical basic basket of services, specified by law, which is updated, usually annually, by a national committee.[18] Services, whose availability differs with location, include doctor visits, diagnostic and laboratory services, hospitalization and discounted prescription medications. The State, through the Health Ministry, is responsible for the supervision, licencing and overall planning of health services.

CAM in Israel has benefited from this National Health Insurance Law. In 1998, the Health Funds were permitted to offer, for supplementary payment, health services additional to those included in the mandatory basic health basket. CAM is among these added services. Within a decade, 73% of those insured had taken out supplementary insurance to cover additional services.[19] By 2011, some two dozen forms of CAM were in frequent use in Israel. The most popular are acupuncture, shiatsu, qigong, reflexology, osteopathy, chiropractic, homeopathy, naturopathy, herbal medicine, aromatherapy, Alexander-Feldenkrais, Paula's technique, *tuina*, biofeedback and medical massage.[20] Their availability is not uniform, and depends on the number and location of practitioners for each.

The number of CAM practitioners in Israel is, however, steadily growing. In 1998, there were some 5,500 nationwide, representing a wide variety of CAM specialties. Only some 2,800 of them were members of professional organisations, making the majority lay practitioners.[21] Four of Israel's medical schools today teach short elective courses in CAM, but none teaches any CAM professions. In other words, medical students learn about CAM, but do not learn CAM itself. Ben Gurion University's Faculty of Health Sciences was the first to open an elective CAM course in Israel. Launched in 2003, it was initiated and guided by the Shaarei Zedek Medical Centre's Centre for Integrative Complementary Medicine. Medical schools affiliated with Tel Aviv and Haifa Universities followed Ben Gurion University's lead, and this year a compulsory CAM course will become part of the curriculum of the Hebrew University's Faculty of Medicine in Jerusalem – as one of the first compulsory CAM courses in the Western world. This is likely a response to the high level of interest in CAM among Israel's medical students: 79% favoured learning about it during their course of study, and 65% expressed interest in applying CAM techniques to patient treatment.[22]

Outside the universities in Israel, CAM professions are widely taught. Some 10,000 people are currently enrolled in CAM courses, which last from several months to four years, most of them taught in one of six large schools.[23] These programmes differ substantially in both their level and quality of teaching. Because they are not formally regulated, entrance requirements are uneven, and the level of education received is questionable.

What of Israel's CAM consumers? Socio-demographically, they are similar to those throughout the Western world. They tend to be women, younger people, with 12 or more years of education, of higher economic status, and living in large cities. There is a significant inverse correlation between levels of satisfaction with conventional medical specialists and use of alternative medicine, a correlation that was far stronger in 2000 than in 1993.[24]

In 1997, the IMA, no longer able to compete with growing public demand for CAM and the increasing number of lay homeopaths, came out with a contradictory response. On one hand, it condemned the unscientific and unproved paradigms of CAM, the absence of acceptable training of CAM practitioners and its potential danger to patients. On the other, it acknowledged the possible usefulness of forms of some forms of CAM, such as acupuncture and chiropractic, under the supervision of conventional physicians. Herbal medicine, too, should be practised only by licenced physicians.[25] This feeble stance was never practically enforced, and the IMA continues to tolerate lay practitioners using CAM, unsupervised by conventional physicians. In 2010, after many unsuccessful attempts, the Organization of CAM Physicians was finally accredited as a full member of the IMA.

Public demand for CAM has also made headway among conventional physicians, with an estimated 42 to 60% of Israel's general practitioners now referring patients to CAM practitioners.[26] While conventional physicians have concerns about the qualifications and standards of individual CAM providers, they tend to be positive about CAM therapy itself.[27] It is believed that conventional physicians in Israel would support national CAM insurance coverage in Israel's clinics and hospitals - were CAM recognized as a specialization acquired by MDs.[28]

Satisfaction with CAM treatment appears to have increased in Israel over the years. In 1993, 60% of CAM consumers reported that the therapy helped them. By the year 2000, that percentage had increased to 75%.[29] There are clear differences among the populations who use CAM in Israel. A 2006 study, which compared the characteristics of CAM consumption among urban Arabs and Jews in northern Israel, found that 40% of the Jewish population had experienced at least one CAM intervention, compared with 31% of the Arabs.[30] Among the Jews, more women were exposed to CAM than men, with the reverse true among the Arab population. It should be noted that in these two groups, more Jews than Arabs had higher education. About a third of Jews and Arabs from the towns of Haifa and Nazareth favoured CAM regulation and its teaching in

Israel's medical and nursing schools. While almost a third of Jews believed that CAM providers should have MDs, however, none of the Arabs did so.

Shmueli *et al.* found that, in the public perception, CAM is no longer 'a collection of esoteric, unidentified techniques, suitable for unspecified, possibly psychosomatic "general health" complaints'.[31] Today, it is regarded as a set of specific skills, useful in treating a large array of identifiable medical problems, ranging from digestive and musculo-skeletal ailments to disorders of the blood and the respiratory system.

Conclusion

Taking a narrow perspective of the development of CAM in Israel, it may resemble a ping-pong game or a one-step-forward-two-steps-back type of dance, with no significant overall progress. In the longer view, however, the gradual entry of CAM into biomedicine cannot be ignored. While never, for a moment, endangering the superiority of conventional medicine in this country, there have been profound and lasting changes in the status of CAM in Israel. Not long ago, homeopathic remedies could be purchased in only seven pharmacies countrywide and only by prescription. Today, they can and are obtained in any pharmacy. Not long ago, acupuncture was seen as black magic, performed by a few bizarre physicians or those exploiting public gullibility in order to line their own pockets. Today, hundreds of acupuncturists treat several thousand people daily, many of them referred by conventional physicians. Not long ago, a hospital director who announced the opening of a small outpatient CAM clinic was accused by his board of directors of returning medicine to the Middle Ages. Today, almost all Israel's hospitals have CAM units, which serve the entire institution.

This is very much in line with what has happened elsewhere in the Western world. In the USA in 1990, for example, more visits (427 million) were made to CAM practitioners than to primary-care physicians (388 million), with 36.3% of Americans using CAM, and spending an estimated annual $10.3 billion out-of-pocket on CAM therapies.[32] And that was far from the peak of US CAM demand: a study, carried out by the same group eight years later, demonstrated that CAM consumption continued to increase, with an annual 629 million visits to CAM practitioners, 46.3% of the population using CAM and paying for it.[33] In the 1980s, no American medical school had a CAM course in its curriculum yet by 1996, 64% were teaching CAM courses,[34] and two years after that, the proportion had risen to 88%.[35] (Almost all were electives.) In 2005, the American Institute of

Medicine recommended, in a report which ran to more than 350 pages, that:

> ...health profession schools (for example, schools of medicine, nursing, pharmacy and allied health) incorporate sufficient information about CAM into the standard curriculum at the undergraduate, graduate and postgraduate levels...[36]

As in the US and other Western countries, CAM is slowly entering Israel's biomedical sphere. The reason seems to be less a belief among conventional practitioners in CAM as a therapeutic mode, and more the combined impact of growing consumer demand, economic factors and market competition. For the moment, CAM in Israel plays no more than a supporting role. It acts within conventional medicine and under its auspices, with CAM professions remaining on the periphery, and thus posing no danger to the starring role of conventional medicine.

Israel's suspicious tolerance of CAM will continue as long as it does not imperil conventional medicine and restricts itself to treating incurable diseases or conditions for which conventional treatment is insufficient. The burning question is what will happen as CAM's embrace extends. How will biomedicine react as CAM research advances? What will happen to the boundaries between MDs and their long and demanding years of study, and CAM therapists whose training is short, unregulated and unsupervised?

If conventional medicine displays some curiosity and opens its educational system to a CAM syllabus, it may discover that some of its practices can be useful, and that integrating them into conventional medicine may resolve issues to which there is no sufficient conventional solution. In an ideal world, CAM will be eased into a transformed field of medicine that is both pluralistic and multi-faceted.

Notes

1. Available at: http://ayush.gov.in/ Accessed 20 April 2018.
2. Fulder, S., *The Handbook of Alternative and Complementary Medicine,* 3rd edn (Oxford: Oxford University Press, 1996)
3. Ernst, E., Resch, K.L. and Mills, S. et al., 'Complementary Medicine: A Definition', *British Journal General Practice* 1995; 45: pp.506; NCCAM. 2002, *What Is Complementary and Alternative Medicine (CAM)?* [Online]. Accessible on 10 June 2004, at http://nccam.nih.gov/health/whatiscam/index.html; Defining and describing complementary and alternative medicine. 1997. Panel on Definition and Description,

CAM Research Methodology Conference. *Alternative Therapies in Health and Medicine,* 1995, 3: pp.49-57; Gevitz, N., *Other Healers: Unorthodox Medicine in America* (Baltimore: Johns Hopkins University Press, 1998; Hufford, D.J., 'CAM and Cultural Diversity: Ethics and Epistemology Converge' in: Callahan, D. (Ed.), *The Role of Complementary and Alternative Medicine: Accommodating Pluralism (Washington, DC:* Georgetown University Press, 2002), pp.15-35.

4. Barel, D., *An Ill Wind: Cholera Epidemics and Medical Development in Palestine in the Late Ottoman Period,* (Jerusalem: Bialik Institute, 2010) [Hebrew].

5. Cohen-Gil, M., *The Israelis who Wished to Cure the World: Feldenkrais, Paula, Nezah, Hoppe* (Keter Books, 2013) [Hebrew].

6. Ibid.

7. Almog, S., 'Basic Law: Freedom of Occupation; Basic Law: Human Dignity and Liberty', *Law and Rule* (ממשל), 1992, vol.A, (1), pp.185-195 [Hebrew].

8. Ibid,, pp.185-195.

9. Physicians Ordinance [New Version], 5737-1976, http://fs.knesset.gov.il/%5C8% 5Claw%5C8_lsnv_318068. PDF [Hebrew].

10. Rees, L. and Weil, A., 'Integrated Medicine', *British Medical Journal,* 2001, 322, pp.119-20.

11. Shmueli, A,. Igudin, I. and Shuval, J., *Change and Stability: Use of Complementary and Alternative Medicine in Israel,* 1993, 2000 and 2007.

12. *Report of the Committee to Examine the Subject of Alternative Medicine in Israel,* http://98.131.138.124/articles/conference2/R9981353.asp [Hebrew].

13. Ibid.

14. State Comptroller's Report No. 46 for 1995. P. 238. http://www.mevaker.gov.il/ he/Pages/default.aspx

15. Protocol No. 584 of the Labour, Welfare and Health Committee, 15th Knesset, 24 October 2004.

16. Protocol No. 439 of the Labour, Welfare and Health Committee, 16th Knesset, 27 June 2005, pp.8-12.

17. Belizovski, A., The Challenge of Rationality: The Council for Higher Education Rejected a Proposal by https://www.hayadan.org.il/victory-of-rationalism-1612091. Regulation of alternative medical professions-the Knesset- http://fs.knesset.gov.il/ globaldocs/MMM/0b566b58-e9f7-e411-80c8-00155d010977/2_0b566b58-e9f7-e411-80c8-00155d010977_11_6810.pdf [Hebrew]

18. Rosen, B., Waitzberg, R. and Merkur, S., 'Israel: Health System Review', *Health Systems in Transition,* 2015,17, p.6.

19. Shmueli, A., Igudin, I. and Shuval, J., *Change and Stability.*

20. Research Centre of the Knesset, Data on 'Complementary Medicine' Patients, http://knesset.gov.il/mmm/data/pdf/m03488.pdf

21. Sela, O., Chairman, Association of Complementary Health Care Organizations, (HaLishka Lemikzto'ot Briut Maslimim), May 2011, personal communication quoted from Chen, S., 16 January 1997, Alternative medicine in Israel, *Yediot Aharonot* (Hebrew daily newspaper), p.25.

22. Oberbaum, M., Notzer, N. and Abramowitz, R. et al., 'Attitude of Medical Students to the Introduction of Complementary Medicine into the Medical Curriculum in Israel', *Israel Medical Association Journal,* 2003, 5 (2), pp.139-142.

23. Bernstein, J.H. and Shuval, J.T., 'Nonconventional Medicine in Israel: Consultation Patterns of the Israeli Population and Attitudes of Primary Care Physicians', *Social Science & Medicine* 1997, 44: pp.1341-1348; Shuval, J.T. and Mizrachi, M., 'Changing Boundaries: Modes of Coexistence of Alternative and Biomedicine', *Qualitative Health Research* 2004, 14, pp.675-690.

24. Shuval, J.T. and Mizrachi, M., 'Changing Boundaries: Modes of Coexistence of Alternative and Biomedicine', pp.675-90.

25. IMA (1997), Letter to the members [Hebrew] in *Bulletin of the Israel Medical Association*, 59, pp.9-12.

26. Shmueli, A., Igudin, I., Shuval, J., Shuval, J.T. and Mizrachi, M., 'Changing Boundaries', pp.675-90; *IMA* (1997). Letter to the members [Hebrew], pp.9-12; Borkan, J., Neher, J.O. and Anson, O. et al., 'Referrals for Alternative Therapies', *Journal of Family Practice*,1994, *39*, pp.545-50; Schachter, L., Weingarten, M.A. and Kahan, E.E., 'Attitudes of Family Physicians to Nonconventional Therapies', *Archives of Family Medicine*, 1993; 2, pp.1268-1270.

27. Bernstein, J.H. and Shuval, J.T., 'Nonconventional medicine in Israel: Consultation Patterns of the Israeli Population and Attitudes of Primary Care Physicians', *Social Science Medicine*,1997, 44, pp.1341-1348.

28. Ibid., pp.1341-1348.

29. Schachter, L., Weingarten, M.A. and Kahan, E., 'Attitudes of Family Physicians to Nonconventional Therapies', pp.1268-1270.

30. Krivoy, N., Habib, M. and Azzam, Z.S., 'Ethnic differences in Population Approach and Experience Regarding Complementary-Alternative Medicine (CAM)', *Pharmacoepidemiology Drug Safety*, 2006, 15, pp.348-353.

31. Shmueli,A., Igudin, I. and Shuval, J., 'Change and Stability'.

32. Eisenberg, D., Kessler, R. and Foster, C. et al., 'Unconventional medicine in the United States – Prevalence, Costs, and Patterns of Use', *New England Journal of Medicine*, 1993, 328, pp.246-252.

33. Eisenberg, D.M., Davis, R.B. and Ettner, S.L. et al., *Journal of the American Medical Association (JAMA)*, 1998, 280, pp.1569-1575.

34. Wetzel, M.S., Eisenberg, D.M. and Kaptchuk, T.J., *JAMA*, 1998, 280, pp.784-787.

35. *Curriculum Directory*, Association of American Medical Colleges, 27th Edition, 1998-1999.

36. Complementary and Alternative Medicine in the United States. Committee on the Use of Complementary and Alternative Medicine by the American Public (Free Executive Summary) http://www.nap.edu/catalog/11182.html.

13

Medicine in Israel Today

Judy Siegel-Itzkovich, Stuart Stanton and Kenneth Collins

This book has covered the story of medicine and aspects of health in the Holy Land from earliest times to the present day. It has looked on the many influences which have shaped that medicine as the country has been settled and fought over for the past three millennia. Standing at a strategic crossroad between Babylon and Egypt, political and military conquerors have crossed its borders many times and traces of their presence form part of the medical story. The book tells the story of medicine in contemporary Israel looking at themes such as medical ethics, delivery of health care and rehabilitation. The inclusion of material on the uptake of complementary medicine indicates the need to examine the national Israeli openness to new and sometimes alternative ways of achieving the best health-care outcomes.

Israel has been described as the 'Start-Up' nation with very many more research-based start-ups than many larger industrialized nations. A lack of natural resources and positive funding initiatives allied to a skilled and well-educated workforce has driven many fields of innovation forward. This ability to think and react in a creative way has extended into every advanced technological area including medicine and health care.[1] This matched the development of computer science and technology in the 1980s and enabled Israel to move from its previous small manufacturing base. Investment in the defence and aerospace industries produced innovative technologies and its new presence in high-tech industries, including many with medical applications.

The large wave of Russian immigration in the early 1990s brought a major element to the workforce skilled in engineering and science. In turn, foreign interest in Israeli innovations developed rapidly with massive inward investment of venture capital and some spectacular buy-outs of

Israeli-developed technology stocks. One of the first of these medical innovations was the development of PillCam, a miniaturized camera system which could be utilized for examining lesions in the small intestine related to Crohn's disease or to identify the source of obscure blood loss which was producing an iron deficiency anaemia. Initial studies showed its effective and ease of use for oesophageal lesions also. The concept was remarkably simple. The patient swallowed a capsule containing a miniaturized camera which could transmit images to be assessed by a gastroenterologist. Suspicious tissue that might need a biopsy could be followed up with endoscopy.

PillCam was developed by Given Imaging which was founded in 1998 by Dr. Gabi Iddan and Dr. Gavriel Meron and initial funding for the company was provided by Elron Electronic Industries, Israel's leading technology holding company, in cooperation with Rafael Advanced Defence Systems. Dr. Iddan, who had been working in the missile division of Rafael, reckoned that missile technology could be miniaturized to create a medical product.[2] By October 2001 Given Imaging had an Initial public offering on NASDAQ. Given Imaging was sold to Covidien in 2014 and purchased by Medtronic the following year.

An article on the Israel 21C media website in 2013 identified a dozen companies in the health sector that it considered would prosper in the years ahead. These companies have all survived and prospered over the past seven years in the highly competitive international biotechnology field.

1. **ApiFix** system to correct severe curvature of the spine (scoliosis) minimizes risks, scar size, complications, recovery time and cost. It cuts down on pain and enables many children to be freed from wheelchairs. Its parent company is now OrthoPediatrics, an American company founded in 2006 to focus on the neglected field of orthopedic implants for children.

2. Argo Medical Technologies' **ReWalk** robotic exoskeleton has enabled paraplegic runners in London and Tel Aviv to complete marathons. The ReWalk Rehabilitation model currently is used by patients in rehabilitation centres around the world, but its total bulk, around 50kg, and cost has been an ongoing problem.[3] The system allows the user to walk, sit and stand, and is controlled from small device worn as a wristwatch.

3. **Gamida Cell** is developing stem-cell therapy products to treat blood cancers, solid tumours, non-malignant blood diseases such as

sickle-cell anaemia, auto-immune diseases and genetic metabolic diseases. As efforts to create effective treatments to date have been hampered by the inability to expand cells in the laboratory while maintaining therapeutic functionality, Gamida is pioneering the expansion of multiple cell types while maintaining their original potency.[4]

4. **GI View Aer-O-Scope** was designed to make colonoscopy cancer screenings cheaper, safer and more accessible worldwide. The self-navigating, flexible Aer-O-Scope removes the risk of perforating the colon, provides superior imaging and can be used by a trained nurse or technician. As the scope is disposable the risk of infection and cross-contamination is removed.

5. **IceCure Medical's IceSense3** has been used since 2012 to remove benign breast lumps in a 10-minute ultrasound-guided procedure that penetrates the tumour and engulfs it with ice without damaging surrounding tissue. It is also indicated for use in the fields of general surgery, oncology, gynaecology and urology. IceCure is currently conducting the ICE3 clinical trial for the non-surgical treatment of low-risk, early-stage breast cancer and there are twenty sites initially participating in this trial where certain small breast cancers will be treated with cryoablation, as an alternative to surgery, then followed for five years.

6. **InSightec's ExAblate OR** uses MRI-guided focused ultrasound to destroy deep tissue in the body tumours and uterine fibroid cysts without the need for incisions without surgery. In 2013 they were beginning studies on ExAblate Neuro for essential tremor Parkinson's disease and neuropathic pain, using the same non-invasive technology and reducing the risk of brain damage. The company was founded by Kobi Vortman, formerly chairman of Elbit Medical Imaging, and Oded Tamir with seed investment from Elbit and GE Healthcare. Now a global company with bases in the USA and Far East the company maintains a strong Israeli presence.

7. **IonMed**, founded by Amnon and Ronen Lam, produces **BioWeld1** which bonds surgical incisions using cold plasma, instead of painful stitches, staples or glue, within minutes, sealing and disinfecting the wound with minimal scarring and recovery time. Studies have confirmed the effectiveness of the product.[5] The Bioweld1 system combines a plasma generating device, including a disposable plasma emitting head and a medical plaster, Chitoplast™, which covers the

wound and assists in approximating the incision edges. To seal the incision and promote coagulation and healing, the Chitoplast 'solder' is affixed to the incision edges, and the plasma jet is applied along the incision edge.

8. **Nano Retina's** Bio-Retina, a tiny implantable device inserted into the retina in a 30-minute procedure, turns into an artificial retina that melds to the neurons in the eye. Activated by special eyeglasses, the device transforms natural light into an electrical impulse that stimulates neurons to send images to the brain.[6] The company is based in Herzliya but has developed extensive international links.

9. **NanoPass Technologies'** MicronJet, founded by Yotam Levin MD MBA from Tel Aviv University in 2002, is a single-use needle for painless delivery of vaccines into the skin using semi-conductor technology. The product has been proven to generate superior immune response with less vaccine, because it does not go past the skin level.[7] The company is based in Nes Ziona and is actively pursuing additional partnerships with vaccine developers worldwide.

10. **OrSense** is a medical device company that develops and commercializes innovative non-invasive monitoring technologies for continuous and spot measurements of blood parameters. Their product SpectOLight™ Occlusion Spectroscopy technology enables easy and accurate measurements of blood indices. Their current focus is non-invasive haemoglobin testing for the detection of anaemia in different clinical settings. OrSense has a multidisciplinary staff including scientists, mathematicians and engineers. The company's intellectual property portfolio consists of 51 granted patents and over 20 additional applications in process.

11. **Surpass Medical's NeuroEndoGraft** redirects blood flow from a brain aneurysm, so that a stable clot can form, and the potentially fatal aneurysm no longer is in danger of rupturing. US medical device manufacturer Stryker, a leader in the field of medical technology with extensive interests in less invasive therapies through innovative ischaemic and hemorrhagic stroke products and services, acquired Surpass for $100 million in October 2012.

12. **VitalGo Systems'** Total Lift bed is the world's only hospital-grade bed that can elevate a patient from a lying to a fully standing position, and all points in between, for treatment and transfer with no lifting required of the care giver. The company now has an extensive American base operating from Fort Lauderdale, Florida.

The most successful Israeli innovation, based on market capitalization, is Mobileye whose founders had already set up OrCam Technologies. OrCam is the maker of a device, OrCam MyEye, that gives blind people 'vision' and OrCam Read, which helps readers with dyslexia and other reading disorders using artificial intelligence technologies. It won a Best of Innovation Award in January 2020 at the International Consumer Electronics Show for its new device OrCam Hear for hearing impairment. OrCam was founded by Amnon Shashua, Professor of Computer Science at the Hebrew University of Jerusalem with Ziv Aviram, a graduate in industrial engineering and Management from Ben Gurion University of the Negev. Professor Shashua's field of expertise is computer vision and machine learning and his academic achievements, have brought him many awards. Shashua and Aviram were also co-founders of Mobileye which is already installed in millions of cars making the vehicles safer to drive. The system provides warnings to prevent or mitigate collisions and Mobileye's autonomous driving technology is already changing the way people drive cars. In August 2017, Intel acquired Mobileye for a valuation of approximately $15.3 billion, the biggest ever acquisition of an Israeli Hi-Tech company.

Medical Scientists

One of Israel's leading medical scientists is Professor Ada Yonath, of the Centre for Biomolecular Structure and Assembly, Weizmann Institute in Rehovot, who received the Nobel Prize in Chemistry in 2009, with Venkatraman Ramakrishnan and Thomas A Steitz, for her studies on the structure and function of the ribosome, focusing on ribosomal crystallography.[8] Her understanding of the place of the ribosome in cellular function has helped to clarify the mode of action of antibiotic drugs, particularly those acting against drug-resistant bacteria.[9] In 1970 she established the first protein crystallography laboratory in Israel and from 1979 to 1984 she continued her researches at the Max Planck Institute for Molecular Genetics in Berlin. This work explains the mode of action of many different antibiotics targeting the ribosome, showing how the ribosome plays a key role in clinical usefulness and therapeutic effectiveness, thus paving the way for structure-based drug design. In 2008, she was awarded the Albert Einstein World Award of Science for her pioneering contributions to protein biosynthesis in the field of ribosomal crystallography and her introduction of innovative techniques in cryo bio-crystallography.

Technion Professors Avram Hershko and Aaron Ciechanover received a Nobel Prize in Chemistry, along with Brooklyn-born Irwin Rose (1926-2015) in 2004 for their extensive of work discovering the Ubiquitin System, which explains the mechanism involved in the breakdown of proteins in cells. Ubiquitin, originally known as ubiquitous immune-poietic polypeptide, was first identified in 1975 and named for its ubiquitous cellular presence. A joint publication by Hershko, Ciechanover and Rose on ubiquitin appeared in 1979.[10] Hershko was born Herskó Ferenc in Karcag, Hungary in 1937 and Aaron Ciechanover was born in Haifa in 1947, to parents who came to Palestine from Poland in the 1920s. Ciechanover's research success has led to his presence on the Scientific Advisory Boards of many bio-science companies.

Ciechanover and Hershko elucidated the basic functions and the components of the ubiquitination pathway in the early 1980s at the Technion. Ubiquitin is a regulatory protein responsible for protein recycling that carries out its activity by binding to proteins and marking them for destruction. Without this regulation, immune activation against pathogens may be defective, resulting in chronic disease or death. Alternatively, the immune system may become hyper-activated and organs and tissues may be subjected to auto-immune damage. In addition, because of its very large number of roles in the cell, manipulating the ubiquitin system represents an efficient way for such viruses to block, subvert or redirect critical host cell processes to support their own replication.

Daniel Kahneman, born in Tel Aviv in 1934, is an Israeli-American psychologist and economist notable for his work on the psychology of judgment and decision-making, as well as behavioural economics.[11] He was awarded the 2002 Nobel Prize in Economic Sciences for his work on Prospect Theory, developed along with Haifa-born Amos Tversky in 1979. As Tversky died in 1996, and Nobel Prizes cannot be awarded posthumously, the Nobel Prize could not be shared. Prospect theory aims to explain irrational human economic choices and is considered one of the seminal works of behavioural economics.

One of Israel's innovative young scientists is Hossam Haick, a Professor in the Department of Chemical Engineering and the Russell Berrie Nanotechnology Institute at the Technion, Israel Institute of Technology. He was born Nazareth in 1975 and attended the St. Joseph Seminary and High School in the city. His research interests include nano-array devices for screening, diagnosis and monitoring of disease, nanomaterial-based chemical (flexible) sensors, breath analysis, volatile biomarkers, and molecule-based electronic devices. The technologies developed by his team have led to the production of dozens of patents and patent applications, establishing partnerships between the Technion and international institutions and companies.

Professor Haick invented the Nano Artificial Nose (NA-NOSE) for detection of disease from exhaled breath and early studies he showed that cancer has a unique volatile molecular print through exhaled breath samples. Later his group found that each disease has its own unique volatile molecular print, and this has led to effective and early disease screening and the recognition of a new field of biomarkers.[12] His Artificially Intelligent Nano-Array that allows diagnosis of more than twenty disease states, and can even identify sub-categories of diseases through exhaled breath.[13] His team has also developed 'smart patches' that imitate the senses of human skin, allowing the possibility of creating touch-sensitive robots, medical devices, prosthetic limbs with tactile feedback, as well as, wearable smart patches for sports and rehabilitation.[14] The implementation of these discoveries and has led to his receiving many grants and awards.

Pathology

Artificial Intelligence (AI) has been used to detect diseases such cancer from radiological scans generated by CT and MRI machines and its use, and the need for further research has been validated in many studies.[15] However, Ibex Medical Analytics is the first Israeli Start-up to apply the technique to tissue biopsies.[16] One motivation to produce this innovation was a projected world-wide shortage of pathologists. Another was the presence of a significant error rate in the reading of pathology samples, up to 12% in various estimates, related to small tumour size or to human error. Ibex Medical Analytics worked on developing an AI-driven diagnostic system to help pathologists deliver more accurate diagnoses also employing data science, image analysis, and machine-learning technologies and applies them to cancer diagnostics in digital pathology. The Ibex AI algorithm was used on 60,000 prostate biopsy slides and a similar number for its breast cancer product with slides coming mainly from the Maccabi Health Fund in Israel but also from the United States and Europe.

Ibex's Second Read application uses software algorithms to analyze cases in parallel with a pathologist. It then compares the pathologist's diagnosis and the algorithm's findings and if there is a discrepancy, the pathologist receives an immediate alert. The system has been in use at Israel's Maccabi Healthcare Service since 2018 at their Pathology Institute, the largest in Israel. Ibex has recently demonstrated an AI system capable of identifying almost all cell types and structures in a prostate CNB (cancer of different types and grades, pre-cancerous glands, other clinical findings, and even various normal tissue structures), unlike earlier models that were trained only to detect adenocarcinoma, the most common cancer type in the prostate). In February 2020, it was announced that the Galen™ Prostate solution had received the CE-IVD Mark for its for use in supporting pathologists in identification of suspected cancer on prostate core needle biopsies. (CE marking is a certification mark that indicates conformity with health, safety, and environmental protection standards for products sold within the European Economic Area. IVD = in vitro device.) With this CE-IVD Mark of Galen Prostate Ibex is now partnering with leading institutes across Europe to implement AI and support pathologists in their diagnostic workflow.

Melanoma

Israel has been a leading centre in the field of research into melanoma, the most aggressive of all skin cancers. It is usually caused by ultraviolet light exposure in individuals with low levels of the skin pigment melanin. Especially common in Australia and New Zealand it kills over 60,000 people worldwide annually, though early treatment, before lymph node spread, can be highly effective. Its prevalence has been increasing in recent years as Europeans have moved into more tropical climate zones.

One of the leading figures in melanoma research in Israel is Professor Carmit Levy from Tel Aviv University. Collaborating with researchers in Europe and American researchers, Levy's team discovered that before spreading to other organs, a melanoma tumour sends out tiny vesicles containing molecules of micro RNA. These molecules prepare the skin's dermis to receive and transport the cancer cells and the changes in the dermis caused by the micro RNA, as well as the presence of the vesicles, could help the earlier diagnosis of melanoma. Levy and her colleague Tamar Golan discovered that fat cells transfer a protein that enables the melanoma cells to spread aggressively beyond the skin. Another Tel Aviv University scientist, Ronit Satchi-Fainaro has been working with her team to develop a nano-vaccine against these processes in the development of melanoma and early results proved positive.[17] Molecular biologist Gabi Gerlitz of Ariel University studies what happens to the nucleus of melanoma cells during migration, a key step in metastasis.[18] When melanoma cells migrate, they squeeze themselves, which condenses the chromosomes to pass through blood vessels or tissues. Ongoing studies look for factors at the nuclear envelope that affect chromosome condensation and cell migration.

The studies of Professor Gal Markel, of the Ella Lemelbaum Institute for Immuno-Oncology, have produced new evidence in the process of cancer development, looking at ADAR1 which has a fundamental role in the regulation of cancer cell phenotypes. [Double-stranded RNA-specific adenosine deaminase is an enzyme that in humans is encoded by the ADAR (adenosine deaminase acting on RNA) gene.] His team have found the events leading to the loss of ADAR1 expression in metastatic melanoma cells, which subsequently facilitate the acquisition of an aggressive phenotype. These findings provide insights into the process of cancer development, with potential implications for future translational medicine.

Collaborative studies, involving researchers from Tel Aviv University, Sheba Medical Centre, the Salk Institute and the Yale School of Medicine at the Sheba have looked at fatty acid metabolism in melanoma patients. When fatty acids metabolize slowly, cancer cells have a chance to 'hide' from the immune system's T-cells that are supposed to destroy them.[19] Doctors can therefore identify the best candidates for immunotherapy and look for ways to speed up fatty acid metabolism. Other international collaborative studies have looked at cases where immunotherapy in melanoma has been unsuccessful while researchers at the Laboratory for Applied Cancer Research, at the Sourasky Medical Centre in Tel Aviv University and at the Rappaport School of Medicine, at the Technion in Haifa, also using mouse models for the disease, have looked at the mechanism for understanding melanoma brain metastases.[20]

3-D Sperm Cell Imaging Technology

Israeli scientists have developed a safe and accurate 3-D imaging method to identify sperm cells moving at high speed. This technology could enable doctors to select the highest-quality sperm for IVF treatment, thus increasing its chances of success. Under natural fertilization in a woman's body, the fastest sperm to reach an egg is supposed to bear high-quality genetic material. This is not possible in IVF treatments, where the embryologist selects the sperm that will be injected into the egg according to different characteristics. To overcome this limitation, Professor Natan Shaked and doctoral student Gili Dardikman-Yoffe from Tel Aviv University used CT technology for sperm-cell imaging. They managed to safely obtain a high-resolution image of the sperm in three dimensions in space, as well as the exact time dimension, producing four dimensions in place and time.[21] Shaked and Dardikman-Yoffe recorded a hologram of the sperm cell during ultra-fast movement and identified various internal components creating an accurate, highly dynamic 3-D map without using cell staining that could harm the embryo. The new technology can greatly improve the selection of sperm cells in vitro, potentially increasing the chance of pregnancy and the birth of a healthy baby.

This new method allows live sperm head internal structure and flagellum fine-detail dynamics to be imaged simultaneously during the sperm cell motion, which is very challenging because of the fine-structures and fast-dynamics which characterizes individual sperm cells. The authors believe that this method will eventually allow selecting the best sperm cell for injecting into the ovum in ICSI (Intracytoplasmic Sperm Injection). It is also expected that this method will be used to assess male fertility by 4-D computed tomography of the patient's live sperm, providing an analysis of both the fine-detailed morphology and motility of the sperm on an individual-cell basis. In addition, the imaging can contribute to other medical applications, such as developing efficient biomimetic micro-robots to carry drugs within the body.

Amyotrophic Lateral Sclerosis (ALS)

One of the most devastating neurological conditions is Motor-Neurone Disease (MND) also known as Amyotrophic Lateral Sclerosis (ALS). This devastating and incurable neuro-degenerative disease robs patients of the ability to walk, to speak, to swallow and, ultimately, to breathe. Research into management of this disorder has been carried out by Professor Dimitrios Karussis of the Multiple Sclerosis Centre at the Hadassah-University Medical Centre at Ein Kerem Jerusalem and the Israeli American BrainStorm Cell Therapeutics company. Their use of stem cells and growth factors, while not a cure, has been shown to inhibit the progression of the fatal neurological disease, as measured by the patients' respiratory function or general motor disability, in early clinical trials.[22] Using the NurOWNstem cell therapeutic platform BrainStorm Cell Therapeutics Phase 3 trials were underway at the time of writing (May 2020).[23]

Drug Therapy

Alzheimer's Disease: Rivastigmine, a cholinesterase inhibitor is a semi-synthetic derivative of physostigmine, a highly toxic reversible cholinesterase inhibitor, and in 2006 it became the first product approved globally for the treatment of mild to moderate dementia associated with Parkinson's disease. A trans-dermal Rivastigmine patch was introduced in 2007. Rivastigmine was developed by Professor Marta Weinstock-Rosin of the Department of Pharmacology at the Hebrew University of Jerusalem and sold by the Hebrew University's technology transfer company Yissum to the Swiss drug company Novartis for commercial development as Exelon.[24] (Yissum was founded in 1964 as a bridge between research and the commercial sector. It has registered thousands of patents, licenced more than a thousand technologies, has spun off many companies and its international business partners span the globe and include leading global companies.)

Professor Weinstock-Rosin was born in Vienna in 1935 and graduated in pharmacology in London, with a PhD at St. Mary's Hospital Medical School. She was appointed a Professor in 1981 and headed the School of Pharmacy from 1983. She was awarded the Israel Prize for Medicine in 2014.

Professor Weinstock-Rosin is also the co-developer, with Professor Moussa Youdim of the Technion-Israel Institute of Technology, of Ladostigil, a novel neuro-protective agent being investigated for the treatment of neuro-degenerative disorders such as Alzheimer's disease, Lewy body disease and Parkinson's disease. It combines the mechanisms of action of older drugs like rivastigmine and rasagiline into a single molecule.[25] In addition to its neuro-protective properties, Ladostigil may be capable of reversing some of the damage seen in neuro-degenerative diseases via the induction of neurogenesis. Ladostigil also has antidepressant effects and may be useful for treating comorbid depression and anxiety often seen in such diseases as well.

Illana Gozes is Professor Emerita of Clinical Biochemistry at the Sackler Faculty of Medicine, Tel Aviv University, Chair for the Investigation of Growth Factors and Director of the Laboratory for Molecular Neuroendocrinology. One area of her work concerns the understanding of changes in the brain in Alzheimer's disease producing the familiar symptoms of cognitive decline as amyloid plaques increase accompanied by Tau pathology.[26] It is believed that the tangles in the Alzheimer brain are caused by the hyper-phosphorylation of the microtubule protein known as Tau, causing the protein to dissociate from microtubules and form insoluble aggregates. It is still not clear whether tangles are a primary cause of Alzheimer's disease or merely play a peripheral role.

This work is important as Alzforum, where news about Alzheimer's is shared, reported in 2019 that Phase 3 trials of aducanumab, a monoclonal antibody that helps clear Aβ from the brain, for early Alzheimer's disease were being terminated.[27] One conclusion was that removal of amyloid in people with disease, even in the early symptomatic phase, is too late and that tau and inflammation are probably more important. Her studies have shown the role of a mutation of ADNP, activity-dependent neuro-protective protein, originally studied in autism, in the development of such diseases as schizophrenia, Parkinson's disease and Alzheimer's.[28] ADNP levels can be easily monitored in routine blood tests and the study also found that ADNP levels in the blood correlate with higher IQ in healthy older adults. With this clear connection between ADNP levels in the blood and amyloid plaques in the brain, from her pioneering study which assessed ADNP in elderly individuals at risk for Alzheimer's disease, she considers that this opens the door for further validation in larger, more informative studies and may lead to new understandings and treatment.[29]

Parkinsons's Disease: Rasagiline (Azilect), developed as noted by Professor Youdim in Haifa, boosts dopamine levels in the brain and is used as a monotherapy to treat symptoms in early Parkinson's disease or as an adjunct therapy in more advanced cases.[30] The racemic form of the drug was invented by the British pharmaceutical company, Aspro Nicholas, in the early 1970s and Professor Moussa Youdim's team identified the R-isomer as the active form of the drug. The Israeli drug company Teva brought it to market in partnership with Lundbeck in Europe and Eisai in the US and elsewhere when it was approved in Europe (2005) and in the US (2006).

Multiple Sclerosis: Possibly the best-selling drug to have come out of Israel is Glatiramer Acetate, also known as copaxone or copolymer 1. Glatiramer acetate (also known as Copolymer 1, Cop-1, or Copaxone) is an immuno-modulator medication currently used to treat multiple sclerosis, administered by subcutaneous injection. It is approved in the United States to reduce the frequency of relapses, but not for reducing the progression of disability as a Cochrane Review indicated that it was not approved for reducing the progression of disability although observational studies suggested otherwise.[31] Glatiramer acetate was originally discovered by Michael Sela, Ruth Arnon and Dvora Teitelbaum at the Weizmann Institute of Science in Rehovot, Israel. Following clinical trials and regulatory assessments in the United States and Britain, Glatiramer acetate has been approved for marketing in most countries worldwide.

Gaucher's Disease: Bar-Ilan University's Dr. David Aviezer and colleagues at the company he established, ProtalixBioTherapeutics based in Karmiel in northern Israel, developed the drug Taliglucerase Alfa (Uplyso), a plant based enzyme-replacement therapy for the long-term treatment of type-1 Gaucher's Disease.[32] This rare, genetic disorder, which is more common in Jews, causes lipids to collect and impair proper functioning in the spleen, liver, kidneys and other organs. Patients are deficient in glucocerebrosidase, which breaks down a certain type of fat molecule. As a result, lipid-engorged cells, called Gaucher cells, amass in different parts of the body, primarily the spleen, liver and bone marrow causing anaemia, excessive bleeding and bruising, bone disease and a number of other symptoms.

Given the perceived economic benefits over existing therapy, while using plant-based therapy rather an animal-based one for the condition, Protalix were able to sign a deal with the US pharmaceutical giant Pfizer on 1 December 2009, giving Pfizer exclusive worldwide licencing rights while Protalix retains commercial rights in Israel. However, the new drug still continued to face competition from Sanofi-Genzyme who continued to market the main competition drug Imiglucerase (cerezyme). Other work by Dr. Aviezer, who holds a PhD. in Molecular Biology and Biochemistry from the Weizmann Institute of Science and an MBA from Bar Ilan University's School of Business. includes studies in immunotherapy for Crohn's disease, achondroplasia and cartilage repair.[33]

Diabetes: Miriam Kidron and Hanoch Bar-On at the Hadassah-Hebrew University Medical Centre's Diabetes Unit have been researching methods, for many years, of producing an oral insulin pill that would free patients from having to inject themselves with insulin possibly several times a day.[34] They established a company, Oramed, on the Hebrew University Givat Ram campus, but also with an office in New York, to produce the pill ORMD-0801. Details of its effects, so far only on Type-2 diabetes, were presented, virtually, at the annual meeting of the American Diabetic Association in June 2020. The presentations did not include an oral insulin for Type-1 diabetes but covered the effects of oral insulin on:

- glucose levels in patients with uncontrolled Type-2 diabetes on oral antibiotics
- reduction in liver fat content in patients with Type-2 with non-alcoholic fatty liver
- effect on blood sugar in uncontrolled Type-2 diabetes of evening oral insulin.

Oramed's website indicates that ORMD-0801, their oral insulin capsule, is anticipated for use as a complementary agent to insulin injections in the treatment of Type-1 diabetes. This, they indicate, would let patients to reduce the number of daily injections and achieve better control in unstable diabetes. Also, in their pipeline is ORMD-0901, an oral glucagon-like peptide -1 capsule (GLP-1) which is indicated for Type-2 diabetes and has already acquired a Canadian patent.

Cell Therapy: A Haifa-based biotech company named Pluristem Therapeutics, whose CEO is Zami Aberman, has developed a cell therapy to treat patients exposed to radiation such as experienced after the Chernobyl nuclear plant disaster in 1986 using placenta-based cells (PLX-R18). These cells were initially developed with Professor Raphael Gorodetsky and colleagues at Hadassah Hospital.[35] Other applications include peripheral arterial disease and bone marrow regeneration. Experimental use, on compassionate grounds, have successfully treated a seven-year old Romanian girl with bone marrow aplasia and a forty-five-year-old with acute myeloid leukaemia and pancytopenia, both at Hadassah Hospital. In 2020 it was announced that the European Investment Bank is to give Israel's Pluristem Therapeutics a €50 million venture debt loan toward advancing the clinical development of its cell therapies.

Natural Killer (NK) cells are an important part of the body's immuno-surveillance system, which can recognize and kill cancerous cells and viruses.[36] Treatments offer the potential for an effective and safer treatment option compared to most current cancer immuno-therapies, which target T-cells in an efficient yet sometimes toxic approach. Professor Ofer Mandelboim's team at the Hebrew University's Lautenberg Centre for Immunology and Cancer Research at the Faculty of Medicine, has recently demonstrated that the NK activating receptor, NKp46, is a major engager of NK cells including infiltrating cells in solid tumours.[37]

This work on NK cells has attracted sponsorship from Cytovia Therapeutics as they look for better disease control without harming healthy cells. Cytovia formed a collaborative partnership in March 2020 with Yissum, the University's technology transfer company, to develop precision medicine for haematological and solid tumours in what is becoming a growing field. The company is committed to the development of novel cancer immuno-therapies, addressing the challenging needs in the prevention of cancer relapse and metastasis. Cytovia focuses on Natural Killer (NK) cell biology and applies precision medicine tools to develop the right therapy for the right patient at the right stage of the disease. Cytovia has secured access to multiple advanced technologies, including allogeneic cell therapy, multi-specific antibodies and cytokines.

The understanding of inhibitory receptors on NK cells has even allowed Mandelboim's team to generate novel checkpoint inhibitors, including one which is currently in pre-clinical development (NectinTX), bringing monoclonal antibody to a group of receptors that have major roles in cancer immunotherapy. Nectin Therapeutics was established by Integra Holdings in 2017 based on the discoveries of Professor Mandelboim and Professor Stipan Jonjic of the University of Rijeka, Croatia.

Cardiac Disease: A technology which holds out hope for treatment of degenerative diseases affecting the heart is being pioneered at Tel Aviv University involving Departments of Molecular Cell Biology and Biotechnology, Materials Science and Engineering and the Centres for Nanoscience and Nanotechnology and Regenerative Biotechnology. An unmet challenge in cardiac tissue engineering is the generation of thick vascularized tissues that fully match the patient.

Professor Tal Dvir's team has reported a simple approach to 3-D – print thick, vascularized and perfusable cardiac patches that completely match the immunological, cellular, biochemical and anatomical properties of the patient.[38] The technique has the potential for organ replacement after failure, but major challenges remain requiring strategies to image the entire blood vessels of the heart and to incorporate them in the blueprint of the organ.[39] Finally, advanced technologies to precisely print these small-diameter blood vessels within thick structures will have to be developed. The current size of the 3-D heart is that of a rabbit. A truly artificial human heart generated in this way with the patient's own cells would be on a completely different scale, so its implementation is some time away as is Professor Dvir's research interest in engineering a 3-D neuronal network for spinal cord and brain regeneration.

Gynaecology

Stem Cell Research: The Hadassah hESC Research Centre is a supplier of clinical and research-grade human embryonic stem cell (hESC) lines. One focus of its research includes the development of novel stem cell-based therapies for the advancement of women's health and for the treatment of infertility.[40] Research includes improving surgical outcome in women with Pelvic Floor Disorders using systemically transplanted Mesenchymal Stem

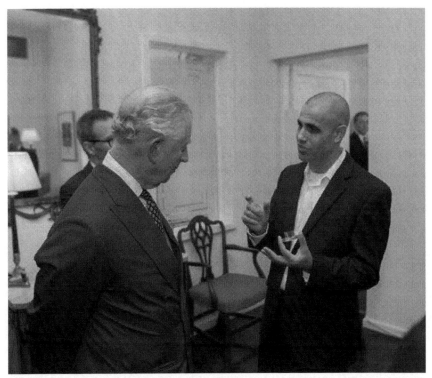

18. Professor Tal Dvir presents his 3-D printed heart to Prince Charles at the British Ambassador's Residence, Ramat Gan, January 2020 (courtesy of FLASH 90)

Cells, which encourage improved blood flow and may also show benefit in other conditions, including retinal disorders and multiple sclerosis.[41]

Vaginal Prolapse: Shveiky and Parkes have described early use of minimally invasive sacrocolpopexy and vaginal mesh colpopexy for vaginal prolapse treatment.[42] In 2018 Shveiky showed that laparoscopic utero-sacral ligament suspension is an option for some forms of uterine prolapse, preserving the uterus and giving good clinical results.[43]

Vaginosis: Another experimental study tests the use of vaginal microbiome transplantation (VMT) from healthy donors as a therapeutic alternative for patients suffering from symptomatic, intractable and recurrent bacterial vaginosis.[44] The study was a small one and the therapeutic efficacy of the procedure in women with intractable and recurrent bacterial vaginosis will need to be tested in randomized, placebo-controlled clinical trials.

Cervical cancer screening can be a great challenge for clinicians across the developing world. In many countries, cervical cancer screening is done by visualization with the naked eye and advanced imaging technologies, such as multi-spectral imaging systems, are seldom deployed in low resource settings where they are needed most. To address this challenge, the optical system of a smartphone-based mobile colposcopy imaging system was refined, using components required for low cost, portable multi-spectral imaging of the cervix. This technology has been developed by MobileEDT, a Tel Aviv based company which produces EVA COLPO described as a portable, internet-connected colposcope which is simple to use. Other products include EVA WELL which is an FDA-cleared and HIPAA compliant digital visualization tool for gynaecologic exams. Data can be recorded, and images and video can be shared in real-time with patients for with colleagues for remote consultation.[45]

Medical Clowning

Medical clowning has been extensively studied in Israel and much of the literature on the topic has come from Israeli sources. One of the best-known practitioners is Amnon Raviv, a graduate of the Graduate School of Creative Art Therapies at Haifa University and the first person in the world to be awarded a PhD in Medical Clowning.[46] His book, *Medical Clowning: the Healing Performance* (University of Chicago Press, 2016) describes his history with the Dream Doctors Project and going into the mind of the medical clown. He offers an in-depth explanation of how medical clowning works in Israel and why it has been so effective with a broad spectrum of patients.

Medical clowning is a growing paramedical practice in various health care settings worldwide, often integrated into health care teams to mitigate stress, loneliness, fear and helplessness in hospitalized patients. Using humour, games and improvisation, medical clowns create a more positive atmosphere and trust between the health care team and the patient. Previous studies have demonstrated a significant positive effect of medical clowns on pre-operative and post-operative anxiety and self-reported pain while it has been clear that clowns are especially appreciated by paediatric patients.

A recent Israeli study, by Gomberg, Raviv et al., from the perspective of the health care team on the medical clown, has shown that there are many unexpected benefits including cost-saving measures for the hospital, increases in staff efficiency, better patient outcomes and lower stress in medical staff.[47] Clowns were reported to lessen the trauma of treating sick children on a day-to-day basis from the medical staff. Having to treat a

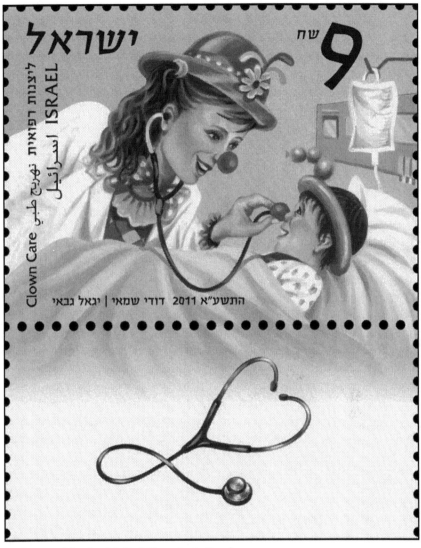

19. Stamp celebrating Medical Clowning in Israel.

smiling child playing a game with the clown is far easier emotionally than being forced to treat or sedate a hysterical one. Parents also benefit. Decreased parental stress in turn decreased the stress of the medical staff. Given that most of the limitations on medical clowning are financial, Gomberg and colleagues suggest that these findings have substantial implications for the future of the field.

Future Trends

It has not been possible to mention every new medical research project, development or initiative being undertaken at Israel's universities, science centres and industrial research hubs. Many likely breakthroughs do not achieve their potential while other innovations reach the market and have considerable commercial success. Before concluding we should review just a few areas of promising research. Many other innovative medical research and development programmes are currently underway in Israel, sometimes as part of international collaborations.

One important neurological study has identified genetic mutations in the Ashkenazi Jewish population and is working with teams in New York to understand the implications of this Parkinsons' Disease phenotype.[48] Another genetic study looks at methods of non-invasive pre-natal diagnosis (NIPD) showing that next-generation sequencing (NGS) can be used for the diagnosis of a wide range of monogenic diseases, simultaneously, instead of present methods which limits the testing to one genetic disorder at a time.[49].

The Israeli medical device company Body Vision Medical was founded in 2014 by Dorian Averbuch, who developed a novel electromagnetic bronchoscopy. The company specializes in lung cancer diagnostics through augmented real-time intra-body navigation and imaging. It has received three FDA clearances for its imaging systems which can reach suspicious deep lung tissue. Further refinements will include surgical markers for radio-surgery and, later, for minimally invasive treatment tools such as radiofrequency or microwave ablation. Another device with much potential is DaRT (Diffusing alpha-emitters radiation therapy) which uses radio-active seeds that continually release short-lived alpha-emitting atoms to treat cancer. Researchers in Israel have now published the positive results of a first-in-human clinical study evaluating the feasibility, safety and efficacy of this novel radio-therapy technique. Protocols in process include those for indications such as vulvar cancer in the UK, skin cancer in Thailand and prostate cancer at multiple locations.[50]

A team headed by Papo and Shifman has developed a powerful tool to simultaneously evaluate thousands of mutations in protein-protein complexes and to map their effect on protein binding affinity, turning what was formerly a lengthy process into one that takes just a few days. Currently, in the pharmaceutical industry, most of the promising new drugs in production are proteins that destroy certain disease-associated protein-protein interactions. The new method of quantifying the effect of thousands of mutations allows researchers to design protein drugs that are both potent and specific, causing minimal side effects.[51]

The Covid-19 virus pandemic which caused world-wide morbidity and mortality from early 2020 unleashed a wave of Israeli creativity. Novel treatments and methods of rapid testing were examined and there was research in vaccine production in several centres around the country. Many new and existing drugs held out hope for ameliorating the condition. It was reported that researchers at the Israel Institute for Biological Research (IIBR) had found that analogues of two drugs for Gaucher's disease are effective against the Coronavirus. Israeli startup Respinova has been developing Pulsehaler, a novel medical device to help chronic obstructive pulmonary disease patients improve their lungs and avoid ventilation. Based on data from their COPD studies, Respinova believes that Pulsehaler can complement other therapies used to treat moderate Covid-19 patients, improving oxygenation, reducing mucus and the risk of secondary infection, and helping to avoid deterioration to a state requiring mechanical ventilator support.

Conclusion

This story began with the first elements of the regional medical story and has concluded with some of the latest developments in Israel's contribution to innovation in the medical world. *Medicine: From Biblical Canaan to Modern Israel* has shown the various influences on medicine in the Holy Land over almost three millennia and is a tribute to that human spirit which has always striven to bring health and well-being to all. Through all its twists and turns it is a truly inspiring story.

Notes

1. https://www.israel21c.org/topic/health/
2. Tong J., Svarta, S., Ou, G., Kwok, R., Law, J and Enns, R. (October 2012), 'Diagnostic yield of capsule endoscopy in the setting of iron deficiency anemia without evidence of gastrointestinal bleeding', *Canadian Journal of Gastroenterology,* 26 (10), pp.687–690; Yuce, M.R. and Dissanayake, T. (2012), 'Easy-to-swallow wireless telemetry', *IEEE Microwave Magazine,* 13 (6), pp.90–101; Slawinski, P.R., Obstein, K.L. and Valdastri, P. (October 2015), 'Capsule endoscopy of the future: What's on the horizon?', *World Journal of Gastroenterology,* 21 (37): pp.10528-10541; Adler, S.N. and Metzger, Y.C. (July 2011), 'PillCam COLON capsule endoscopy: recent advances and new insights', *Therapeutic Advances in Gastroenterology,* 4 (4), pp.265-268; Liao, Z., Gao, R., Xu, C. and Li, Z.S.(2010), 'Indications and detection, completion, and retention rates of small-bowel capsule endoscopy: a systematic review', *Gastrointestinal Endoscopy.* 71 *(2),* pp.280-286.

3. A candidate for ReWalk must be in good general health, have healthy bone density and be free of fractures. The hands and shoulders must be able to support crutches or a walker and not suffer from severe spasticity.

4. https://www.gamida-cell.com/our-rd/; Anand, S., Thomas, S., Hyslop, T. and Adcock, J. (2017), 'Transplantation of Ex Vivo Expanded Umbilical Cord Blood (NiCord) Decreases Early Infection and Hospitalization', *Biology of Blood Marrow Transplant*ation, 23 (7), pp.1151-1157; Mitchell, E., Horwitz, S.W., Blackwell, B., Valcarcel, D. and Frassoni, F. et al (2019), 'Phase I/II Study of Stem-Cell Transplantation Using a Single Cord Blood Unit Expanded Ex Vivo with Nicotinamide', *Journal of Clinical Oncology*, 10, 37 (5), pp.367-374.

5. N. Schwaiger, J., Wu, B., Wright, L., Morrissey, M. and Harris, R. (2010), 'Rohanizadeh, BioWeld® Tube and surgical glue for experimental sutureless venous micro-anastomosis', *British Journal of Surgery*, 97 (12), pp.1825-1830; Boyko, V., Kryvoruchko, I., Parhomenko, K., Firsyk, T.M. and Bozhko, Yevtushenko. D. (2019), *Health Care Sciences* (Ukraine), Surgical Treatment of Rectal Fistulae Using Biowelding, print ISSN: 2618-0553; online ISSN: 2618-0561; DOI: 10.26697/ijes

6. Professor Yael Hanein is the co-founder of Tel Aviv University's Micro and Nano Central Facilities and is the Vice-President, Scientific Affairs at Nano Retina. She has a special interest in neuro-engineering particularly in developing wearable electronic technology and bionic vision. Professor Hanein has been part of Nano Retina since its inception in 2009 and is responsible for providing the Nano Retina team with scientific training and technical leadership. Her research includes: Gautam, V., Rand, D. and Hanein, Y. (2014), 'A Polymer Optoelectronic Interface Provides Visual Cues to a Blind Retina', *Advanced Materials*, 26, pp.1751-1756; Eleftheriou, C.G., Zimmermann, J.B., Kjeldsen, H.D., David-Pur, M. and Hanein, Y. and Sernagor, E. (2017), 'Carbon nanotube electrodes for retinal implants: A study of structural and functional integration over time', *Biomaterials*,112, pp.108-121.

7. Levin, Y., Kochba, E. and Kenney, R. (2014), 'Clinical evaluation of a novel microneedle device for intradermal delivery of an influenza vaccine: Are all delivery methods the same?', *Vaccine*, 34 (4), pp.249-52.

8. Yonath, A., 'Hibernating Bears, Antibiotics, and the Evolving Ribosome', (Nobel Lecture),9 June 2010, accessed at https://onlinelibrary.wiley.com/doi/abs/10.1002/anie.201001297 (Copyright: The Nobel Foundation 2009).

9. Yonath, A., (2005), 'Antibiotics targeting ribosomes: resistance, selectivity, synergism, and cellular regulation', *Annual Review of Biochemistry*, 74, pp.649-679.

10. Hershko, A., Ciechanover, A. and Rose, I.A. (1979), 'Resolution of the ATP-dependent proteolytic system from reticulocytes: a component that interacts with ATP', *Proceedings of the National Academy of Sciences USA*, 76 (7), pp.3107–3110.

11. 'In The Inner Physician: Why and how to practise big-picture medicine', (Royal College of General Practitioners, 2016), Roger Neighbour shows how Kahneman and Tversky's insights apply to medical decision making, p.193.

12. Peng, G., Tisch, U., Adams, O. and Haick, H. et al. (2009), 'Diagnosing lung cancer in exhaled breath using gold nanoparticles', *Nature Nanotechnology*, 4, pp.669-673; Haick, H., Broza, Y.Y., Mochalski, P. and Ruzsanyi, V. (2014), 'Assessment, origin, and implementation of breath volatile cancer markers', *Chemical Society Reviews*, 43, pp.1423-1449; Hakim, M., Broza, Y., Barash, O., Peled, N. and Haick, H. et al. (2012), 'Volatile organic compounds of lung cancer and possible biochemical pathways', *Chem.*

Reviews, 112, (11), pp.5949-5966; Konvalina, G. and Haick, H. (2014), 'Sensors for breath testing: from nanomaterials to comprehensive diseasedetection', *Accounts of Chemical Research*, 47 (1), pp.66-76; Haick, H. and Cahen, D. (2008), 'Making contact: Connecting molecules electrically to the macroscopic world', *Progress in Surface Science*, 83 (4), pp.217-261.

13. Vishinkin, R. and Haick, H. (2015), 'Artificially intelligent nanoarrays for disease detection via volatolomics', IEEE International Electron Devices Meeting (IEDM), Washington, 7-9 December 2015 Electronic ISSN: 2156-017X Accessed at https://ieeexplore.ieee.org/abstract/document/7409821/authors#authors 21/5/2020

14. Jin, H., Abu-Raya, Y.S. and Haick, H. (2017), 'Advanced Materials for Health Monitoring with Skin-Based Wearable Devices', *Advanced Healthcare Materials*, 6 (11), accessed on 21/5/2020 athttps://onlinelibrary.wiley.com/doi/abs/10.1002/adhm.201700024

15. Louis, D.N., Feldman, M., Carter, A.B., Golden, J.A. and Becich, M.J. et al. (*2016*), 'Computational Pathology: A Path Ahead', *Archives of Pathology and Laboratory Medicine*, 140 (1), pp.41-50.

16. https://www.israel21c.org/the-israeli-technology-that-helps-pathologists-spot-cancer/

17. Müller-Decker, K., Stein, R., Tsarfaty, G. and Satchi-Fainaro, R., 'Incipient melanoma brain metastases instigate astrogliosis and neuroinflammation', *Cancer Research*, 76 (15), pp.4359-4371 (This work was performed in partial fulfillment of the requirements for a PhD. degree by Hila Schwartz, Sackler School of Medicine, Tel Aviv University); Brocchini, S., Zloh, M., Peppas, N.A. and Satchi-Fainaro, R. et al. (2018), 'α-Galactosylceramide and peptide-based nano-vaccine synergistically induced a strong tumor suppressive effect in melanoma', *Acta Biomaterialia*, 76, pp.193-207.

18. Luboshits, G., Ashur-Fabian, O., Pinhasov, A. and Gerlitz, G. et al. (2017), 'Toward the development of a novel non-RGD cyclic peptidedrug conjugate for treatment of human metastatic melanoma', *Oncotarget*, 8 (1), pp.757-768; Minnes, R., Nissinmann, M., Maizels, Y. and Gerlitz, G. (2017), 'Using Attenuated Total Reflection–Fourier Transform Infra-Red (ATR-FTIR) spectroscopy to distinguish between melanoma cells with a different metastatic potential', *Scientific Reports*, 7, Article number:4381, Accessed on 21/5/2020 athttps://www.nature.com/articles/s41598-017-04678-6#citeas; Sandrusy, O., Rosenberg, A. and Gerlitz, G. (2017), 'Increased chromatin plasticity supports enhanced metastatic potential of mouse melanoma cells', *Experimental Cell Research*, 357, (2), pp.282-290; Gerlitz, G., Livnat, I., Ziv, C., Yarden, O., Bustin, M. and Reiner, O. (2007), 'Migration cues induce chromatin alterations', *Traffic*, 8 (11), pp.1521-1529.

19. Harel, M., Ortenberg, R., (2019), 'Proteomics of Melanoma Response to Immunotherapy Reveals Mitochondrial Dependence', 179 (1), pp.236-250.

20. Amit, M., Laider-Trejo, L., Shalom, V., Shabtay-Orbach, A., Krelin, Y. and Gil, Z. (2013), 'Characterization of the melanoma brain metastatic niche in mice and humans', *Cancer Medicine*, 2 (2), pp.155-163.

21. Dardikman-Yoffe, G., Simcha, K., Mirsky, I.B. and Shaked, N.T., 'High-resolution 4-D acquisition of freely swimming human sperm cells without staining', *Science Advances*, 10 April 2020, 6, (15), essay7619. DOI:10.1126/sciadv.aay7619Accessed on 21/5/2020https://advances.sciencemag.org/content/6/15/eaay7619.

22. Petrou, P., Y., Argov, Z. and . (2008), 'Safety and Clinical Effects of Mesenchymal Stem Cells Secreting Neurotrophic Factor Transplantation in Patients With Amyotrophic

Lateral Sclerosis: Results of Phase 1/2 and 2a', *Clinical Neurology and Neurosurgery*, pp.889-896.

23.	USA National Library of Medicine: https://clinicaltrials.gov/ct2/show/NCT03280056

24.	Weinstock, M., Luques, L.,Poltyrev, T., Bejar, C. and Shoham, S. (2011), 'Ladostigil prevents age-related glial activation and spatial memory deficits in rats', *Neurobiology of Aging*, 32 (6), pp.1069-1078.

25.	Weinstock, M., Bejar, C. and Wang, R.H. et al. (2000), 'TV3326, a novel neuroprotective drug with cholinesterase and monoamine oxidase inhibitory activities for the treatment of Alzheimer's disease', *Journal of Neural Transmission*. Supplementum (60), pp.157-69; Weinreb, O., Mandel, S. and Bar-Am, O. et al. *(January 2009),* 'Multifunctional neuroprotective derivatives of rasagiline as anti-Alzheimer's disease drugs', *Neurotherapeutics, 6 (1), pp.163-74;* Weinstock, M., Luques, L., Bejar, C. and Shoham, S. (2006), 'Ladostigil, a novel multifunctional drug for the treatment of dementia co-morbid with depression', *Journal of Neural Transmission*. Supplementum *(70)*, pp.443-6.

26.	Matsuoka, Y., Jouroukhin, Y., Gray, A.J., Gozes, I. and Aisen, P.S. et al. (2008), 'A Neuronal Microtubule-Interacting Agent, NAPVSIPQ, Reduces Tau Pathology and Enhances Cognitive Function in a Mouse Model of Alzheimer's Disease', *Journal of Pharmacology and Experimental Therapeutics,* 325 (1), pp.146-153.

27.	https://www.alzforum.org/news/research-news/biogeneisai-halt-phase-3-aducanumab-trials. Aβ(Amyloid beta) denotes peptides of 36–43 amino acids that are crucially involved in Alzheimer's disease as the main component of the amyloid plaques found in the brains of people with Alzheimer's disease.

28.	Malishkevich, A., Marshall, G.A,. Schultz, A.P., Sperling, R.A., Aharon-Peretz, J. and Gozes, I. (2016), 'Blood-Borne Activity-Dependent Neuroprotective Protein (ADNP) is Correlated with Premorbid Intelligence, Clinical Stage, and Alzheimer's Disease Biomarkers', *Journal of Alzheimer's Disease*, 50 (1), pp.249-260.

29.	Pachima, Y.I., Zhou, L. and LeiI Gozes, P. (2016), 'Microtubule-Tau Interaction as a Therapeutic Target for Alzheimer's Disease', *Journal of Molecular Neuroscience*, 58, pp.145-152; Gozes, I., Iram, T., Maryanovsky, E., Arviv, C., Rozenberg, L., Schirer, Y., Giladi, E. and Furman-Assaf, S. (2014), 'Novel Tubulin and Tau Neuroprotective Fragments Sharing Structural Similarities with the Drug Candidate NAP (Davuentide)', *Journal of Alzheimer's Disease*, 40 (s1), pp.S23-S36.

30.	Parkinson Study Group (2004), 'A Controlled, Randomized, Delayed-Start Study of Rasagiline in Early Parkinson Disease', *Archives of Neurology,* 61 (4), pp.561-566.

31.	La Mantia, L., Munari, L.M. and Lovati, R. (2010), 'Glatiramer acetate for multiple sclerosis', *The Cochrane Database of Systematic Reviews*, 5 (5), CD004678.

32.	David Eliezer has published widely on this topic. The following papers outline some of the research behind the treatments: 'Plant based oral delivery of β-glucocerebrosidase as an enzyme replacement therapy for Gaucher disease', *Plant Biotechnology Journal*,13 (8), 2015; Shaaltiel, Y., Gingis-Velitski, S.,Tzaban, S., Aviezer, D., Brill-Almon, E., Shaaltiel, Y. and Zimran, A. (2010), 'Novel enzyme replacement therapy for Gaucher disease: Phase III pivotal clinical trial with plant cell expressed recombinant glucocerebrosidase (prGCD) – taliglucerase alpha', *Molecular Genetics and Metabolism*, 99 (2) DOI: 10.1016/j.ymgme.2009.10.026.

33.	Shaaltiel, Y., Ben Ya'acov, A., Shabat, Y., Ilan, Y. and Eliezer, D. et al. (2014), 'Tu2029 A novel method for anti-TNF based-oral immunotherapy: Oral administration of a plant cell-expressed recombinant anti-TNF fusion protein for treating of Crohn's disease', 2014, *Gastroenterology,*146 (5), pp. s-901; 'Fibroblast Growth Factor Receptor-3 as a Therapeutic Target for Achondroplasia - Genetic Short Limbed Dwarfism', August 2003, *Current Drug Targets*, 4 (5), pp.353-65 DOI: 10.2174/1389450033490993; Aviezer, D., Golembo, M. and Yayon, A. (2002), 'Mechanical Resistance of Biological Repair Cartilage: Comparative in vivo Tests of Different Surgical Repair Procedures', *The International Journal of Artificial Organs*, 25 (11), pp.1109-15, DOI: 10.1177/039139880202501111

34. Ziv, E., Kidron, M., Raz, I., Krausz, M., Blatt, Y., Rotman, A. and Bar, H. (1994),-O 'Oral administration of insulin in solid form to nondiabetic and diabetic dogs', *Journal of Pharmaceutical Studies*, 83 (6), pp.792-794; Arbit, E. and Kidron, M. (2009), 'Oral Insulin: The Rationale for This Approach and Current Developments', *Journal of Diabetic Science and Technology*, 3 (3), pp.562-567.

35. Ofir, R., Pinzur, L., Levent, A., Aberman, Z., Gorodetsky, R. and Volk, H.D. (2015), 'Mechanism of Action of PLX-R18, a Placental-Derived Cellular Therapy for the Treatment of Radiation-Induced Bone Marrow Failure', *Blood*, 126 (23), p.2417; Gaberman, E., Pinzur, L., Levdansky, L., Tsirlin, M., Netzer, N. and Aberman, Z. et al (2013), 'Mitigation of Lethal Radiation Syndrome in Mice by Intramuscular Injection of 3-D Cultured Adherent Human Placental Stromal Cells', *PLoS ONE 8,* (6), e66549. https://doi.org/10.1371/journal.pone.0066549.

36. Porgador, A. and Mandelboim, O. (1997), 'Natural killer cell lines kill autologous β2-microglobulindeficientmelanoma cells: implications for cancer immunotherapy', *PNAS Proceedings of the National Academy of Sciences (USA)*, 94 (24), pp.13140-13145; Koch, J., Steinle, A., Watzl, C. and Mandelboim, O. (2013), 'Activating natural cytotoxicity receptors of natural killer cells in cancer and infection', *Trends in Immunology*, 34 (4), pp.182-191.

37. Glasner, A., Levi, A., Enk, J. and Mandelboim, O. et al (2018), 'NKp46 Receptor-Mediated Interferon-γ Production by Natural Killer Cells Increases Fibronectin 1 to Alter Tumor Architecture and Control Metastasis', *Immunity,*48 (1), pp.107-119.

38. Noor, N., Shapira, A., Edri, R., Gal, I., Wertheim, L. and Dvir, T. (2019), '3-D Printing of Personalized Thick and Perfusable Cardiac Patches and Hearts', *Advanced Science*, 6 (11). Accessed on 3/6/2020 at https://onlinelibrary.wiley.com/doi/full/10.1002/advs. 201900344

39. Shapira, A., Noor, N., Asulin, M. and T Dvir, T., 'Stabilization strategies in extrusion-based 3-D bioprinting for tissue engineering', *Applied Physics Reviews*, 3DB. https://doi.org/10.1063/1.5055659@are.2019.3DB.issue-1

40. Shelly, S.E., Tannenbaum, Singer, O.,Gil, Y., Berman-Zaken, Y., NiliIlouz, B. and Reubinoff, E. (2020), 'Hadassah, provider of "Regulatory-Ready" pluripotent clinical-grade stem cell banks', *Stem Cell Research*, 42, 101670

41. Ben Menachem- Zidon, O., Michal Gropp, M., Ben Shushan, E., Reubinoff, B. and Shveiky, D. (2019), 'Systemically transplanted mesenchymal stem cells induce vascular-like structure formation in a rat model of vaginal injury', *PLoS One*, **14** (6): e0218081Published online June 13 2019. doi: 10.1371/journal.pone.0218081

42. Parkes, I.L. and Shveiky, D. (2014), 'Sacrocolpopexy for Treatment of Vaginal Apical Prolapse: Evidence-Based Surgery', *Journal of Minimally Invasive Gynecology*, 21, (4), pp.546-557; Shveiky, D., Iglesia, C., Sokol, A.I., Kudish, B.I. and Gutman, R.E. (2010), 'Robotic Sacrocolpopexy Versus Vaginal Colpopexy With Mesh: Choosing the Right

Surgery for Anterior and Apical Prolapse', *Female Pelvic Medicine and Reconstructive Surgery*, 16 (2), pp 121-127.

43. Yahya Rani, H., Chill, H.H., Herzberg, S., Asfour, A., Lesser, S. and Shveiky, D. (2018), 'Anatomical Outcome and Patient Satisfaction After Laparoscopic Uterosacral Ligament Hysteropexy for Anterior and Apical Prolapse', *Female Pelvic Medicine and Reconstructive Surgery*, 24 (5), pp.352-355.

44. Lev-Sagie, A., Goldman-Wohl, D., Cohen, Y., Yagel, S. and Elinav, E. (2019), 'Vaginal microbiome transplantation in women with intractable bacterial vaginosis', *Nature Medicine*, 25, pp.1500-1504.

45. Bolton, F.J., Weiser, R., Kass, A.J., Rose, D., Safir, A. and Levitz, D. (2016), 'Development and bench testing of a multi-spectral imaging technology built on a smartphone platform', *Proceedings Optics and Biophotonics in Low-Resource Settings*, 9699, II; 969907 https://doi.org/10.1117/12.2218694; Research papers on MobileEDT products can be accessed at https://www.mobileodt.com/medical-research/

46. Raviv, A. (2012), 'Still the Best Medicine, Even in a War Zone My Work As a Medical Clown', *The Drama Review*, 56 (2), pp.169-177; Pendzik, S. and Raviv, A. (2011), 'Therapeutic clowning and drama therapy: A family resemblance', *The Arts in Psychotherapy*, 38 (4), pp.267-275. See also The Dream Doctors Project: Medical Clowning in Action at https://dreamdoctors.org.il/. The project was founded by Yaacov Shriqui, who serves as Executive Director. In 2011, the Dream Doctors Project's First International Conference on Medicine and Medical Clowning was held in Jerusalem with 250 guests from 22 countries.

47. Gomberg, J., Raviv, A., Fenig, E. and Meiri, N., 'Saving Costs for Hospitals Through Medical Clowning: A Study of Hospital Staff Perspectives on the Impact of the Medical Clown', *Clinical Medicine Insights, Pediatrics*, accessed on 25/4/2020 at https://journals.sagepub.com/doi/full/10.1177/1179556520909376, For an overview of the topic see Finlay, F., Baverstock, A. and Lenton, S. (2013), 'Therapeutic clowning in paediatric practice', *Clinical Child Psychology and Psychiatry*, 19 (4), pp.596-605.

48. Alcalay, R., Mirelman, A., Gurevich, T., Orr-Urtreger, A. and Giladi, N. et al. (2013), 'Parkinson disease phenotype in Ashkenazi Jews with and without *LRRK2*', *G2019S* mutations, 28 (14), pp.1966-1971.

49. Rabinowitz, T., Polsky, A., Golan, D. and Shomron, N. et al. (2019), 'Bayesian-based noninvasive prenatal diagnosis of single-gene disorders', *Genome Research*, 29: pp.428-438.

50. Popovtzer, A., Rosenfeld, E. and Keisari, Y. et al. (2020), 'Initial Safety and Tumor Control Results From a "First-in-Human" Multicenter Prospective Trial Evaluating a Novel Alpha-Emitting Radionuclide for the Treatment of Locally Advanced Recurrent Squamous Cell Carcinomas of the Skin and Head and Neck', *International Journal of Radiation Oncology*, 106, 3, 1, pp.571-578.

51. Shifman, J.M. and Papo, N. (2017), 'Editorial overview: Engineering and design: New trends in designer proteins', *Current Opinion in Structural Biology*, 45, pp.iv-vi; Heyne, M., Papo, N. and Shifman, J.N. (2020), 'Generating quantitative binding landscapes through fractional binding selections combined with deep sequencing and data normalization', *Nature Communications*, 11, Article no. 297: https://www.nature.com/articles/s41467-019-13895-8

Index